fluent bodies

Body, Commodity, Text

Studies of Objectifying Practice

A SERIES EDITED BY ARJUN APPADURAI,

JEAN COMAROFF, AND JUDITH FARQUHAR

JEAN M. LANGFORD

fluent bodies

Ayurvedic Remedies for Postcolonial Imbalance

Duke University Press Durham and London 2002

Printed in the United States of America on acid-free paper ∞

Designed by Rebecca M. Giménez Typeset in Carter & Cone Galliard with Ex Ponto display by Keystone Typesetting, Inc.

Library of Congress Cataloging-in-Publication Data appear on the last printed page of this book.

This book is gratefully

dedicated to my father,

Joseph Walton Langford Jr.,

and to Vd. Someshwar Bhatt,

in loving memory

contents

acknowledgments

My greatest thanks go to my teachers. This project was first conceived through conversations with my dissertation adviser, Lorna A. Rhodes, who thereafter insightfully commented on every stage of the work. Marilyn Ivy and Ann Anagnost guided me through many thorny theoretical problems. David Spain and Frank Conlon were both unfailing supports to me in the early years of this project. In addition, I owe thanks to many other teachers who have helped in the conceptualization of this project over the years, especially John Pemberton, T. N. Madan, David Lelyveld, and Stacy Leigh Pigg.

Then there is my reading, writing, and hiking group: Sara Van Fleet, Sara Nelson, Rebecca Klenk, Peter Moran, and Ann Sheeran, who shared many moments of creativity, angst, and wildflowers. I am particularly grateful to Sara V. for pointing out the Wizard of Oz structure of chapter 6. I also thank my Hindi teachers, Michael Shapiro, Naseem Hines, and the late Alan Entwistle, as well as Dinkar Rai, Rakesh Nautiyal, Girish Joshi, and Urmila Raturi, none of whom, however, should be blamed for my language errors. Alan was especially patient in spending an entire quarter with me poring over Hindi texts on appropriate bowel movements and other such topics, not only without complaint, but even with interest. Charles Leslie was kind enough to loan me his copy of the Madras Report on indigenous medicine.

Valuable critiques and comments on parts of this work were generously given at various times by Gloria Goodwin Raheja, Purnima Mankekar, Lawrence Cohen, Judith Farquhar, E. Valentine Daniel, Ken Wissoker, and anonymous reviewers.

To all of the practitioners who may recognize parts of themselves in these pages and to their families, I express my deepest gratitude for their time, patience, friendliness, and wisdom, not to mention their cold remedies. Beyond them I thank Prerna Raturi for her two months' companionship as interpreter, transcriber, and chief chapati maker; Prem and Anjani Bijalwan for their familial care; and most of all the Dr. Narendra Bhatt family for an assistance and affection that went far beyond what any researcher could hope for. In addition, I thank Professor R. K. Mutatkar of the Department of Anthropology at the University of Poona for his advice on this project. I also thank my research adviser, Professor M. B. Mandke, of the same department for his warm support, his ability to discuss the five types of vāyu, and his reminder that our thoughts also must be properly digested.

Tremendous thanks go to close friends and family who have given me encouragement and support, sharing in every elation and difficulty, especially Judith Clarke, Kathy Ross, June Gabriel, Gina Ryken, Gail Smith, Marie-Louise Pauson, Francesca Profiri, James Langford, Judith Augustson, and Sally Ridgeway. Portions of chapters two, six, and seven were published in the journals *Cultural Anthropology* 10, *Political and Legal Anthropology Review* 21, and *American Ethnologist* 26 (Langford 1995, 1999, and 1998). I am grateful to the journal editors for making it possible to publish these sections in their present form.

The fieldwork for this book was funded by the National Science Foundation, the Wenner-Gren Anthropological Foundation, the American Institute for Indian Studies, and Fulbright-Hays. Analysis and writing was supported through the Foreign Language Area Studies Program, a University of Washington Dissertation Grant, and summer research funds from the University of Minnesota.

Last but not least, I thank all the teachers of the heart who sustained me throughout this project, most concretely during fieldwork but no less essentially during the years of writing.

one (Re)inventing Ayurveda

I was sitting with Dr. Vijayan in my room, shaded with coconut fronds, at the small hospital run by him and his family in a South Indian fishing village-cum-suburb.[1] We were discussing my treatment. I was sodden and fragrant with herbal oils, skin silky from gritty daily massages. The night before, rain had drummed in a steady rhythm against the hospital roof. Now the morning air was yellow and steamy, full of smoke and rain and milky gold sunshine. It was monsoon, the best time, according to received wisdom and classical texts, for Dr. Vijayan's specialty, *pancakarma,* a purification regimen that is part of the centuries-old set of South Asian healing practices known collectively as Ayurveda.[2] Yet there was only one other patient at the clinic, a South Indian man. The Europeans and North Americans to whom Dr. Vijayan increasingly directed his practice came only during the cool winter months. When we had finished talking about my treatment, I asked him whether his experience with foreign patients had changed the way he thought about Ayurveda. I was startled by his answer. "Yes definitely," he replied. "Now I know the true essence of Ayurveda." What might this mean? How had he discovered the "true essence" of Ayurveda through his work with foreign patients, whose treatments were timed not by the recommendations in ancient texts, but rather by the seasonal attractions of a nearby beach resort?

Dr. Vijayan's treatment of foreign patients is a very recent and transnational moment in a much older story about the modernization of Ayurveda, a story that is the subject of this book. Nonetheless, his comment starkly directs us to a central question threaded through this story. How does it happen that Ayurveda, with all its claims to antiquity, is being most clearly delineated in its cultural distinctiveness in an era when it is also most intensely marked by encounters with other medical understandings? Over the course of the last two centuries, Ayurvedic practitioners, like other healers around the globe, have confronted their marginalization in the face of the global ascendance of modern European medicine, or biomedicine, as it is called by anthropologists. Practitioners have met this challenge by reinterpreting and reshaping their knowledge and practice for a modern era. Yet simultaneously, like Dr. Vijayan, they have turned their very marginalization and their struggle against it in into an opportunity to (re)invent Ayurveda.[3] This book, then, is partly concerned with the paradoxical process through which Ayurvedic practitioners recover the "true essence" of Ayurveda even as they define its modern relevance. In illuminating certain moments in this process, I am not suggesting that contemporary definitions of Ayurveda fall short of "true" Ayurveda; nor am I arguing that there is or is not any such thing as "true" Ayurveda. Instead I am arguing that what needs to be understood is not what "true" Ayurveda might or might not be but rather what is involved in establishing a realm of Ayurvedic "truth."

To some extent the recovery of Ayurvedic essence is linked to a recovery of Indian "culture." For instance, during my many conversations with Dr. Vijayan, I realized that his account of Ayurveda's "true essence" was intricately intertwined with an account of Indianness. Like tourist-industry entrepreneurs everywhere, he strategically employed a discourse of authenticity and antiquity, seeming to understand that for foreigners, the healing power of Ayurveda rests not only in its medicinal powders and extracts, but also in its cultural difference. His explanations of his practice therefore worked to sustain a neo-orientalist mystique of India as a land of spiritual esoterica. He told me, for instance, that only certain foreigners manage to overcome all the obstacles necessary to come to India. These obstacles are not the superficial obstacles of geography or plane fare, but more obscure obstacles that filter out those who are less sincere and less ready for what India has to offer. In this way, he said, Indian thought patterns are protected from too much foreign influence. Indians, he asserted, "function on specific energy levels." While Western thinking is very rational, Indians' thinking is more "subtle." Those foreigners who do manage to come, he continued, are changed forever. On returning home, they are less consumerist, less competitive.

In such comments it becomes clearer that what is at play in Dr. Vijayan's treatment of Westerners is not only a story of Ayurvedic essence and

Indian subtlety, but also a story of Western shallowness and fragility. "Westerners," Dr. Vijayan said, "have a lot more psychological problems than Indians. These problems sometimes surface during treatment." Pancakarma, he went on, touches "something on a development level." Many of his foreign patients recall painful incidents from their past on the massage table. Such "psychological" reactions, he emphasized, are not seen in Indian patients or mentioned in the Ayurvedic texts. Therefore it is only through his work with foreign patients that he has realized that massage can have effects that go beyond the bodily tissues, to the "subtlest level." Notice how fluidly the figure of "subtlety" moves through this discourse. It is Indians whose thought patterns are most subtle. Yet on the massage table it is only foreigners who can make visible the subtle effects of Ayurvedic treatment. For Indians themselves apparently have no need of these subtle effects.

Why not? Dr. Vijayan explained that Westerners, unlike Indians, do not receive proper attention as children. Therefore, as adults, they are in constant states of "stress" or "worry" or "helplessness." "Westerners' laughter," he said, "often sounds like crying." Interestingly, then, even as Dr. Vijayan's healing theories construct an Indian and Ayurvedic essence, they also work to unravel an orientalist logic within which such an essence is often located. Indian irrationality becomes, in his talk, not a sign of weakness but a sign of strength, whereas Western independence becomes not strength but weakness. Moreover, the Western universalism that needs no cultural essence to supplement its all-too-real and globalized power appears in Dr. Vijayan's talk as a form of impoverishment, an absence of cultural nourishment. I will return to Dr. Vijayan's treatment of foreign patients in the epilogue. For now, however, his discourse of Ayurvedic essence and foreign emptiness helps to crystallize a crucial concern of this study. For even as Ayurvedic practitioners involved in recovering a "true essence" of Ayurveda seem to participate in colonial and neocolonial modes of knowledge, such as the framing of Ayurveda as Indian tradition, they also, at unexpected moments, work to subvert such modes of knowledge in inventive ways. Redefinitions of Ayurveda over the course of the twentieth century can therefore be interpreted in part as ways of creatively addressing an epistemological "imbalance" of late colonial and postcolonial times. This is the larger story I want to tell in this book.

Before beginning this story, a few words are needed about the word Ayurveda itself and its vast and expanding field of referents. Ayurveda can be translated simply as knowledge of life or of long life, although for strategic reasons having to do with its promotion as medicine, it is more often translated now as the science of life. For thousands of years the name has been used across South Asia to refer to an eclectic range of healing practices.[4] While there is some discussion of healing practices in the early Vedic texts collectively known as the *Atharvaveda,* the word Ayurveda is associated today with three ancient Sanskrit texts that are the extant works most fully devoted to praising and prescribing Ayurveda. These three texts are *Caraka Saṃhitā, Suśruta Saṃhitā,* and *Aṣṭāṅga Saṅgraha.* (Caraka and Suśruta are the authors of the first two texts.) Of these the *Suśruta Saṃhitā* is oriented toward surgical treatment, while the other two are oriented more toward other therapies, ranging from herbal and mineral medicines to Dr. Vijayan's specialty, pancakarma, which classically includes oil massages in preparation for cleansing enemas, emesis, and purgation, as well as nasal drops and bloodletting.

The ancient texts provide a baseline, setting certain parameters for Ayurvedic practice. For the most part, however, this book is concerned with contemporary Ayurveda rather than with the Ayurveda of the ancient texts. In the world today the practices that a particular patient or healer might consider Ayurvedic range from urban South Asian home remedies based on an understanding of "hot" and "cold" foods; to medicinal herbal lore of the countryside; to standardized Ayurveda as taught in Indian or Sri Lankan colleges; to eclectic practices taught in workshops in Europe, North America, and elsewhere and geared to an international clientele. At least one common thread running through these diverse practices is the idea that illness develops through the aggravation or increase of one or more of the three bodily *doṣa* (often translated as humors)—*vāta, pitta,* and *kapha.* As discussed further in chapter 5, the doṣa are treated alternately as substances (loosely associated with air, bile, and phlegm), processes, or principles. While the doṣa are bodily forces, they are closely related to forces in the environment and can be influenced by food, climate, seasonal changes, and even social activities. A central purpose of most treatment that is considered to be Ayurvedic is to calm or remove the aggravated doṣa that is responsible for the illness. The chapters to follow offer glimpses of the complexity and flexibility of this pursuit.

A telling entry point for our story of Ayurvedic modernity is in 1836, when British officials ordered a fifty-round cannon salute to celebrate the first dissection of a cadaver by a group of Indians at Fort Williams Medical College in Calcutta (B. Gupta 1976). What significance did this celebratory blast of cannon fire hold for Ayurveda? For one thing, the event marked the end of a brief period of British sponsorship of Ayurveda, which had been studied side by side with European medical science at the Native Medical Institution during the previous decade. This dual educational program had been legitimated by a scholarly interest in classical Indian texts, including important Ayurvedic works.[5] Now it was overturned by T. B. Macaulay's 1835 *Minute on Indian Education*, which declared that all Indian higher education would be conducted in English and modeled on the British system. The *Minute* is sometimes represented as a victory of Anglicism over orientalism, a dramatic about-face in British policy, when a sympathetic interest in Indian knowledge gave way to an insistence on the superiority of European knowledge. The event is, however, better understood as an adjustment in colonial tactics than a turning point in colonial policy, which was, in any case, always ambivalent. Both before and after the *Minute*, British intention was to champion European medicine and expose the errors of indigenous knowledge. The purpose of teaching Ayurveda alongside European medicine had never been to develop Ayurveda per se, but rather to allow Indians to observe for themselves the superiority of European medicine. The superintendent of the indigenous medical college, Dr. John Tytler, explained this superficially tolerant position in 1834, noting that "Coercion always produces the direct contrary effect to what is intended" (quoted in Arnold 1993, 55). The *Minute* thus marked a shift from a noncoercive to a coercive policy, which indeed, as Tytler predicted, motivated prominent *vaidyas* (Ayurvedic practitioners) to organize against the increasing dominance of European medicine.

Nonetheless, the cannon blast memorialized an important moment in the colonial enframing of indigenous science. It decisively ended a brief period during which an Indological interest in classical medicine was allowed to intermingle with the introduction of modern medicine. It placed British military might behind an order of academic disciplines in which the study of Ayurveda and other indigenous healing practices was Indology or ethnology but not medicine. Orientalism had not been so much displaced as more strategically placed to differentiate Indian knowledge. Even as Ayurvedic practitioners began to resist the invalidation of Ayurveda as medicine, they also, as I will elaborate in the coming chapters, judiciously began to accommodate the validation of Ayurveda as culture.

The cannon fire is, therefore, a more complex sign than it first appears, marking both the confinement of Ayurveda to the realm of cultural belief systems and the opening of European medicine to creative appropriations by Indian scientists, including Ayurvedic practitioners. Modern medicine and its bodily disciplines would be enforced by the economic and military might of the colonial regime. Both before and after the cannon salute Indian bodies were subjected to hospitalization, vaccination, quarantine, inoculation, and autopsy.[6] Yet simultaneously and paradoxically, like other colonial exercises of science, the practice of European medicine in the subcontinent would also recruit and require Indians as co-knowers (Prakash 1992). Indeed many of the students attending the new nineteenth-century medical colleges were sons of vaidyas (Leslie 1976a, 362). In the mid-nineteenth century there was also a group of hereditary practitioners in Bombay who referred to themselves as "English doctors" and who dispensed European medicines without formal medical education (Leslie 1973, 219). Over time, then, those who had been recruited as scientific co-knowers began to position themselves to revise scientific knowledge.[7] Later generations of Ayurvedic practitioners would argue, for instance, that Ayurveda was the original medical science, influencing Greek and later European medicine. British celebrations of the "first Indian dissection" notwithstanding, contemporary practitioners often point out that Suśruta, considered the father of Indian surgery, described a method of dissection a few thousand years ago.

Homi Bhabha (1984) has suggested that the motive behind Macaulay's *Minute* was to create a "mimic man," an Indian elite that would be almost the same as the English ruler but not quite, not white. In the medical field this mimic man was to be the Indian practitioner of European medicine. The military salute explicitly inaugurates this medical mimicry, which is intended to confirm the universality of European science. Yet if the official mimic was to be the Indian biomedical doctor, another "mimic" soon arose. By the end of the nineteenth century Ayurvedic practitioners widely recognized that in order to combat the increasingly widespread mimicry of European bodily practice, it would be necessary to copy certain forms of European institutional practice. They therefore began to found professional associations, colleges, and pharmaceutical firms (Leslie 1973, 1974, 1976a, 1992; Brass 1972). In establishing parallel institutions, Ayurvedic practitioners established a parallel medicine, a parallel science, a professional Ayurveda that was increasingly separated from a wider field of healing practices.

Initially, a newly professionalized Ayurveda seemed too out of step with modernity to appeal to the elite who were designing the independent nation. One practitioner, Vd. (Vaidya) Shukla, who had joined the nationalist movement in the 1930s, bitterly recalled to me that most of the original members of the Indian National Congress favored European medicine over Ayurveda. Nonetheless, by the 1920s the Indian National Congress had already passed its first resolution in support of Ayurvedic medicine. The inclusion of Ayurveda in the nationalist program exemplifies that peculiar ambiguity of nationalism, the contradictory need to fashion institutions commensurable with those of other nations while simultaneously constructing a unique national–cultural identity (Chatterjee 1986; Anderson 1991). For Ayurvedic practitioners this ambiguity was both an opening and an imperative to create a medicine that was not only parallel to modern medicine, but also in contrast to it. Vd. Shukla told me that when he joined the Indian nationalist movement, he quit dispensing quinine and other European medicines despite their effectiveness because he was determined that his Ayurvedic treatments would reflect his political sentiments. His story, like others that will be told in these pages, suggests how Ayurveda was gradually transformed from an eclectic set of healing practices to a quintessentially Indian medicine.

Around the same time that he stopped dispensing quinine, Vd. Shukla joined one of the first professional associations for the advancement of Ayurveda. The founders of this association recognized that in order to qualify as a medical system Ayurveda had to be arranged into college courses, institutionalized in hospital procedures, scientifically proven in clinical research, and ordered into new taxonomies of drugs and disease. Like most modern citizens, the association members treated such activities as transparent and rational instruments through which any knowledge could be organized and conveyed. Yet in his later years Vd. Shukla and other practitioners became concerned that such institutional forms, no less than the use of quinine, were interfering with the distinctiveness of Ayurveda. For over a hundred years and still today, Ayurvedic practitioners have been working to sustain the uniqueness of their practice even as they give it a modern edge.

Bhabha has observed that one effect of mimicry of the colonial power by the colonial subject was to mock the "monumentality of history," its "power to be a model" (1984, 128). He is interested in the consequences of this mockery for the colonizer, whose fullness of presence is necessarily shattered by the partial mirrorings of the colonized. I suggest here that it is not only for the colonizer that the monumentality of history or science or other master narratives is mocked, but also for the colonial and postcolonial subject. In the hand of colonial subjects, the fetishistic glints of the tools of history or science or the state often become more visible. They can no longer be (mis)understood as simply functional (indeed many seem clumsy in their new environments) but must be understood also as evocative of the power of the modern. Regardless of whether Ayurvedic drug companies, colleges, and textbooks actually improved Ayurvedic knowledge, they unquestionably gave it a new authority.

As Bhabha argues, the mimicry of the colonial or postcolonial subject is metonymic in that it only partly reproduces the (always already no longer intact) original. In metaphorical signification a sign substitutes for and represents a clearly separate referent. In metonymic significations, on the other hand, the sign borrows only part of the essence of the now fragmented referent.[8] For Ayurvedic medicine to be metaphorically like European medicine would confirm biomedicine's priority, separateness and "power to be a model." For Ayurvedic medicine to be metonymically or partially reproductive of European medicine tends rather to challenge that medicine's systemic integrity. To redefine Ayurveda as a medical system did not, therefore, simply give it a place in the World Health Organization's compendium of ethnomedicines; it also opened up and exposed the signs of medicine to metacolonial plays and appropriations. It allowed Vd. Shukla's colleagues to redefine science itself. The resulting challenge to medical paradigms offered by contemporary Ayurvedic practice is a central theme of this study.

Gyan Prakash has argued that the articulation of the Indian nation was not mimicry since it did not produce a "failed imitation" but rather a "culturally rooted moral community" (1999, 199). In these pages, however, I draw attention to another sense of mimicry—not as failed imitation but as an embodiment of power in which the terms of power can possibly be rewritten (Taussig 1993). The (re)invention of Ayurveda as a system of medicine in parallel to biomedicine serves to highlight certain peculiar features of a modern organization of knowledge. I argue that even as practitioners give Ayurveda a modern institutional framework, they also implicitly critique many of the philosophical premises underlying that framework.[9] Ironically, then, in modernizing Ayurveda, practitioners often succeed in subverting certain latent assumptions of modernity.

Using the Name of Ayurveda

Dr. Upadhyay, an Ayurvedic practitioner, research consultant, and friend, once complained to me that one of his colleagues whom he considered a quack (and whom I introduce more fully in chapter 6) was "using the name of Ayurveda." In Dr. Upadhyay's view, Ayurveda was a coherent system that should not be confused with the eclectic mix of healing theories and therapies of his colleague. While I was sympathetic to his complaint, I could not help noticing that we were all "using the name of Ayurveda," the quack to sell his miracle drugs; my friend to organize various precepts and practices into a medical system; I to argue certain insights about the cultural politics of healing practice; other scholars to argue other insights about medical syncretism, pluralism, holism, tradition and modernity, secularism and the sacred, professional and folk sectors, history versus culture. The name Ayurveda has a powerful polyvalence, whether in the economy of health and illness, the politics of culture, or the theoretical projects of the academy. In framing Ayurveda as a medical system or even a unitary medical praxis, we familiarize the strange (Ayurveda) at the cost of failing to make the familiar (medicine) strange. The earliest colonial framings of Ayurveda were dominated by an orientalist intellectualism that located "authentic" Ayurveda in the ancient texts rather than in the field of actual Ayurvedic practice. These texts were assumed to represent a set of rules, guidelines, and schema for Ayurvedic diagnosis and treatment, while the field of practice was assumed to reflect the decline of Ayurveda from its early empirical glory. Yet

Ayurvedic texts were collections of cases and accounts of colloquia overlaid with centuries of commentary. They were composed of cryptic aphorisms in poetic phrasings oriented toward mnemonic and mimetic learning practices guided by experienced vaidyas. Reframing Ayurveda as a medical system meant interpreting these texts as normative and exhaustively expository, rather than deliberately evocative or even provocative documents.[10]

The vast project of codification that was an orientalist longing became a nationalist imperative. Cosmopolitan practitioners turned to the task of systematizing and standardizing Ayurveda. In the twentieth century, with which this study is mostly concerned, Ayurveda has been (re)invented as a medical system in what can be read as a strategically essentialist move to both compete with European medicine and offer a corrective for it. The (re)invented Ayurveda is a supplement, in the Derridean sense, that both represents a presumed field of healing practices and knowledge and fills a gap of missing presence, the lost science of antiquity (Derrida 1976). The construction of Ayurveda as a *system* of medicine, whether through practitioners' testimonies to government committees on the condition of indigenous medicine or through Ayurvedic college textbooks, clinical research reports, and doctor self-promotions, is not, however, seamless. There are within it countercurrents that subvert modern commonsense medical understandings of, for example, the relationship between symptom and illness, the distinction between the real and the imaginary or counterfeit (the placebo), and the separation between logos and cosmos, word and world.

In addition, if pressures in colonial and postcolonial South Asia have prompted a construction of Ayurveda as medicine, they have, with equal urgency, prompted the construction of Ayurveda as culture. As suggested above, the cannon fire ordered by the British defined by default the cultural arena within which Ayurveda could be valorized. Ayurveda has been developed as a sign of Indian culture since the early days of the independence movement. Whether Ayurveda's status as culture undermines or amplifies its status as medicine depends on how the desires of practitioners, patients, and a wider populace are conceived. These desires are not simple; the desire to cure or be cured of illness mingles easily with sundry and often contradictory desires: hegemonic desires to emulate Europe and counterhegemonic desires to reject things European; desires for professionalism and desires for folk tradition; desires to be modern and desires to cure or be cured of illnesses associated with modernity.

Bodies of Knowledge

The nationalist project to read Ayurveda as culture dovetails with an anthropological project to read Ayurveda as "ethnomedicine," a distinctive medical system embedded in a particular cultural matrix that can then be compared to other medical systems embedded in other cultural matrices. There is a large and persuasive literature that argues that the phenomenology of health in Ayurveda, particularly its formulations of person and illness, is culturally distinct from that of biomedicine (also referred to as modern medicine, cosmopolitan medicine, or allopathy).[11] Scholars have observed that psychic and somatic components of health that are isolated from one another in most biomedical paradigms are integrated in Ayurvedic paradigms (Obeyesekere 1976; Kakar 1982; Zimmermann, 1987). These scholars also note that while biomedical practitioners generally conceive of the body and person as solid and bounded, Ayurvedic practitioners conceive of the body and person as fluid and penetrable, engaged in a continuous interchange with the social and natural environment. Medical anthropologists have convincingly argued that in Ayurveda, illness is frequently framed as socio-psycho-somatic distress, and patients are understood as part of an enclosing social, climatic, or cosmic field (Nichter 1981b, 1981a; von Schmadel and Hochkirchen 1987). It has also been clearly demonstrated that if biomedical practitioners configure illness as a discrete entity, then Ayurvedic practitioners, by contrast, configure illness as a disruption in delicate somatic, climatic, and social systems of balance (Zimmermann 1987; Kakar 1982). According to the anthropological literature, if biomedicine generally understands body, person, and illness as objects, Ayurveda generally understands body, person, and illness as processes and patterns of relationships. Within a comparative frame such assertions are indisputable. In this book, however, I join more recent work that moves outside of this comparative frame to compose questions about how Ayurveda or other health practices figure in local political discourses (e.g., Nichter 1992a, 1992b; Cohen 1995; Trawick 1991). My intention is to consider Ayurveda not taxonomically, as a type of medicine, but dialogically, as a strategic sign evoked in political and cultural maneuvers. I ask not so much how Ayurveda as a system has absorbed elements of biomedicine or even whether Ayurveda actually constitutes a system, but rather how and why Ayurveda came to be framed as an ethnomedical system.[12] Even more important, I seek out the moments when Ayurveda slips out of this frame, moments that allow an interrogation of the frame itself.

Earlier research has laid essential groundwork for this study by documenting the response of Ayurvedic practitioners to the complex medical field of twentieth-century South Asia. Political and historical studies have addressed the standardization of Ayurveda through the introduction, early in the twentieth century, of institutions such as medical colleges, professional associations, and hospitals, which increasingly replaced the guru–disciple apprenticeships and practice in noninstitutional settings that were prevalent in the early nineteenth century (Brass 1972; Leslie 1976a). These political and historical accounts have been complemented by ethnographic accounts, which have examined how Ayurveda interacts with other healing ideologies in local contexts of medical pluralism (Nichter 1978, 1980; Nichter and Nordstrom 1989; Nordstrom 1988; Waxler 1984). Such ethnographies explore the ways that Ayurvedic patients and practitioners strike a balance between accepting elements of competing medical systems and maintaining the distinctiveness of Ayurvedic insights and methods. Anthropologists have frequently argued that biomedical beliefs, practices, and substances are absorbed into contemporary Ayurvedic practice without disturbing underlying paradigms of body and illness (Nichter and Nordstrom 1989; Nordstrom 1989; Tabor 1981).

Following in the wake of such work, the question originally motivating this study was whether and in what ways modern teaching hospitals and clinics and their attendant methodologies might be actually reworking underlying Ayurvedic paradigms. In the anatomo-clinical method of the modern teaching hospital doctors locate disease at particular sites in the interior of the body (Foucault 1973). This perception of disease shifts attention from readily observable manifestations of disease to signs that are solicited from the interior of the body by mechanical instruments. Symptoms playing on the surface are no longer considered simply facets of the illness, or even the primary and exhaustive signifiers of the illness, as they were in earlier phases of European medicine. The temporal suffering of the patient becomes epiphenomenal; it is the spatially described organic dysfunction that is now the central object of medical knowledge. Diseases are no longer nosological categories spread across a natural historical landscape; instead they are entities enclosed in an individual body. Medical sociologists and anthropologists have observed that the technologies and organization of the modern hospital permit disease to be separated from the social environment and discovered in passive bodies (Armstrong 1987; Taussig 1980; Sullivan 1986). They suggest that modern clinical methods continually reinforce the formulation of the body and person as isolated, solid, and acted on rather than acting. Such studies suggest that modern medical institutions cannot be introduced into Ayurveda without altering underlying formulations of person and illness.

My original research intent, then, was to study the ways that Ayurvedic knowledge had been changed by or preserved from modern disciplinary modes of knowledge.[13] My proposed method was a comparison of the practices of physicians ranging from older-generation vaidyas who had been trained by their gurus to vaidyas who had been trained in modern university settings. My conversations and observations were designed to collect data about diagnosis and treatment procedures that would reveal the underlying models of body and illness being used by each group of practitioners. In this way I expected to trace the effect of modern institutional procedures on Ayurvedic phenomenology. In a sense my research was intended to diagnose the extent to which the disease of modernity had invaded the corpus of Ayurvedic knowledge. What I had planned was a sort of clinical trial in which I would compare a body of knowledge that had not been exposed to the virus of modern institutions with one that had. In that way I expected to find out whether Ayurvedic phenomenology was immune to modern medical paradigms or whether in fact it was affected/infected. The biomedical metaphor here is useful because it reveals that such a methodology is itself deeply embedded in a modern epistemological framework that depends on a division between history and culture, modernity and tradition, as decisively as it depends on a division between viral invaders and intact bodies. This framework insinuates itself easily into discussions of modernization. The modernization of Ayurveda, for example, can be considered a process in which modern institutional forms reshape patients' and practitioners' conceptions of the body.

My aim in this book is to problematize this framework, if not to escape it. I was originally guided in this purpose by fieldwork experiences, recounted in chapter 2, that dismantled my original research question. If Ayurveda is not considered a cultural artifact modified by historical forces, then it can be understood as itself a force of change. Then the question becomes not how modern modes of knowledge affect Ayurvedic ideology and practice but how modern modes of knowledge are reworked through Ayurvedic ideology and practice. The use of the word "modern" to even fuzzily denote a complex of epistemological practices is itself problematic, however. Even the most critical usage of the word tends to hold vestiges of evaluative and chronological connotations. It is also questionable how completely its meanings in academic discourses can be insulated from its meanings in development and world-capitalist discourses. In using this term, I want to at least acknowledge its strange tautological twist. For it is the modern episteme itself that is responsible for constructing the dichotomy between the modern and the premodern or traditional. Despite this awkward (il)logic, it seems that we can no more talk ourselves entirely outside of the modern than we can talk ourselves entirely outside of signification (see Derrida 1976) or entirely outside of history (see Chakrabarty 1992a).[14]

Beyond the Seduction of Systems

Suppose we as scholars refuse to take for granted the categorization of Ayurveda as a medical system. Suppose we resist the temptation to fix Ayurveda in a discourse of order as a classical medicine operating according to a strict logic. We still may have difficulty disentangling our studies from a paradigm that has informed anthropological analyses of healing since Victor Turner's (1967) work on rites of passage. In this paradigm, not only seemingly formalistic practices such as Ayurveda, but also the most riotous "shamanic" treatments are said to restore social, cosmic, and/or somatic order. Illness is framed as a liminal time in which ordinary social meanings are interrupted by unintelligible pain and incapacity, while healing is framed as the symbolic reconstitution of social meaning through ritualized cure (e.g., Lévi-Strauss 1963a; Comaroff 1983). If Michael Taussig (1987) has succeeded in upsetting this paradigm at least for "shamanic" healing, in which the hallucinogenically induced tearing apart of signifier from signified disallows an orderly conclusion, it still seems to map only too well onto Ayurvedic healing, in which the signifiers can apparently be apprehended along their chain as surely and methodically as beads along a *mālā*. In fact, in his detailed anthropological examination of ancient Ayurvedic texts, Francis Zimmermann has suggested that ancient Ayurvedic scholars ordered their topic not in terms of taxonomic hierarchies, but in terms of "garlands of names (*nāmamālā*)" (1987, 96).

Yet how closely does such an ordering fit the liminality-communitas paradigm of anthropology? As I discuss in chapter 4, up until the beginning of the twentieth century the grouping of topics in Ayurvedic texts was one that scarcely did obeisance to modern differentiations between historic and mythic, natural and supernatural, entity and activity, representation and reality. While the liminality-communitas paradigm seems to offer resolution, summary, or totalization, these texts seem rather to offer endless elaboration, ambiguity, and never completed predication. Modern Ayurvedic textbooks, on the other hand, offer closure to such open-endedness. Contemporary urban practitioners, at least those working in hospitals, are largely committed to a representation of Ayurveda as a tidy system satisfying even the most structuralist desire for a narrative in which diseased oppositions are (re)solved through synthesizing cures. There are, however, rifts in this native discourse breaking open at several levels: in the rumors of rampant corruption prying apart the signifiers of Ayurvedic status from any certain meaning of medical competence; in the ruptures in institutional procedure that mock the power of form to enframe function; in the awkward disjunctures between a biomedical anatomy and a seemingly mythographic physiology; in the explosive miracles of apparent quacks whose cures are unexplainable by medical logic; and in the noninstitutionalized memories and mimetic reenactments of "folk" practices drenched in mystique, which are both marginalized as non-Ayurvedic and desired as an originary knowledge. These rifts run like cracks, now widening, now narrowing, through twentieth-century Ayurveda, complicating and fragmenting what has sometimes been read as a straightforward narrative of (re)rationalization and revival.

In texts discussing Ayurveda that were produced prior to the twentieth century, a clear demarcation between magical and rational is missing. Spirits and the doṣa that resemble medieval European humors are equally empirical, moving together across the same somato-climatic landscape. Mantras and herbal distillations are equally tangible and material, manipulating the same physio-mental substance. When British orientalist scholars became interested in Indian *cikitsā* and *upacāra* (treatments and remedies), they sought and isolated the vestiges of an Indian "classical" age that would serve their own narratives of civilization. They dismissed the references to "fabulous" animals unlocatable in a Linnean taxonomy or lengthy mantras or recipes for amulets or illnesses that manifested as the presence of demons, gods, fairies, celestial musicians, and a host of other entities whose reality was scorned by modern European science. They dismissed all these as the superstitions gathered during a period of medieval decline from the pure rationalism of the classical age. They thus set the parameters of an Ayurvedic secularism that would facilitate Ayurveda's inclusion in a national-cultural program.

The narrative of decline was easily assimilated into native discourses on the *yug,* in which the *satyayug,* or era of truth, has given way to the *kāliyug,* or era of darkness, when *adharma* (a word carrying a sense of unrighteousness, neglect of duty, and disruption of the proper arrangement of the world) is rampant. Twentieth-century histories of Ayurveda often lament the descent into magical practices during the colonial era and call for a return to the scientific Ayurveda of the "classical" age (e.g., Banerji 1981). Zimmermann (1978, 1987) points out, on the other hand, that early Ayurvedic therapy was a mix of "rational" and "ritual" theories and therapies. Even more to the point, as I will discuss in chapter 3, is the contingency of such histories, in which the construction of an Indian classical past followed by a medieval decline echoes European historiographic projects. In the orientalist project of preservation there was in fact a refurbishing, decontextualization, and polishing that prepared Ayurveda as a museological object, a sign of an illustrious antiquity separated from current medical practices that were thought to be permeated with irrationality. The orientalists of the eighteenth and nineteenth centuries thus orchestrated the split of the "great" and "little" traditions, the classical and the folk, that was so readily accepted by the anthropologists of the twentieth century. This dichotomy, which still shapes scholarly interpretations of South Asian religious practices, has also shaped interpretations of South Asian healing. The great tradition, into which the name Ayurveda was absorbed, has become a sign of civilizational glory, while the little traditions have become rather a sign of Indian backwardness. Twentieth-century Ayurveda had therefore to be cleansed of esoterica, cleared of contradictions, sanitized of ghosts. The marginalization of healing mantras, supramental curing powers, and "magical" rather than "rational" uses of substances, no less than the marginalization of miracles, devotional ecstasy, and caste-indifferent charismatic movements, has lent such practices a powerful and mysterious alterity that can then be exploited by political reactionaries and charlatans. For Ayurveda would lose its value in the national-cultural imaginary if it was totally assimilated to the modern.

A further aim of this book, therefore, is to demonstrate that contemporary Ayurveda is simultaneously modern and in tension with the modern, invoking, like other signs of antiquity, an ever deferred authenticity. It is in the margins, fringes, and even failures of official Ayurveda that the power of Ayurveda to satisfy a national (and transnational) nostalgia for tradition comes most clearly into focus. For the promises of twentieth-century Ayurveda extend from calming the overexcited doṣa to easing the excessiveness of industrial lifestyles and from curing illness to healing modernity itself. To fulfill such promises, practitioners employ potent neo-orientalisms, promoting Ayurveda as spiritually attuned, antimaterialist, and nonviolent, in contrast to biomedicine. Its therapies are advertised as antidotes for the severe and toxic side effects of both modern lifestyles and modern pharmaceuticals. The healing of modernity, whether at the somatic or social level, is enveloped by and yet always escaping a rhetoric and a discipline of the restoration of order. This healing spills out into wilder hopes, less structured longings for the miraculous, the unexplainable, the "traditional." For it is in these, finally, that the cure for modernity seems most compellingly to lie—not in plant extracts, but in a newly fashioned antiquity, Dr. Vijayan's "true essence" of Ayurveda.

To take on the forms of the modern while simultaneously retaining the promise of redemption from the modern involves intricate maneuvers. Contemporary Ayurveda is packaged in modern institutions. Yet here and there in pharmaceutical advertising and private practices, in magazine articles and the conversation of practitioners, strategic signs of "folk" medicine work their magic against the modern. One of the most recurrent of these signs of "folk" medicine is the popular mystique of an elaborately predictive pulse diagnosis, which speaks the insufficiencies of official Ayurveda. While pulse reading to detect the predominant and aggravated doṣa is considered part of "classical" Ayurveda and taught in Ayurvedic colleges, more elaborate pulse reading, to detect a patient's specific complaints or personal history, is not. In this way Ayurveda differs from Tibetan, Chinese, or even Unani or Siddha healing practices, in which a complex semiotics of pulse is integral to contemporary medical programs and not simply haunting their edges.[15] Ayurvedic colleges profess to mass-produce vaidyas but not pulse readers. Like the "authentic" works of art discussed by Walter Benjamin (1968), pulse diagnosis carries an "aura," an association with "ritual." It possesses a uniqueness in time and place as the specific province of practitioners linked to gurus in particular lineages. The popularity of a noninstitutionalized pulse diagnosis can be understood as the nostalgia for tradition that often thrives in counterpoint to the drive toward modernity. This nostalgia is oriented not so much toward the actual past as toward the aura itself, toward the very idea of authenticity. To borrow a phrase from Susan Stewart (1993, 143), nostalgia is enamored of its distance from the referent (e.g., "traditional" Ayurveda) and not of the referent itself.[16] Thus the popular fascination with pulse-reading vaidyas rests as much on their distance from institutional Ayurveda as on their actual skills or connection with a lineage.

Yet it would be a mistake to suppose that it is only such emblems of "folk" medicine as pulse reading that can enchant Ayurvedic healing practice. For, in some contexts, the signs of professional science possess a magical charge of their own. In the tent of an itinerant vaidya we will meet in chapter 6, for example, jar labels of major pharmaceutical companies and gilt-framed certificates impress the vaidya's authenticity on the patient just as compellingly as a six-hundred-year-old book of formulae and the claim to read pulse. Ayurvedic authenticity is thus given definition through a mimetic and countermimetic reverberation of paradoxical cultural imaginaries. The Ayurvedic elite appropriates institutionalized forms of scientific knowledge introduced by the British, even as they simultaneously evoke the authority of ancient texts to anticipate or even surpass modern science. Miracles of modern medical technologies such as inoculation and X rays are recognized alongside the marvelous paranormal powers of professional folk healers that render these technologies superfluous. Meanwhile, the romance of modernization manifest in the immaculate pharmaceutical factory of an urban pulse reader works in mysterious tandem with the nostalgia for tradition motivating the patients who crowd his waiting room. Ayurvedic practices ever refer / defer beyond themselves to orientalist / colonial imagery reverberating in indigenous imagery reverberating in turn in postcolonial / neo-orientalist imagery (see Taussig 1987). Here the sign of authenticity always already precedes the referent, which is itself another sign reflecting particular desires for the healing of tradition, in every sense of the phrase. In this book, then, I follow the current of contemporary desires for a traditional healing that conjures the very tradition it promises to heal and restore.

From Genealogies to Orientations

The idea of "authenticity" is one feature of a modern mode of knowledge that understands persons, social spaces, and knowledge itself through an opposition between reality and its representations, between content and form, between the private and the public. In the modern world this opposition is so taken for granted and ingrained as to be self-evident. It is embedded in modern scholarship, including the ethnographic enterprise in which anthropologists read the statements of our interlocutors as representations of cultural reality. Yet anthropology, with its frequent experiences of incomprehension, miscommunication, and raw frustration also offers rare opportunities to detach from deeply ingrained ways of knowing. In chapter 2 I will show how I was led to abandon the comparative frame in which this ethnography was first conceived as certain aspects of a modern epistemology were disrupted through my encounters with three Ayurvedic practitioners. I went to the field affecting detachment from the very modern knowledge whose infiltration I wanted to document. Yet my own modern assumptions were reflected back to me through answers to my questions that resisted their epistemological thrust. One of these assumptions was that medical phenomena can be mapped onto the space of the body; another assumption was that local / regional medical practices can be isolated and delineated; a third assumption was that a particular instance of illness is a private rather than public concern. In my observation of Ayurvedic practice these three aspects of illness and of medicine eluded me, made quixotic flash appearances, but ultimately opened out into spaces I could not easily enframe.[17]

In subsequent chapters I will continue to pursue this theme, tracing the challenges posed to a modern epistemology by contemporary Ayurvedic practice—whether at the level of institutions, bodies, psyches, remedies, diagnostic methods, or practitioner competence. Chapter 3 traces the genealogy of contemporary Ayurveda as a sign of Indian culture, focusing in particular on a pivotal historic moment in which Ayurvedic practitioners began to lament not simply the malaise of the human body, but also the malaise of the national body. From that turning point onward the name Ayurveda stood not simply for knowledge of life or long life (the literal meaning), but also for *Indian* knowledge of life. The sign took on the task not just of healing disease, but also of healing a newly conceived Indian tradition. Before this moment the turn-of-the-century books on Ayurveda cranked out by the new printing industry lamented the loss of health and of Ayurvedic knowledge. They attributed these losses to poor health habits due to the imitation of European lifestyles. After this genealogical moment books on Ayurveda began to lament the loss of Ayurvedic status. They began to sustain a rhetorical redefinition of Ayurveda on the grounds of both its scientificity (running parallel to European medical science) and its resonance with Indian culture (running counter to European medical science).

The redefinition was bolstered by the restructuring of Ayurvedic training and scholarship into teaching hospitals modeled on European biomedical institutions. This disciplinary project, discussed in chapter 4, demonstrates not so much the impact of modern institutions on indigenous tradition as the reification of indigenous tradition through the medium of modern institutions. The most potentially transformative event here is not so much the introduction of specific institutional forms and their attendant methodologies (such as anatomy) and phenomenologies (such as docile bodies) (Foucault 1979). Rather it is the introduction of an episteme whereby an institutional structure is understood to contain and represent a particular content or function, as discussed above. In the context of my fieldwork this epistemic operation results in an expectation that an Ayurvedic teaching hospital represents Ayurvedic knowledge. While this expectation is shared, if somewhat awkwardly, by practitioners, professors, administrators, patients, and anthropologists alike, it also, at certain moments, gives way to an admission that hospitals utterly fail to represent Ayurvedic knowledge. Moreover, when I attempted to penetrate and "thickly describe" (Geertz 1973) the inner workings of an

Ayurvedic hospital, I was deflected by what I experienced as an aggravating thinness. The college schedule, for instance, rarely reflected the daily activities. The degree offered rarely reflected the professional intentions of the students. The subject matters into which Ayurvedic knowledge had been organized were not easily read as an intelligible corpus.

Historical memories of elderly vaidyas suggest a reason for this thinness. The institutional signs, such as degrees and examinations, required for a nationalist agenda, were disseminated in a political field that elicited different kinds of significance. In the context of colonial and postcolonial India such signs became less avowedly constative, in the linguistic sense, than performative, asserting professional status without, however, assuring professional expertise. It is not so much that these educational signs are deceptive, or falsely representative of reality, as that they are creative, or powerfully productive of reality. In the establishment of a modern Ayurveda such educational signs were crucial to creating a class of registered professional Ayurvedic practitioners. Yet for the most part there seems to be no necessary linkage between such formal markers and the actual process of transmitting Ayurvedic knowledge. What the Ayurvedic institutions I visited make almost embarrassingly obvious is the brazen performativity of modern institutions, which are routinely posited rather as the ground of performativity, a neutral syntax or medium. Modern institutional structure is then revealed as not just representing knowledge but performing authority.

Beginning in chapter 4 and continuing into chapter 5, I investigate other disturbances in the form and content relationship at the level of physical bodies. The distinction between symptom and disease that informs a modern diagnostic semiotics, though enforced by the modern medical technologies of Ayurvedic hospitals, is only partially reproduced in contemporary clinical practice. In much Ayurvedic practice the signs of disease have a contiguity with their presumed referents that is close to unity. The ontological hierarchy wherein symptom is simply an indicator and disease an objective entity, the focal point of treatment, is therefore not easily sustained. Diseases themselves are signs, metonyms of aggravated doṣa, while so-called symptoms such as fever are treatable in themselves, even without being traced to a seemingly more final referent. The binarism of symptom and disease, though invoked in clinical discourse, is nonetheless often irrelevant to clinical practice.[18]

Moreover, if the structure of Ayurvedic training seems out of alignment with its function, contemporary Ayurvedic anatomy seems similarly out of alignment with Ayurvedic physiology. The body that lies passively on the dissection table as a positivistic object is difficult to reconcile with the body that courses with angry or calm doṣa. This latter body is, I argue, not the disciplined body of modern medicine, but rather a fluent body, streaming with temperatures and aromas, eloquent with densities and moistures, where illness is communicated in a teeming polysemic lexicon of air currents and blockage, emotions, and digestive fire. In modern Ayurvedic hospitals, however, techniques of quantification are being applied to discipline this body, to map and tabulate the transformations of *dhātu* (bodily tissues) and flow of doṣa. As the poetics of the body is translated into scientific equations, so the rhythmic aphorisms of Ayurvedic texts are translated into textbook explanations. The wisdom that as recently as a hundred years ago was most often rendered in a complex verse that proliferated meanings is now rendered in textbook expositions and research hypotheses that affix meanings. Yet I argue that a certain creative polyvalence remains vital to clinical work.

Furthermore, even within this new regime of scholarship the imaginations of students and practitioners alike are stirred by the stories of practitioners outside of the modern institutional system who escape and sometimes mock its disciplinary powers. One pivotal image of traditional medicine, as I mentioned above, is that of a practitioner who reads the intricacies of personal health through the pulse. Practitioners who claim this talent are found not only in villages and small towns or in the colorful tents of itinerant vaidyas on urban street corners, but also in efficiently streamlined clinics in arboreal suburbs. Here the site of longing also becomes the site of suspicion, as the desire for authentic traditional cures is complicated by the desire for professional legitimacy and the tropes of an ascetic discipline compete with the tropes of a modern regimental discipline. Chapter 6 focuses on a controversial urban pulse reader, investigating the conflicting rhetorics of authenticity spun by the practitioner himself, the colleagues who consider him a quack, and the anthropologist who is trained to scrutinize cultural efficacy even more closely than medical efficacy. The quack's medical mimicry borrows, empties out, and exaggerates the signs of both "folk" and "professional" practitioners, directing attention to a social world in which these signs circulate in a dizzying mimetic and countermimetic display. In an environment where professional doctors imitate folk doctors who imitate professional doctors and so on, the genuine practitioner or pure referent of either category becomes unrecoverable. This chapter interrogates the rituals of signification by which we distinguish medicine from placebo, doctor from quack, expertise from gimmickry, and authentic cultural object from consumer-oriented copy. Contemporary Ayurveda emerges as a play of simulacra that effectively parodies the relationship between sign and natural object central to modern science.

I continue the theme of postcolonial parody of imported disciplines in chapter 7, which explores the disruption of one of modernity's key assumptions, the interiorized self, at what would ordinarily be a key site in its deployment, the confessional form of psychotherapeutic consultations. The use of group psychotherapy at an Ayurvedic university exposes the ordinarily mystified mechanism whereby a modern interiorized self is posited at the same moment as and by means of its perceived repression and attempted recovery. The practice of Ayurvedic psychotherapy in its partial replication of a European medical model draws attention to the hollowness of that model. In the Ayurvedic context psychotherapy is recruited to new ends that undermine not only its utility as a transposable sign, but also the priority of the interiorized self it is designed to apprehend. The modern narrative of individual identity, in which the self is constructed by means of the epiphany of its repression and the move toward its recovery, reminds us again of the modern narrative of national-cultural identity. These are twin folktales, the first serving to mystify the invention of the modern individual and the second to mystify the invention of culture. The (re)invention of Ayurveda as a primordial Indian essence is accomplished through the discovery of its decline and a move toward its revival. The word revival, when applied to this (re)invention, disguises the continuity of indigenous healing practices, in which textual and oral erudition, "rational" and "irrational" procedures, were freely intermixed. The word also, ironically enough, disguises the radical newness of an Ayurveda that has been assimilated not only to orientalist, but also to neo-orientalist claims about Indian culture, as touched on early in this chapter and again in the epilogue.

In the pages that follow, then, I explore the ways that various Ayurvedic practitioners engage, transform, or circumvent the modes of medical knowledge introduced through modern institutional procedures. I find that contemporary Ayurvedic practice tends to disturb and reinterpret such monumental divisions as those between science and miracle, symptom and disease, private and social selves, institutional form and academic content, professional and folk sectors. I suggest that such binaries, when transposed into the Ayurvedic context, operate paradoxically as both signs and parodies of modernity.[19] I trace how a modern semiotics is transformed in local settings to accomplish different work.

There are two key dangers in such an enterprise. The first is the danger of enframing or seeming to enframe an alter-semiotics, permitting it to be absorbed again in a modern epistemology of representation and enclosure. It is, after all, tempting to assimilate the seeming resistance to European semiotics to differently nuanced philosophies of signification perhaps rooted in South Asia before the British ever arrived.[20] A second danger is that of simply using the indigenous subversions of modernity as a base from which to launch a critique of modern European knowledge practices.[21] My intention here is to understand Ayurvedic responses to modern knowledge not as signs of cultural essence but rather as resonances of colonial and postcolonial encounters (see Taussig 1993, 1987). My concern is not to use indigenous semiotic projects either to undermine a modern episteme or to heal it. Rather my concern is to interpret parts of the dialogue reverberating from certain political encounters. Nonetheless, these two dangers remain a constant tension in the following historical and ethnographic accounts, in which I skirt but try to defer the enframing of Ayurveda.[22] In this way I endeavor to resist satisfying a modern desire for authentic culture or healing a modern sense of cultural emptiness with "ethnomedicine."

two Ayurvedic Interiors

In chapter 3 I will trace the development of Ayurveda in early twentieth-century texts from a set of health behaviors to a sign of Indian culture. Before doing so, however, I would like to draw attention to some of the effects of this development in current Ayurvedic practice. In this chapter I recount a series of ethnographic moments with each of three private practitioners. The first, Vd. Sharma, in his eighties, was trained largely in the context of a guru-disciple relationship, although he also interned briefly with a biomedical doctor. The second, Dr. Karnik, in his sixties, was trained and worked for many years in modern-style Ayurvedic teaching hospitals. The third, Dr. Upadhyay, in his forties, is the son of an Ayurvedic physician; like Dr. Karnik, however, he was trained in modern-style teaching hospitals. All three of these practitioners are residents of an urban metropolis. All three have been involved in Ayurvedic professional associations to one degree or another. They are each in their own way concerned with the fate of Ayurveda. In both their discourse and their practice they participate in a dialogue not only with their anthropological interlocutor, but also with a larger field of voices and forces. Together they make it clear that Ayurveda is being (re)invented in ways that answer not merely to requirements of modern science, but also to problems of postcolonial cultural identity.

I find Timothy Mitchell's (1988) concept of enframing useful for understanding the epistemological collisions that occurred between me and these practitioners. In his study of the colonization of Egypt, Mitchell demonstrates how modern epistemology establishes a binary split between reality and its representations, private and public, content and form. This epistemology is evident, for example, in an urban architecture of facades that represent their interiors to an outside observer. Mitchell points out that the spatial split between facade and interior, architectural sign and institutional referent, did not exist in precolonial Egyptian towns. He calls this modern binarism enframing and shows how it conflicted with precolonial ways of organizing the world on many fronts, from architecture to scholarship to the use of language.

While Mitchell's account focuses on a process of colonization, it documents an epistemological collision that still occurs in postcolonial encounters. In this chapter I focus on three practitioners' points of engagement with particular projects of enframing. It should not be inferred that their interpretations of Ayurveda are collapsible into an encounter with European modernities. Nonetheless, their interpretations are certainly shaped by an encounter with these modernities that takes place on various fronts, from the purely medical to the socio-moral. Their interpretations of Ayurveda are not determined by a cultural domain of "ethnomedical beliefs," but rather dialogically directed by a politically charged field of actors that includes biomedical doctors, government agencies, ambivalent patients, social researchers, and non-Indian consumers of Indian "culture." I argue that each of these physicians resists modern modes of knowledge at different levels: Vd. Sharma at the level of medicine itself, Dr. Karnik at the level of social science, and Dr. Upadhyay at the level of neo-orientalist commodification. Each of these practitioners, therefore, strategically constructs his medical knowledge in a way that addresses the epistemological imbalance by which a European universalist knowledge would enframe Ayurveda as a bounded and limited knowledge. In this chapter, then, I trace a few of the possible ways that contemporary Ayurvedic knowledge is shaped by the discursive maneuvers of Ayurvedic doctors who seek to evade the tidy (en)closures of modern European epistemological frames. The stories I tell here serve to underscore both the problematic meanings and the practical and political usefulness of Ayurveda as a category.

Going Deep

Dressed in a white dhoti and carrying a black umbrella, Vd. Sharma led me through the streets toward what he refers to as his dispensary. On the way we kicked off our sandals at a temple to do *pūjā* (loosely translatable as ritual prayer) at a *mūrti* (sacred image) of Vishnu and Laksmi. The temple consisted of a roof supported by pillars and a marble floor raised off the street by two or three stone steps. There were no walls or doorways. The threshold was marked by the rows of muddy shoes left by the temple-goers. I stood in a queue of muttering men facing the mūrti, while off to one side a circle of women sat chanting. Conditioned to prayer as a private act, I wondered how the worshippers could pray in such a noisy and unenclosed place, open to the surrounding marketplace. From the temple we passed through a narrow lane lined with stalls selling brass incense holders, mūrtis of gods and goddesses, and gaudy silk cloths fringed with gold tinsel. As we wound our way through the stalls, Vd. Sharma told me that this was the dirtiest and most crowded part of the city. We passed into a narrow street barred from taxis or bullock carts by the sheer press of pedestrians. From there we turned into a dirt alley.

The rickety stairs leading to his dispensary begin in a corner of the alley that is the workshop of a metal polisher who was hard at work shining silver chains. Above one of the doors opening off the dark hallway at the top of the stairs is a Hindi sign painted with Vd. Sharma's name. He unlocked a padlock, led me into a tiny entryway, and from there showed me into the dispensary, which consisted of one large room with a window at the end opening onto a balcony overlooking the street. Vd. Sharma sat in a chair at the end of the room. The chair is wedged between a counter where he and his assistants mix up medicines and a small table where he scribbles notes. Patients sit at this table, kitty-corner from Vd. Sharma, detailing their complaints above the sounds of street vendors and honking horns. On the other side of the desk is an examination couch, which was, however, never used as such during any of my visits. The outer portion of the room is lined with cupboards crammed with bags and bottles of medicinal substances. The day of my first visit a fan suspended from the ceiling whirled slowly. On a wooden bench along one wall patients awaited their turn. The consultation area can be separated from the waiting area by a sliding partition, but this is always left open. Since there is no air conditioning, the outer doors are always ajar as well. Occasionally children from neighboring homes wander in to watch or interact with the vaidya, his assistants, or his assistants' children.

By beginning my account of Vd. Sharma's practice with a familiar trope of anthropological (or colonial) arrival, I do not mean to simply add my voice to an unreflective orientalist discovery of Indian chaos.[1] Rather I wish to draw attention early on in this story to the modern perspective underlying my research intent, whereby I looked for an organized Ayurveda that would be arranged before me like a cultural exhibit. Vd. Sharma's dispensary is a space virtually without a facade in Mitchell's terms. One approaches it through twisting passages that offer no vantage point from which the dispensary or its building can be viewed. Much like early travelers and anthropologists, I accompanied my "informant" with the expectation of taking an ethnological snapshot of his practice. Thus my initial frustration at understanding his practice was very much akin to the frustrations of European travelers and colonialists with the supposed chaos of Indian cities, Indian social relations, and Indian minds.

If it seemed to me that the categories of public and private continuously overlapped in the ordering of space around Vd. Sharma's dispensary, then it also seemed that the categories of interior and exterior overlapped in his orderings of health and illness. In answer to my first question about diagnosis Vd. Sharma emphasized the importance of "going deep with the patient." For him, "going deep" does not imply penetration to the malfunctioning organ but rather penetration into a network of forces unknown to modern anatomy. Vd. Sharma provided an impromptu translation of a passage in one of the ancient Ayurvedic texts as follows: "Only the vaidya who goes deep to the root of the soul and *mana* [usually translated as mind but also including much of the connotation of the English heart in its nonanatomical sense] of the patient is the real vaidya." The purpose of "going deep" is to find out "which doṣa are there, which dhātu are affected, which organ is affected, and what the *prakṛti* of the patient is."

Of these four factors affecting the illness, only two, the dhātu (which is usually translated as tissue, though the inadequacy of the translation can be seen in the fact that one of the dhātu is semen) and the organ, can be clearly thought of as contained within the body. Prakṛti is usually translated as constitution. The patient's prakṛti can be defined as the predominant doṣas manifest in his or her body type and behavior, affinities, and aversions. According to Vd. Sharma, a person's prakṛti can change slowly due to the influences of medicine, food, and climate. Prakṛti, therefore, is less a feature of the patient than of the relationship between the patient and her environment. As noted in chapter 1, the word doṣa is usually translated as "humors," while the three doṣa, vāta, pitta, and kapha, are usually translated as "air," "bile," and "phlegm" respectively. These translations can be misleading, however, in their identification of doṣa with substances inside the body. As I will discuss at more length in chapter 5, doṣa are more often understood today as principles that are linked through an elaborate system of correspondences not only to somatic processes, but also to processes in the environment. Even that phrasing is misleading insofar as the idea of doṣa bypasses the conceptual split between body and world altogether. In many versions of Ayurvedic phenomenology, body, society, and world seem to be folded into one another in convoluted ways. Vāta, pitta, and kapha, for instance, correspond also to types of behavior and to the astrological elements of air, fire, and water/earth. Thus the state of the doṣa may be manifest not only in physical phenomena such as pulse movement or skin color, but also in habits such as athleticism or lethargy and in the positions of the planets at the time of the patient's birth.

Vd. Sharma's diagnosis consists primarily of *darśan* and of talking to the patient. Darśan literally means "seeing" but in many contexts also carries the connotation of imbibing another's presence. For Vd. Sharma darśan includes an examination of tongue, eyes, skin color, and so on. He explained, "Darśan—look at a patient and you come to conclusions. . . . We see the tongue, eyes—yellowish, bright or not . . . dry or not, burning or not." It is only when he reaches across the tiny table to take the patient's pulse that Vd. Sharma seems to try to solicit signs from the patient's interior. Yet he uses pulse diagnosis not so much to assess the state of the heart or arteries as to determine prakṛti. The qualities of the pulse vary according to the predominant doṣa. In texts discussing pulse diagnosis the vāta pulse is compared to the movement of a leech or snake, the pitta pulse to the movements of a frog, and the kapha pulse to the movements of a goose or swan. When Vd. Sharma practices darśan, he does not seem to be reading signs that refer to the hidden essence of the patient's illness. Rather he seems to be observing the visible aspects of the patient's illness in order to construct a narrative that includes the less visible aspects. Pulse motion and tongue color are not so much symptoms of a disease entity as glimpses of a disease process unfolding between patient and world.

Vd. Sharma is not averse to using modern diagnostic technology, particularly to measure the efficacy of his treatments. In our conversations, however, he cautioned that modern diagnostic tools will not always give an accurate account of a patient's state of health. He compared two patients, one with a good hemoglobin count who is always exhausted and the other with a low hemoglobin count who "does his good work." Vd. Sharma told me that in the second case the patient's "general vitality and the strength in the blood cells, hear me, is so good that he can digest . . . and do his life's work. . . . So here the comparison [between Ayurvedic and modern diagnosis] won't help us." Moreover, Vd. Sharma says that he "will accept what the patient says" over the results of modern tests. In Vd. Sharma's practice the interior medical gaze traced by Foucault (1973) is used for corroborative purposes only. Although Vd. Sharma does ask the patient about his complaints, he tends to emphasize darśan more than interrogation.

Vd. Sharma's treatment, like his diagnostic method, "goes deep" into the patient's life and not necessarily deep into his or her body. He recited to me the prescriptions for health in the oldest Ayurvedic texts. According to these prescriptions, he told me, one should rise before sunrise, perform breathing and other yogic exercises, and pray. He correlated this prescription with the English aphorism "Early to bed, early to rise," although this aphorism, of course, does not include yoga, which is arguably as much a form of mental discipline as a form of exercise, let alone prayer. "Preventive medicine," according to Vd. Sharma, involves three considerations: hygiene, seasons and environment, and diet. He defined health broadly as a state in which the doṣa are balanced, the dhātu are in "required form and energy," the digestive system and *mala kriya* ("the whole eliminative function") are in order, and the mind is happy. He quoted and translated an Ayurvedic verse: "Who is very satisfied, easily at enjoyment and peace, in *ātmā* [soul or self, but not in the sense of personality], *man* [mind/heart], and *indriya* [organs], . . . full of joy, he is the only healthy man." He continued, "Again I come to my religious philosophy, Ayurvedic philosophy, or philosophy. If one doesn't control the attachment to food, the attachment to taste—if I advise you not to eat chilis, but you are fond of chilis, suppose, and you eat them against my advice, then you are going to meet suffering."

This philosophy manifests in very specific advice for particular patients. "In Ayurveda it is said, 'Who is the best vaidya? [The one] who can counsel the patient,'" Vd. Sharma informed me. His own counseling most often takes the form of advice about diet, as in the above example. Yet diet is not only a matter of likes and dislikes, but also of social and religious affiliations. He told me the story of one patient with "hot yellow" urine, "red inflammation in legs," and only "four grams [of] hemoglobin." He prescribed four to eight ounces of honey per day with one lime and water in which dried grapes had been soaked. The patient stayed on this diet for two months. In addition, he was treated with various Ayurvedic medications. After a year and a half of treatment the hemoglobin count doubled. Then, because the patient was a Parsi (and therefore a meat eater), Vd. Sharma told him, "If you want to get better earlier, take fresh liver of goat, crush it, put it in one or two liters of water, cook [down] to one-quarter of it, prepare it nicely, and then drink with lime and sugar." He concluded, "So I am not against even all these things." In other words, despite his own vegetarianism he is willing to prescribe meat where appropriate to the social situation of the patient.

Considerations of treatment also extend beyond the patient's social world to the climate. A patient with a lung problem was told to continue his course of antibiotics but also to take *tulsī* (basil) brewed in boiling water as a nerve stimulant and general tonic. Vd. Sharma explained that because the patient lives in a moist climate, antibiotics are appropriate. In a drier climate antibiotics would not be necessary. In Vd. Sharma's practice, antibiotics have been swallowed into a classificatory schema of substances, both somatic and environmental, whose properties interact to produce various harmful, indifferent, or curative effects.[2] Antibiotics are understood, like all medications, not only according to their specific effect, but also according to more general properties that participate in a vast organization of *rasa,* translated as "taste" or "savor," and *guṇa,* translated as "quality." Zimmermann (1987, 9) suggests that rasa are not merely "flavors" accessible to the senses but "essences" circulating in the landscape. Vd. Sharma's treatment may be thought of as a matter of orchestrating or directing a flow of savors and qualities through the cosmic and somatic terrains. He performs this orchestration from his small counter by reaching over his head for various glass jars filled with brown, ochre, orange, and red powders.

It is apt that Vd. Sharma refers to his private practice as a dispensary since a great deal of his time is spent preparing medicines. Each medicine prescribed is mixed while the patient waits. After removing some powder from a jar on a flat knife, he taps the powder off the knife into a small pile on a page torn out of a magazine. He lines up a specific number of such piles for each herb or mineral according to the recipe scribbled on a piece of paper at his elbow. Then he pours the contents of this paper into a mortar. Either he or one of his assistants pounds and mixes the powders and finally pours out small amounts of the finished compound onto two-inch-square pieces of brown paper, which are then folded into neat envelopes. Each of these packets is one dose. I asked once if he repeats mantras as he mixes the medicine (as is recommended in some of the Ayurvedic texts). He said no, that he had to concentrate on mixing the medicine accurately. But later he said, "If you go on concentrating on God, that does help here . . . spontaneously." He said also that each vaidya is different, "like two bakers preparing bread." Even though the ingredients are the same, the "judgment, efficiency, experience, and knowledge" of the person preparing the medicine has a large effect. Certainly Vd. Sharma's units of powder balanced on the flat surface of the knife do not conform to a strict standard of measurement. When I complained of a sore throat, he gave me a powder that tasted strongly of cardamom. Later another doctor gave me what I was told was the same medicine, but the cardamom flavor was missing. When I asked Vd. Sharma's opinion of the prepackaged Ayurvedic drugs now on the market, he replied, "I am not so much in favor but there is no alternative. . . . We have to accept realities here." For Vd. Sharma the ideal of standardization holds no particular glamor. A method of mixing medicines that a modern pharmacist would be constrained to call inaccurate is for Vd. Sharma an act of carefulness born of devotion, exactitude born of concentration. The seeming subjectivity of a practice whereby every vaidya brews a different potion is not a problem. Moreover, the seeming objectivity of a practice whereby Ayurvedic products are mass-produced according to scientifically repeated (and, more important, repeatable) formulae is not necessarily desirable.

Vd. Sharma partly falls into a category that some Ayurvedic practitioners working within modern institutional settings call "the traditional practitioner." Not having been trained in the anatomo-clinical method, he seems to work with a model of the person that is rather different from that described in an anatomical text. At the end of our first conversation I had planned to request that he draw me a picture of the person as conceptualized by Ayurveda. Before I even attempted this question, however, I developed a deep perplexity about how I was going to get it across. I was not at all sure I could explain what I meant by "person," with all of its social science nuances. The Hindi / Sanskrit word most frequently given as a translation for English "person" is *vyakti*. It is far from clear, however, that the two terms cover the same semantic terrain.[3] Vyakti is also given as a translation for English "individual." Yet in English "individual" has a definite modern tinge, conjuring up the cluster of rights, motives, interests, and responsibilities associated with citizenship in a nation-state. "Person," on the other hand, is less specifically connotative, more encompassing, more presumably capable of crossing cultural boundaries. Anthropologists have published innumerable discussions of the concept of person in various cultures. In South Asian studies, Marriott (1976) is often cited for his assertion that the Indian person is a "dividual" rather than an individual. Other South Asian researchers have also argued that the South Asian person, as conceptualized and as lived, is less discrete, less bounded, more permeable by the environment than the European/North American "individual." Moreover, I was doubtful that either "person" or "vyakti" would be meaningful to Vd. Sharma as a generic term outside of any reference to a *particular* person.

Sidestepping this abstraction, therefore, I asked Vd. Sharma if he could diagram for me the relationships among the doṣa, dhātu, and organs. He waved his hand dismissively and said, "In Jamnagar [a city in Gujarat where there is a college and teaching hospital known for being relatively free of biomedical influence] they have some maps of all this. . . . I belong to the old school of thought." He referred me to another Ayurvedic doctor, a "modernist" who could explain how these things are "interpreted in the modern technology." I persisted: "You don't think of these relationships in a visual way?" "I think, but in my way," he replied. "I cannot satisfy you in that." I tried shifting my terms, saying, "I'm not looking for anything in particular. I'm just curious about whether the way Ayurveda looks at the body could be diagrammed." Vd. Sharma responded, "Now suppose you are here for three months. My way is to prove to you the results. . . . Because instead of reading very deeply, I experienced and experimented nicely in my life and found results." Vd. Sharma would not (or perhaps could not) sketch the doṣa or dhātu, but he would track them over a period of months along a particular course of treatment.

Zimmermann notes that in ancient Sanskrit texts, "The listing and description of living beings do not constitute an end in themselves but are subordinated to a normative aim of some kind, whether it be ritual or political, astrological or medical" (1987, 130). He argues that such a knowledge, in which the effects of physical substance are intertwined with strategies of life and health, is "anthropocentric." Therefore, "India proceeded no farther than the bestiary, whereas others managed to escape from the enchantments of the dharma [in this context, cosmic order], that ritualistic vision of the universe, and invent the natural sciences" (1987, 196). Yet the question arises of whether a modern ordering of phenomena that claims to be autonomous from the situation of the knower deserves to be privileged over an ordering of phenomena that is precisely oriented by the situation of the knower. I suggest, along with other scholars, that a knowledge that asserts its own positivity rests on a historically contingent dichotomy between observer and the object-world.[4] For Vd. Sharma, doṣa and dhātu have meaning not within a phenomenological museum but within a particular trajectory of healing. The next time I asked if doṣa and dhātu can be diagrammed, my respondent replied, "Very difficult." The gist of his answer was in close parallel to Vd. Sharma's: doṣa and dhātu have to be observed; they are processes happening over time, not objects in space.

Having not visited the Ayurvedic college at Jamnagar, I do not know how the diagrams there portray the relationships among doṣa and dhātu. In any case it is clear that Vd. Sharma viewed the diagrams I was requesting as producible only through the language of "modern technology." Every Ayurvedic anatomy department I visited displayed countless anatomical sculptures, with organs duly exposed and labeled in Sanskrit, as well as shelf after shelf of jars containing pickled brains and hearts and malformed fetuses. In the dissection rooms small groups of students stood over cadavers, separating the muscles of the foot, for example, with precision tools. Yet in these places I did not see a single diagram of the doṣa that are considered so central to Ayurvedic diagnosis and treatment. In fact, the only diagrams of the doṣa I have encountered have been schematics. Figure 1, for example, is the cover of an Ayurvedic textbook about the fundamentals of Ayurvedic thought. Here the names of the doṣa are written along the sides of a triangle that is nested within a pentagon, the five sides of which underscore the names of the five elements of Ayurvedic cosmology: *pṛthvī* (earth), *jal* (water), *agni* (fire), *vāyu* (air), and *ākāśa* (ether). The pentagon in turn is nested inside of

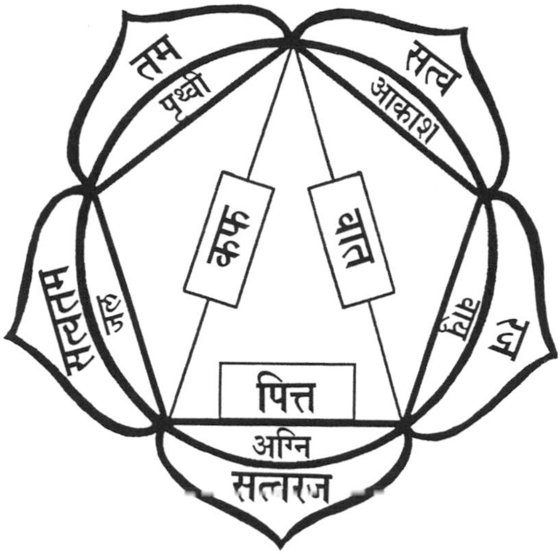

Figure 1. Mandala of Names. Diagram of the names of the doṣa, the five basic elements, and the three guṇa from the cover of an Ayurvedic textbook on basic principles (Tripāṭhi 1994).

a lotus, the petals of which are inscribed with the names of the three guṇa—*sattva, rajas,* and *tamas*—along with two hybrid guṇa, *sattvatamas* and *sattvarajas.*[5] Here what are illustrated are names and their relationships to other names, rather than the entities those names apparently represent. The question then arises as to whether the entities and the names are equivalent, a question to which I return in chapter 5.

When E. Valentine Daniel (1984) asked his informants to draw a picture of the Tamil *kirāmam* and the Tamil *ūr,* either one of which might be translated as village, he received two very different sets of drawings. The kirāmam had fixed, standardized, state-determined boundaries that were exactly known only to surveyors and government officials. The ūr had more elastic boundaries, marked by sacred landmarks and open to various interpretations by the members of the ūr. The kirāmam is analogous to the anatomical diagram in which the shape and position of the organs is fixed, standardized, and determined by the canons of scientific positivism. The hypothetical diagram of the doṣa and dhātu would be analogous to the ūr. My consultants, however, were reluctant to conceptualize these in spatial terms.

These Ayurvedic phenomena also escape another type of description. In the notes Vd. Sharma keeps on particular patients, there are long lists of physical and emotional complaints interspersed with biomedical disease terms. Nowhere, however, is there a record of prakṛti or of the particular aggravation of the doṣa. When I asked Vd. Sharma about this omission, he replied in much the same way he had replied to my request for a diagram: "I am a simple practitioner, not working in institute or hospital, so I'm not expected to write down all these things. They are in my mind." It is true that prakṛti is recorded in hospital charts; in the wards I visited, however, it was relegated to the bottom and seldom consulted page of a clipboard containing a thick sheaf of papers. The bulk of the case records kept in both private clinics and hospitals contain detailed reports of physical complaints, biomedically defined conditions, test results, and drugs or therapies administered. There are at least two possible interpretations of the relative absence of attention to doṣa or prakṛti in the written record. One is that the concept of prakṛti may be considered less crucial than the other items recorded. While this is quite conceivable in some of the modern-style Ayurvedic hospitals (as we will see in chapter 5), it is clearly not the case in Vd. Sharma's dispensary. He reiterated more than once the importance of prakṛti to diagnosis and treatment. Another interpretation is that the concept of prakṛti is not easily framed within the modern instrument of the medical chart. Vd. Sharma informed me that in the past a vaidya would have kept all of his knowledge of a patient in his mind. In his view, the medical record is a modern device appropriate to modern categories of information. If prakṛti refuses to be contained within the patient, constantly referring the observer to a flow of energies between patient and environment, perhaps it also refuses to be contained within a standardized record of illness. In Vd. Sharma's practice, at least, it seems to require narration rather than listing, measurement, and classification. The relative omission of prakṛti from medical records has the curious effect of both privileging and erasure. By its exclusion it is marked simultaneously as information that eludes scientific methods of data collection and as information that is peripheral, even diaphanous. Yet for Vd. Sharma the key point is that the knowledge of prakṛti is "in his mind." The doṣa that evade modern surveillance, including the surveillance of the anthropologist, remain vital to Vd. Sharma's diagnosis and treatment.

Vd. Sharma assumed my alliance with the modern world, as well he should. When he explained to me the quality of concentration required in mixing medicines, he offered the example of Napoleon awaking from a nap just in time to join the last man of his army. He added that he was using the example of Napoleon "because you can understand, but our *ṛṣi* [sages] were of that type." At another time he compared empiricism with his philosophy as bases for medical knowledge. He told me, "Now you are come from America. . . . Principles, lines of treatment have been always changing in your [medicine], according to research. . . . We appreciate these things, but there are some eternal principles, not changing; in Ayurveda there are some eternal principles. So until those eternal principles are understood and practiced, by theory or practical things, man cannot get good health." Once again Vd. Sharma was identifying me with the modern, the progressive, against which he defended the value of Ayurvedic "eternal principles." When I asked whether students of allopathy should learn Ayurveda and vice versa, he ignored or failed to hear the first question, perhaps because of its sheer unexpectedness, and answered only the second. "Suppose for India, just as you say, Ayurvedic students must be given modern education also, compulsory; well what happens then. . . ." He went on to predict that Ayurvedic students would "completely neglect Ayurvedic principles." For Vd. Sharma, whatever else I am, I am also a representative of modern medicine and of the modern in general. No matter how hard I tried to phrase my questions in a way that aligned me with the truths and interests of Ayurveda, no matter how I aspired to the "native's point of view," I remained the spokesperson for an opposing epistemology in all of our conversations.[6] It is hardly surprising, therefore, that the syntax in which I wanted to find Vd. Sharma's rejection of the anatomo-clinical method still reflected my own modern bias of reality and its framework. My effort to draw a contrast between the methods of Vd. Sharma's "ethnomedicine" with the methods of biomedicine was thwarted in a very simple, and yet to the modern thinker mysterious, way. Anatomy is an orderly representation of the reality of blood and muscles, bones and guts, inside the skin. But there is no similar binary of representation and reality in Vd. Sharma's talk about Ayurveda. The doṣa are not contained, nor are they depicted or arrayed in a modern display of natural phenomena. Vd. Sharma offers no enframing of the forces of disease, no map of the person. For such an enframing he was only too happy to refer me to modern-style medical colleges and younger "modernist" vaidyas, excusing himself from the obligation to build modern models with the explanation that he was of the "old school," a "simple practitioner." With such phrases he invoked the imagined chronology of Ayurveda's march into the modern world while also firmly separating his own practice from that parade. He simultaneously asserted both his tolerance of and his resolute nonparticipation in modern epistemologies. Whenever my scrutiny seemed to require a split between representation and Ayurvedic reality (diagrams of doṣa, written records of prakṛti) he deflected my attention toward those forms of Ayurvedic practice that he believed could satisfy this peculiarly modern need.

Whole Body, Half Body

In contrast to the lack of facade at Vd. Sharma's dispensary, there is a clearly lettered sign for Dr. Karnik's clinic hung on the side of a building and visible from the quiet and tree-lined street. On my first visit I passed through a gate into a small private courtyard. From there a door with another neatly printed sign led directly into the doctor's waiting room, where a patient sat awaiting his appointment. The door to the consultation room was closed. I sat down on a vinyl-cushioned couch. After a few minutes Dr. Karnik opened the door and invited the patient and then me inside. Dr. Karnik sat down behind a desk opposite two chairs. One of these was occupied by his assistant, who took notes and occasionally assisted in the examination, and the other was occupied by me. The patients and their accompanying friends or relatives sat on the examination couch against the wall. If I had not been there, one of the friends or relatives would have sat in a chair. As it was, some of the friends and relatives had to stand. The consultation room was small and bright and spotlessly clean. There was a small sink on one wall where Dr. Karnik rinsed his hands from time to time but no pharmaceutical supplies. I soon learned that Dr. Karnik treats by prescription only. He advised me that very good standardized Ayurvedic medicine is available from the Ayurvedic pharmaceutical companies.

It was very difficult to ask Dr. Karnik about his practice since he frequently dismantled my questions rather than answering them. My first line of inquiry was his educational background. When I asked if he had received an integrated education of allopathy and Ayurveda (as did many others of his generation), he replied, "The demarcation between modern medicine and Ayurveda is diffuse." He went on to explain the compatibility of Ayurveda and modern medicine. It was not until our second meeting that I noticed that he nearly always used the term modern medicine in preference to allopathy. When I asked him whether the integration of Ayurveda and allopathy was desirable, he responded that at present it was not possible but then threw my term back at me. "What is allopathy?" he challenged. While I hesitated, he supplied the answer: "Allopathy is world medicine." It is, in other words, universally applicable. When I argued that culture shapes science if only in the choice of experiments, he conceded but then asserted that culture does not shape the results of experiments; these are "fact." Very quickly every consultation and every phone call became fuel for the argument that there was no basic antagonism between Ayurveda and allopathy. Integration of the two would become possible as soon as Ayurvedic physicians were willing to adopt the experimental method. He assured me that the Ayurvedic examination and the modern examination were (or should be) the same. He reported a case that had been diagnosed by another doctor as appendicitis. When Dr. Karnik saw the patient, he was able to rule out appendicitis because the patient had no appendix. In any system of medicine, he said, "Appendix is appendix." For him, the anatomical body was the bottom line.

Dr. Karnik accordingly downplayed the importance of doṣa theory. In diagnosis the identification of the disease is more central to him than the identification of prakṛti. He offered the analogy of two persons whose heights differ by a half inch. If they are standing across the room from each other, he asked, "who can tell the difference?" The difference is real but negligible and difficult to discern. Between individuals with the same illness, Dr. Karnik claimed, there can be only minor differences in prakṛti. The identification of disease, therefore, would seem to make the identification of prakṛti almost gratuitous. Dr. Karnik told me that he had been criticized for performing allopathic diagnosis. Curious as to whether this criticism had been leveled by other Ayurvedic doctors or by allopaths, I asked, "Criticized by whom?" He dodged: "That is another point; criticism is there." More than once he aphoristically recited that if disease were not important, there would be only three treatments, one for each doṣa.

In contrast to Vd. Sharma, Dr. Karnik makes no extensive inquiry into his patients' diets. He asserted, moreover, that it is impossible to follow Ayurvedic precepts of life in the contemporary world. Most people, for example, cannot rise early. When I asked if any fundamental principles of Ayurveda could be followed, Dr. Karnik discussed the changed environment, the prevalence of pollution, the noncircadian rhythm of modern schedules. Although Dr. Karnik gave patients detailed instructions as to how to ingest the prescribed medicines, I did not once hear him make dietary suggestions. In fact, another practitioner confided to me that when he had told Dr. Karnik that he now required a diet diary of all his new patients, Dr. Karnik responded that that was all very well for making oneself look good and increasing one's client load. In other words, in Dr. Karnik's opinion, attention to diet has little or no diagnostic or curative significance.

He advocated a heavy reliance on modern diagnostic tools. One morning there was a phone call from a patient with a "urinary tract problem." An endoscopy had revealed a narrowing in the urethra that, Dr. Karnik told me, Ayurvedic diagnosis would not have been able to detect. He mentioned a student who had developed a computerized form for piles diagnosis yet provided no space on the form for an endoscopy. Piles diagnosis cannot be definitive without an endoscopy, Dr. Karnik stated. His examination is far more pursuant of the signs of internal processes than Vd. Sharma's darśan. He spends at least as much time in examination as he does in talking to the patient. Moreover, he pays more attention to the affected parts of the body than to tongue and pulse. He peruses the results of laboratory results and X rays in the files patients bring from biomedical treatment centers. He told me that before modern methods for revealing heart blockage were developed, an Ayurvedic doctor would have treated it according to "symptoms." What Vd. Sharma considers the visible manifestations of aggravated doṣa, then, Dr. Karnik dismisses as "symptoms." For Vd. Sharma the distinction between symptoms and disease, sign and referent, is superfluous if not spurious. For Dr. Karnik, on the other hand, the distinction between symptoms and disease is both pertinent and genuine. Just before he told me that he had been criticized for allopathic diagnostic procedures, he stressed that it is the disease that must be treated, not the symptoms. His confidence in the difference between symptoms and disease is assured by modern diagnostic tools. "Now," Dr. Karnik said, "everything is visual: I can see." For Dr. Karnik, the anatomical gaze into the interior of the body is the very essence of effective medical practice.

Dr. Karnik insisted to me that the purpose of medicine is the same in all systems: to maintain health and to cure the patient. I confronted him with the many literary and conversational assertions by other Ayurvedic physicians that Ayurveda is more concerned with prevention while biomedicine is more concerned with cure. He countered that the World Health Organization has the largest known program for the prevention of disease. For him, the maintenance of health and the prevention of disease are equivalent. Yet for Vd. Sharma the maintenance of health implies also the persistence of joy, not only in one's organs, but also in one's mind and soul, the most transpersonal facets of one's self. Vd. Sharma's conception of the aim of medical treatment seems to follow one of the first sutras in the *Caraka Saṃhitā:* "Ayurveda is that which deals with good, bad, happy and unhappy life, its promoters and non-promoters, measurement and nature" (P. V. Sharma 1981, 1: 6). The aim of medicine, then, seems to encompass longevity, happiness, and the good life generally, not only in Vd. Sharma's perspective, but also in one of the most respected Ayurvedic texts.

With such authorities apparently on my side, I confronted Dr. Karnik with the assertions made by other practitioners that Ayurveda is concerned with the whole body while biomedicine is concerned only with the disease. Ayurveda, he countered, is "not a thing saying, 'whole body, half body.' Everything is there." In psychological ailments, he conceded, the whole body approach is essential, but in the case of a brain tumor, for example, a localized approach is necessary. He repeated, "Ayurveda is a total science; it's not only one concept, whole body or half body." He was severely critical of those who say or imply that the diagnosis of a brain tumor is allopathy. "How can that be allopathy?" In other words, if an appendix is an appendix, surely a brain tumor is a brain tumor. I conceded that in the case of a brain tumor at least part of the medical response was perhaps clear-cut: the doctor should, if possible, operate to excise the tumor. Here Dr. Karnik interrupted me to say that in actual fact an Ayurvedic doctor would not operate: modern Ayurvedic surgeons have neither the facilities nor the skills to operate on a brain tumor. Disregarding this fact, which is crucial to his interests but peripheral to mine, I proceeded with my line of questioning. I asked whether the medical response was not less clear-cut in the case of a patient who has twenty different complaints that do not add up to a clearly identifiable disease. Dr. Karnik replied that he teaches his students that a patient with twenty complaints is a "psychosomatic patient." Sometimes he tells his patients not to ask the diagnosis "because if the patient hears psychosomatic, he thinks all the time psychosomatic and becomes more psychosomatic." Dr. Karnik identified "psychosomatic" ailments with the class of ailments resulting from mana in ancient Ayurvedic texts. Vd. Sharma had also mentioned this class of ailments, though he had not translated them as "psychosomatic." Vd. Sharma stated simply that "when mana is affected, it will affect the organs." In Vd. Sharma's understanding, moreover, multiple complaints do not necessarily indicate a fundamentally mental disturbance. They are just as likely to indicate a doṣic disturbance. Many Ayurvedic practitioners and patients argue that Ayurveda is more effective for chronic illness, while allopathy is more effective for acute illness. Dr. Karnik, however, asserted that with the increase in life span modern medicine would turn its vast resources toward the problem of chronic ailments. He predicted that over the next two decades, allopathy would advance beyond Ayurveda even in the treatment of chronic disease. In his view, then, Ayurveda has no corner on "whole person" medicine.

While Dr. Karnik asserted that today's Ayurvedic surgeons perform only modern surgical procedures, he did confirm that these surgeons perform unique preparations for surgery. Nonetheless, when I repeated one surgeon's assertion that it is essential for the surgeon to become intimate with his patients, he took issue. "I'm supposed to be one of the senior persons in Ayurveda," he said. Therefore, foreigners and allopaths frequently ask him what Ayurveda has to offer that is different. "If I say doctor-patient relationship, they say, we have that also. How much I am practicing doctor-patient relationship; how much he is practicing doctor-patient relationship: it is an individual thing." He concluded that it is useless to practice an intimate doctor-patient relationship if you "miss the disease." Clearly he believes that too many Ayurvedic doctors "miss the disease."

Dr. Karnik seems to be a perfect example of an Ayurvedic practitioner who has been thoroughly modernized by his encounter with modern medical institutions and methods. He attributes his expertise to the excellent "patient experience" he obtained in an Ayurvedic hospital, where, in the outpatient department, he would see one hundred or more patients in a single day.[7] A great number of physicians admitted to me that in such departments it is virtually impossible to pay close attention to doṣa and prakṛti. Throughout our time together I tried to ask Dr. Karnik to define the uniqueness of Ayurveda. He persistently refused, however, to construct this uniqueness. Unlike many Ayurvedic practitioners and authors, he is not interested in promoting Ayurveda as a medical philosophy whose basic principles address the limitations of modern medicine. He is not tempted by neo-orientalist valorizations of Ayurveda as a holistic medicine, a discourse transcending the narrow objectivism of science. For him medicine of any kind is a purely empirical matter: "Everything is visual"; "Appendix is appendix." With the phrase "whole body, half body" Dr. Karnik effectively ruined the assumed dualism of holistic versus atomistic perspectives on the body. In replacing the opposition of whole and part with the opposition of whole and half, he did not so much create a new dualism as mark the meaninglessness of the original.

Frequently our conversations devolved into argument in which I was embarrassed to find myself attempting to save Ayurveda as a form of ethnomedicine. Dr. Karnik seemed to delight in dismissing each example of Ayurvedic essence that I tried to offer. Paradoxically, in his very allegiance to medical modernism, he undermined my anthropological modernism. For he would not permit Ayurveda to fill the empty category of tradition against which modernism is defined. He would not let me claim Ayurveda as a healing balm for modernity's excesses. If Vd. Sharma subverted the enframing of doṣa and prakṛti, Dr. Karnik subverted the enframing of Ayurveda itself. For Dr. Karnik, Ayurveda itself has the status of science: therefore, it cannot be reduced to a scientific object, exhibited behind the glass of an anthropological display case.

Dr. Karnik's resistance to easy characterizations of Ayurvedic principles should not, however, be understood as a wholesale rejection of Ayurvedic principles. When I asked if Ayurveda provides basic concepts that can be adapted to the modern world, he was noncommittal; this, he said, "requires research." He went on to say that Ayurvedic research was about drugs rather than about basic concepts because that is the "simple thing." He repeatedly emphasized to me that research—for example, my own research—should be controlled, quantified, documented. The problem with the aphoristic nature of the ancient texts is that "to read in between the lines is required." The *Caraka Saṃhitā,* for instance, stresses the importance of time and frequency and amount of dosage, without exactly specifying any of these for a given condition. When I suggested that this information may have been passed from guru to student, he agreed, yes, "it must have been, but today it is not." I echoed what I had heard from other practitioners about the disruptive influence of colonialism on the continuity of Ayurvedic practice, and he responded, "If the gap is to be filled, how much work is required." It is not that Ayurvedic principles are disproved by modern medicine; it is rather that Ayurvedic principles remain to be proven through experimentation and precise empirical measurement.

Nor does Dr. Karnik ignore doṣa altogether. After asking one patient if his gastric pain precedes or follows meals, he classified the pain as pitta and then explained to me that pain immediately after eating would be kapha and pain four hours after eating would be vāta. Moreover, although he makes a clear etiological distinction between physical and psychosomatic ailments, he does not make a rigid distinction between the lines of treatment for these two classes of illness. Dr. Karnik does not refer psychosomatic patients to a psychiatrist, as would an allopath. He mentioned that one patient in his mid-thirties, very silent and downcast, with multiple complaints, was suffering from psychosomatic illness. Dr. Karnik felt the man's stomach for colonic tenderness, listened to his chest with a stethoscope, and checked for pain while the patient leaned forward. A short while later he told the patient's relative, "Depression is there." He told the relative to bring the patient again after fifteen days. He said, "I will see him and talk with him. It will help him. It's part of the treatment."

For Dr. Karnik Ayurvedic practice is a vital science, endangered by drastic underfunding, ignorance of new diagnostic technologies, lack of quality research, and (perhaps it is fair to add) a tendency to rest in images of philosophical grandeur. Certainly he fiercely battled any trace of such images in my questions. Medicine, Dr. Karnik argued, is a matter of fact, not belief. He will not allow such Ayurvedic concepts as prakṛti, or the integration of psyche and soma, to be used as evidence of an alternative worldview. He has no interest in witnessing for anthropology's proliferation of contrasting cognitive universes. He holds Ayurveda firmly out of reach of such dichotomies as holism and atomism, prevention and cure, positive health and allopathy. It is as if he suspects that the greater threat to Ayurveda is not so much the encroachment of biomedicine as the enframings of social theory, which would reduce Ayurveda from a science of health or a knowledge of long life to a sign of Hindu or Indian culture.

Toward the end of our final conversation Dr. Karnik informed me that I had forgotten to ask one thing: whether dosage should differ according to prakṛti. In other words, I had forgotten to ask one thing that is integral to my apparent anthropological agenda of essentializing the difference between Ayurveda and biomedicine. I had forgotten to ask one thing that might help me install Ayurveda in the anthropological display case. I said, yes, you are right; *should* dosage differ according to prakṛti? Dr. Karnik smiled and offered a parable for an answer. If he is having fifteen guests over for dinner, he asks his cook to make a meal. The cook will make a meal suitable for all fifteen guests despite their differences. "There is something like common food. There is something like average. Differences are very minute." I told Dr. Karnik that many vaidyas have told me that the dosage definitely must differ according to prakṛti. He smiled again and replied, "My common person [the cook] has common sense."

All Westerners Want to Be Kapha

Dr. Upadhyay's clinic is on a busy street crowded with sidewalk retailers as well as a few glass-enclosed shops. The English sign for the clinic is relatively small and high above the thoroughfare, inconspicuous among the balconies and upper-story windows but legible from the other side of the street. After spotting the sign, one must thread through the dense traffic to the opposite curb, brushing the fenders of cars as they inch forward honking. At the curb one must step gingerly among the wares of the vegetable sellers to enter a dark passage. There one turns a corner and ascends a steep, narrow wooden stairwell to a second-floor verandah with a wooden railing that serves one or two residences as well as the clinic. There someone is often sleeping, wrapped up in a blanket on the floor. Moving toward the back of the building between the stairwell and a vacant area surrounded by wire fencing, one comes at last to the door of the clinic. Just inside the door is a narrow foyer, beyond that a small waiting room with a television, pūjā shelf, a low table covered with magazines, and several chairs. A door to the left opens into the dispensary where Dr. Upadhyay's two pharmaceutical assistants prepare medicines. A door to the right opens into the air-conditioned, immaculate, and well-lit consultation and examination room, where several chairs and stools are arranged around a table. One wall is lined with bookshelves interrupted only by another small pūjā, where Dr. Upadhyay's medical assistant, a young graduate from a local Ayurvedic college, lights a stick of incense at the beginning of the day's office hours. Along another wall is an examination couch. A computer sits on a table in the corner. Behind Dr. Upadhyay's chair is a small sliding glass window that opens on the dispensary and through which prescriptions are passed to his assistants.

I was once present when one of Dr. Upadhyay's friends was joking to another about the clinic. He described the crowded street, the steep stairwell, the dingy hallway, and then the door opening onto the completely "modern" clinic. All three of the friends laughed, but Dr. Upadhyay seemed particularly gleeful. In fact, he seemed as slyly pleased with the contradiction as if he had intentionally designed the chaotic urban Indian scene in order to camouflage his modernity. At the start of his book, Mitchell (1988, 1) describes an "authentic" Egyptian mosque in the 1889 world exhibition whose facade opened into a coffee house. The mosque exemplifies modernity's project of architectural signification, the use of a building facade as a readable sign, not to mention its projects of the commercialization of authenticity and the separation of representation from reality. The street and building around Dr. Upadhyay's clinic, however, resemble one of the labyrinthine urban scenes that frustrated European tourists in nineteenth-century Cairo who "were unable to find any point from which to take the picture" (Mitchell 1988, 27). The thronged street and haphazardly arranged building offer no facade to announce the presence of a modern Ayurvedic clinic—or of anything else for that matter. The modernity of the clinic is hidden, tucked away between vegetable stalls and sleeping derelicts. What is interesting is that this inversion is, for Dr. Upadhyay and his friends, not a problem to lament or to repair, but simply a source of amusement, even delight. The friend's description of the packed street and the ramshackle building is neither flatly visual nor value-free. This description carries the ironic connotation of a European or North American image of India: density and dirt, poverty and disorder. The nonfacade becomes a facade of a stereotypically suffering India.

Behind this facade are other contrasting layers of facade: the modern decor of the foyer, waiting room, dispensary, and consultation chamber. The signs for Indian backwardness and medical modernity jostle one another. The joke between Dr. Upadhyay and his friends is that the reality, the referent, remains elusive. It is as if the three of them were playing with one of modernity's most sincere epistemes, the relationship between form and content, representation and reality. It is this subversive play that justified Dr. Upadhyay's expression of mischief.

The upsetting of the architecture of interior and exterior extends from clinical space into personal space. Dr. Upadhyay's series of rooms seem to gradually lead the visitor from the public space of the street to the most private space of his innermost room, the consultation and examination room. Yet his office and his practice are anything but private in the late twentieth-century North American sense of the word. Patients rarely come to the clinic alone. If they are not accompanied by family members, they are accompanied by friends. Frequently everyone in the group consults the doctor about his/her health problems in turn. When one person's case is discussed, the others chime in with additional information. In addition to friends and family of the patient, there is always an assistant physician and at least once a week an observing physician and occasionally, for extended periods of time, social researchers like me. My acceptance into this context, given sufficient personal contacts, was immediate and complete in a way that took me by surprise. My presence often went unexplained to others. Yet none of the patients (with the exception of the non-Indian patients) seemed hesitant or embarrassed to discuss the details of their diet, physical complaints, and health worries. Sometimes they glanced at me as they spoke, addressing partly to me apologies about their lifestyle or concerns about their condition. During any given consultation, the health of persons mutually known but not present may also be discussed. What at first seems to be a private space, divided from the waiting room by a bolted door and from the dispensary by a window that slides open and shut, eventually comes to seem oddly public.

In Vd. Sharma's dispensary and Dr. Karnik's clinic, patients are also often accompanied by friends or relatives. Yet the confusion of public and private was more problematic for me in Dr. Upadhyay's clinic for the simple reason that his consultations more often included the kinds of information I was conditioned to consider private. When Dr. Upadhyay asked one woman about her late afternoon depression, her daughter interrupted to say, "She's very busy earlier in the day, then she's free. The moment she's free, she gets depression. . . . You can tell when she is depressed by the shape of her mouth. . . . She pouts." From the standpoint of biomedicine depression might be labeled one of the most private illnesses. A primary characteristic of depression, according to the authoritative biomedical text on psychological states, is social withdrawal (American Psychiatric Association 1987). In Dr. Upadhyay's clinic, however, depression and many other emotional states are matters not only of familial commentary, but also of more general roundtable discussion.

If Vd. Sharma's diagnosis privileges darśan and Dr. Karnik's diagnosis privileges modern technologies, Dr. Upadhyay's diagnosis seems to privilege conversation. He may spend from thirty to forty minutes or longer with a new patient, inquiring into health history, including childhood illnesses and allopathic medicines taken in the past, diet, state of mind, and expectations of treatment. The examination of the patient, which routinely includes pulse, weight, blood pressure, tongue, and attention to affected parts of the body, usually takes just a few minutes. He pays close attention to the results of modern laboratory tests. For example, he chose not to begin treatment of a patient with fluctuating blood sugar levels until he received the latest report of his blood sugar. It was clear from his conversation, however, that he would use such information less to assign the patient to a particular disease category than to make a more total assessment of the patient's condition. He told the above patient, for instance, that he did not seem like a typical diabetic and that many factors, including diet, smoking, and drugs, might be affecting his blood sugar.

Dr. Upadhyay's conversation ranges as widely through the language of biomedicine as through the language of textbook Ayurveda. He freely translates Ayurvedic disorders into allopathic disease categories, glossing *āmavāt,* for example, as rheumatoid arthritis.[8] He often explained ailments to me in terms of organ dysfunction—for example, contrasting digestive problems centered in the duodenum with those centered in the stomach. The medical records of Dr. Upadhyay's patients include lists of physical and emotional complaints, chronology of major diseases, results of examinations and outside laboratory tests, lists of medicines administered (organized in categories of herbal compounds in tablets, herbal compounds in powders, and metals), and a track record of improvement registered by a series of pluses and minuses next to each complaint. Dr. Upadhyay has been working to develop an even more systematic, streamlined, and computerized form to assure that he makes no omissions during a consultation. Dr. Upadhyay's language and documentation seem therefore quite consistent with a modern ordering of information.

Missing from Dr. Upadhyay's records, as from those of Vd. Sharma, is any discussion or listing of doṣa and prakṛti. Also missing is another component frequently and strikingly interwoven into Dr. Upadhyay's interrogation of the patient: a moral discourse on proper living habits—that is, not simply diet and seasonal adjustments, but also attitude and ethics, the whole complex nexus of relationships to society and to oneself. A handful of stories can illustrate this discourse. A woman in her twenties came with her parents. For several years she had eaten only fruit and milk. Dr. Upadhyay probed, "Only because of some health problem or something is there in your mind? There must be some reason for suddenly going on fruit and milk." The woman was quiet; she smiled slightly and looked into her lap. He asked, "Have you tried to ask yourself why it is happening?" When he learned that she was a student of economics, he quipped, "So you are economizing your food." He told her he could not start treatment unless she was willing to change her diet and asked, "What are you going to choose, injection or diet?" Later he commented to me that there must be a psychological reason for her strange diet. Gradually, he said, it will come out. Maybe next time or the time after that. Perhaps, he speculated, someone in her family had remarked on her eating the family's food without contributing to its income.

Another woman came to the clinic because of infertility. Dr. Upadhyay could find no physiological reason for her inability to conceive. An allopathic doctor had prescribed sedatives and antipsychotic drugs for her mood swings. At the last visit Dr. Upadhyay had asked her to discontinue these medications, but in the interval she had experienced a bout of anxiety and had begun taking them again. Dr. Upadhyay told her, "To allow a little worry might be part of your treatment. . . . If you look for your escape from medicines, it is not going to help you." He warned, "If you are not able to stop these medicines, I will not be able to go further with you." He went on to tell her that her system was depressed and needed not sedation but stimulation. He told her that only after she had lost weight and discontinued the sedatives would he be able to focus on the problem of her infertility. He reiterated that she may have to experience a little anxiety as part of her treatment. He would not permit her, however, to endure anything as extreme as acute insomnia. He told her to feel free to call him whenever she was feeling anxious.

Another patient reported that he had been free of insomnia for four months without the use of sleeping pills. Dr. Upadhyay said, "That's a good achievement, yes?" and then asked about his general well-being. The patient said that his outlook had improved: he was more philosophical about life. Dr. Upadhyay responded, "I want you to think philosophically also. . . . That is also a part of treatment." Later in the session Dr. Upadhyay advised, "Try to be like a Buddha, not that you have to be a Buddha, but follow what Buddha has said." They agreed that in the city it was difficult to live like a Buddha. Dr. Upadhyay said, "By going to the Himalayas everyone can remain quiet." Staying in the city and remaining quiet "is a bigger challenge."

A large man came to be treated for excess weight and other complaints. He was concerned about his tobacco habit. He used to be a chain smoker—sixty cigarettes a day, he told us. He had quit smoking without difficulty. Yet he could not seem to give up chewing tobacco. Dr. Upadhyay suggested that he reduce his tobacco intake from six times a day to four. Then he brought up the subject of the patient's childhood. The patient had had too many responsibilities thrown on him. Dr. Upadhyay said, "There are people who carry the whole burden." This sympathy prompted the man to tell a story of loaning his brother-in-law money. He was bothered by his brother-in-law's ingratitude. Dr. Upadhyay advised him, "If you do good, forget it." He reminded the patient that he does not remember the times he gives a beggar two rupees. Why, then, should he remember a time when he gave a relative two *lākhs* (lākh = one hundred thousand) of rupees? Dr. Upadhyay: "The minute you expect anything, you suffer. . . . What is success?" He emphasized that peace of mind is the most important thing. The patient confided that he had trouble controlling his temper. If he takes less tobacco, his "nature becomes nasty." Dr. Upadhyay said that if he must express anger, it should be "artificial anger," required by the situation, and not "natural anger." The patient attributed his anger to physical problems such as his high blood pressure. Dr. Upadhyay replied that these were simply excuses. If the patient can be in command of his business and his diet, then he can also be in command of his temper. He recommended that the patient spend fifteen to twenty minutes alone every day. He told him to go to the ocean, sit in his car, watch the waves, and "talk to your driver about *his* problems." The patient listened, then mentioned on his own behalf that he did not party or drink. Dr. Upadhyay told him to go to the park and walk on the beach, not for the exercise, but to "see the beggars, smell the stink." In this way he would reach some peace, some perspective, about his own problems.

Dr. Upadhyay told me the story of a heart patient who had a shop in the neighborhood. He refused to take care of his health. He would not stop eating salt or "junk food." Every day he bought fried food from the stalls on the street corner. He worried incessantly about money. Every year he went into the hospital for one or two months because of "right ventricle failure." Still he continued his destructive lifestyle. Dr. Upadhyay predicted that he would die on the streets someday.

This is Dr. Upadhyay's discourse of health, a discourse that circles out from prakṛti and disease, diet and family relations, to moral philosophy. Dr. Upadhyay demands of his patients not merely the compliance of taking their medications, but also a complete attention to their actions and mental/emotional states. The woman who eats only fruit and milk must free herself from her sense of indebtedness to her family. She must stop using her body as a ledger in which to balance the family accounts. The woman who is infertile must face her anxieties. The man who has recovered from insomnia must practice the philosophical detachment of Buddha. The man who is addicted to tobacco must learn to loan out two lākhs of rupees to his brother-in-law with the same equanimity with which he hands over two rupees to a mendicant. Meanwhile, the man who worries about money and eats junk food will fall dead in the street as an example to the others. A person who wants to be healthy should not escape into antidepressants or Himalayan caves but learn to remain "quiet" in the center of city life, in the center of his or her anxieties. A person who wants to lower his blood pressure should contemplate the vastness of the sea and of other people's problems. What in a contemporary North American context might have been an unearthing of the intimate psychological secrets of illness opens out into a declaration of moral principles. Dr. Upadhyay might as well have been quoting Kṛṣṇa in the *Bhagavad Gita,* when he argued that expectations lead to suffering and disregard for reward leads to peace. My initial discomfort at eavesdropping on a private conversation began to seem misplaced. Just as Vd. Sharma's "going deep" penetrates not so much the patient as his or her network of relationships with the social and natural environment, so Dr. Upadhyay's interrogation investigates not so much the hidden folds and foibles of the personality as problems of human action.

Dr. Upadhyay requires yet a further moral courage from his patients: "faith" or "confidence" in Ayurveda. He first discussed this faith with me while seeing a patient with a very extreme case of eczema. He examined the sore on her leg with a magnifying glass. He told me that the steroids the woman had been taking for her eczema had only made it worse. He also believed a leg operation had affected the "subdermal layer." Dr. Upadhyay practiced with this patient, as with all his patients, a careful and expert interior gaze. After that he talked to me of faith. The evidence of this patient's faith was that since she began Ayurvedic treatment, she had taken no steroids. He recalled another patient with similar faith. This patient asked him one day if she could begin to eat salt again. He had forgotten that he had casually remarked to her ten months earlier that restricting her use of salt would aid in her healing. Patients with such faith, he assured me, make treatment easier.

He went on to explain that Ayurvedic treatment with patients who take allopathic drugs involves more trial and error since the specific effects (including toxicity) of these drugs are often unknown. Because of the difficulty of treating patients who bounce between allopathy and Ayurveda, Dr. Upadhyay sometimes "tests" patients for their "faith" in Ayurveda. One woman came to the clinic twice in three days. She said of the pain from her eczema, "I can't bear it." An allopathic doctor had given her an ointment. Dr. Upadhyay told her she could keep using it but then added, "You are taking too many medicines. I don't know where this will lead." At the time the woman was taking antibiotics and steroids, as well as Dr. Upadhyay's medicine. She volunteered, "I should not go to the allopathic doctor." Dr. Upadhyay warned her that Ayurvedic treatment would take longer. The woman indicated that she was resigned to a longer treatment. Reluctantly Dr. Upadhyay prescribed some medication but then continued to voice skepticism over her treatment, saying, "And you are working. You are continuing to work, which I cannot stop." The woman said that she had taken enough allopathic medicine but then asked abruptly if she should go to a skin specialist. Dr. Upadhyay answered, "You need that in a way. But he will give you steroids only. He cannot give you anything else." Finally he told her, "You choose one"—that is, allopathy or Ayurveda—and then reiterated, "In the present situation with your asthma and this [eczema] flaring up you must choose. Ayurveda will take more time." Again the woman said she was willing to take the extra time. Dr. Upadhyay, however, became even more resistant. He told her to get a recommendation for a dermatologist from her general practitioner and to follow his treatment plan. When the "problem is less severe," she can return for Ayurvedic treatment. He stressed that he could not offer acute relief but that the dermatologist could not offer a long-term cure. After she left, he told me that "in a way" he had been testing her sincerity. He was not sure she was committed to Ayurveda. One patient initially tried to hide the fact that he had been to an allopathic heart specialist. After he left, Dr. Upadhyay told me that the man claimed to have confidence in Ayurveda but actually did not.

Ayurveda is treated by anthropologists as an indigenous system of medicine that is deeply ingrained in Indian society. Researchers have often suggested that Ayurveda has persisted, despite the enormous competition from biomedicine, precisely because it encodes deep-seated cultural experiences and values that extend beyond medical diagnosis and cure (Nordstrom 1989; Weiss et al. 1988; Obeyesekere 1976). Yet Dr. Upadhyay spends a good deal of his consultation time educating his patients about Ayurveda in order to sell it to them. In a sense he is forced to essentialize Ayurveda, to package it, simply in order to practice it. Dr. Upadhyay, however, cannot count on invoking a set of cultural essences with which Ayurveda is supposedly suffused. Instead he must improvise cultural essences, drawing on whatever ideologies are at hand, ranging from orientalist-reminiscent constructions of Indian spiritual wisdom to international trends of holistic health.[9] At a time when the confidence of urban and many rural Indians seems to have turned away from Ayurveda toward biomedicine, Ayurvedic physicians employ different strategies to win it back. Dr. Karnik attempts to erase the differences between Ayurveda and biomedicine. Dr. Upadhyay, however, assembles those differences into a marketable commodity.

Dr. Upadhyay teaches his patients that Ayurveda is a systemic approach to health. During the session with the anxious, infertile woman he explained to her that her "whole metabolism had to improve." He offered an analogy with the office fan, which had a mysterious problem. To start the fan running one must first manually turn the blades. Each part of the fan is intact; there is no mechanical reason for its difficulty, but there is "some small problem somewhere in the system." Similarly there is no physiological reason for the patient's infertility; there is, rather, some small problem in her system. Even though Dr. Upadhyay compared her system to a fan, he was arguing that her body was not a mechanism but a system that was more than the sum of its parts. The patient whose faith in Ayurveda must be tested was told at one point that her body was not "some machine." He told the infertile woman, "If I were going to treat all cases of infertility in the same way, then there is no difference between allopathy and Ayurveda." Dr. Upadhyay teaches his patients that while allopathy isolates disorders and counters them with standard remedies, Ayurveda links disorders to a complex system and adjusts that system with particularized remedies.

Another patient complained of some discomfort as a result of taking Dr. Upadhyay's medicines. He responded, "See, we don't have a suction machine to take things out. Things have to go out of your system in some way." He told her that as an Ayurvedic doctor, he does not sanction drastic measures. He said, "Here we are trying to change the whole system." Then Dr. Upadhyay and the woman's husband discussed the importance of faith in Ayurveda. Without faith, the husband said, "you should not come." Dr. Upadhyay predicted that gradually the literate class would return to Ayurveda. The conversation turned then to Ayurveda's assets and liabilities. The husband mentioned that Ayurveda required more time. Dr. Upadhyay responded, "Normally you would feel Ayurveda is slow. I will strongly deny this thing." He noted that illness arises through processes that have evolved over many years. When we single out a specific disease, "we are not identifying our ill health as such; we are identifying some manifestation." Acute treatments such as antibiotics may suppress a given manifestation. "But still disease is being changed to something else." According to Dr. Upadhyay, he is fully capable of treating acute illness. "But I am not doing [so] because my *śāstra* [the precepts in Ayurvedic texts] is not allowing me to do that." Ayurveda's advantage over allopathy is its ability to address the systemic disorder and not simply to suppress the manifestation. Acute Ayurvedic treatment would undermine the systemic principles that give Ayurveda its unique value.

In one conversation Dr. Upadhyay asserted that Ayurvedic research should be less oriented toward specific diseases and drugs and more oriented toward "therapies." At present such a development is impossible, he said. I knew what he meant, having seen the wall chart in the office of a research director of a prominent Ayurvedic drug company. The chart listed at least a dozen research projects, all of them testing the effects of a particular product on a particular biomedically defined disease such as osteoarthritis, diabetes, or schizophrenia. At times Dr. Upadhyay seemed to believe that research that is less reifying of disease would inevitably develop. He explained that biomedical understandings of disease themselves are already shifting from "infections" to "metabolic disorders," — in other words, to more systemic models. While Dr. Karnik foresees that biomedicine's attention to chronic illness will efface the last apparent stronghold of Ayurvedic uniqueness, Dr. Upadhyay hopes that this attention will help to legitimate it.

Unlike Dr. Karnik, Dr. Upadhyay does not compartmentalize physical and psychosomatic disorders. After the departure of one patient with chronic bowel problems and several other complaints, Dr. Upadhyay informed me that modern medicine would label his case "IBS," Irritable Bowel Syndrome. Since biomedicine recognizes no physiological cause for IBS, it treats it as a "mental" (i.e., psychosomatic) disorder. Allopathic treatment therefore targets the nervous system. Dr. Upadhyay, however, would treat the problem as simultaneously physical and psychological. For Dr. Karnik, multiple complaints always signal a psychosomatic problem. For Dr. Upadhyay, however, multiple complaints are understood as the many manifestations of a systemic problem that is both physical and psychological. Similarly, Dr. Upadhyay suggested that Ayurvedic attention to the whole person should result in a more sensitive doctor-patient relationship. We discussed my observations of an Ayurvedic practitioner whom he also knows. He said that she lacked the "human touch." Like Dr. Karnik, he said that this was a matter of personal temperament. Yet when I commented that some scholars argue that biomedical education actually undermines the "human touch," Dr. Upadhyay said that he was more disturbed when an Ayurvedic physician lacked this touch because he had been taught to examine the affected part *and* the patient, the body *and* the mind, the illness *and* the doṣa.

Ayurvedic literature published in English in the last several decades is a medley of ideological voices. At different moments the authors seem to be involved in selling Ayurveda to North Americans, Europeans, and cosmopolitan Indians either as holistic medicine (taking advantage of the international trend toward holistic health care—e.g., Thakkur 1965; Dhyani 1987) or as a source of new drugs for biomedicine (taking advantage of the endless expansion of the biomedical pharmaceutical repertoire—e.g., Udupa et al., eds. 1970; Olok 1987). The literature often highlights Ayurveda's emphasis on positive health and preventive care, its use of nontoxic herbs, its concern with the whole person, while it paradoxically also plays up the wonder drugs it can offer for certain biomedically defined diseases (e.g., Savnur 1984; Central Council for Research in Ayurveda and Siddha 1988). Biomedical practitioners who take an interest in Ayurveda are also attracted either by the possibility of new drugs (witness the booming business of marketing Ayurvedic medicines for pharmacists and allopaths) or by holistic wisdom (e.g., Lele 1986). Dr. Upadhyay himself embraces this paradox, eloquently defending Ayurvedic principles while also taking an avid interest in research on Ayurvedic drugs. Yet he is critical of allopaths who court Ayurveda only to appropriate its medicines. It is significant that because of my own biases and background in health care I am more responsive to Ayurvedic philosophy than to Ayurvedic pharmaceutics. Dr. Upadhyay freely admitted that with me and with other cultural anthropologists, he is more apt to discuss Ayurvedic principles, while with biomedical researchers, he is more apt to discuss physiological processes. Dr. Upadhyay is in the difficult position of both appreciating the interest in Ayurveda stirred by biomedical trends and protecting Ayurveda from being absorbed by those very same trends.

Dr. Upadhyay's promotion of Ayurveda as a systemic medicine must be understood, at least partly, in the context of the increasing demand for such medicine among European and North American consumers. Yet how well his practice of Ayurveda in fact matches this demand for holism was partly revealed when a North American woman visited his clinic. Unlike the Indians who must be educated about Ayurveda, she had already read at least one book, by another North American, on the subject. Indian patients who have some education about Ayurveda have certain expectations of Ayurvedic cure. They commonly believe, for example, that Ayurvedic medications have less dramatic results and less negative side effects. The North American woman, however, had expectations not just of Ayurvedic cure, but also of Ayurvedic diagnosis. After her first visit, for example, she confided in me (I had offered her the extra mattress in my flat) that she was surprised Dr. Upadhyay had not asked her about her psychological history, which she was sure would be central to a correct diagnosis. Moreover, before she first arrived in the clinic, she was already convinced from what she had read that her constitution was predominantly vāta. After examining her, Dr. Upadhyay commented to me that she had a very "peculiar pulse." Then he said, "It's very rare that you find a pure prakṛti." I asked, "Is she a pure prakṛti?," and he said that yes, in his opinion she was almost totally pitta. Out of earshot on the examination couch, where Dr. Upadhyay's assistant was taking her blood pressure, the woman asked with interest if she was vāta. Dr. Upadhyay misunderstood and commented to me that "Every Westerner wants to be kapha." When the woman understood that he had pronounced her pitta, she asked, "What's that? Fire?" He answered yes, but then turned to me and confided that he preferred not to refer to the doṣa as wind and bile and so forth. Upon taking Dr. Upadhyay's medication, the woman experienced almost immediate relief from two of her most pressing complaints. She remained mystified, however, about her diagnosis as pitta. When she told him again just before she left India that she seemed to have all the characteristics of a perfect vāta, he simply said, "We will see."

What is striking about Dr. Upadhyay's comment that all Westerners want to be kapha is not the doubtful assertion that Westerners want to be predominant in the doṣa usually glossed as phlegm and associated with a fleshy figure. What is striking is his observation that Westerners want to be predominant in *some* doṣa, that they want to be categorized as a particular prakṛti. I never observed an Indian patient voicing curiosity, let alone desire, about his or her prakṛti. In his remark Dr. Upadhyay seemed to be commenting on a specific North American craving for individuality served up in an Ayurvedic recipe. The "Westerner" transforms prakṛti from a particular relationship with foods and climate to a personality trait. The North American woman had trouble accepting herself as pitta because she already had recognized herself within the complex of adjectives associated with vāta. The book she had read about Ayurveda reads like many other self-help books published in the United States. It presents Ayurveda as a simple, elegant, and well-organized system. It translates Ayurveda into terms that are readily assimilable by experienced consumers of holistic health. Chapter 3 is entitled "Constitutional Examination: How to Determine Your Unique Psycho-Physical Nature"; chapter 5, "Balancing the Humors: The Ways of Holistic Living"; and chapter 6, "Ayurvedic Diet: Personalizing Your Dietary Regime" (Frawley 1989). The book may be used as an Ayurvedic self-healing program or as preparation for visiting an Ayurvedic practitioner. My intent here is not to criticize the book itself; translations of Ayurveda into the terms of North American holism are inevitable, and as such translations go, this one is clear, inclusive, and respectful of intricacies. My intent is rather to locate the North American patient's interest in her prakṛti within late twentieth-century formulations of expressivism.

In the United States, the enthusiasm for holistic health care exists within a context of the valorization of the individual, who is to be developed to his fullest "human potential" through elaborate and eclectic self-attention and self-expression. In this context holism implies an in-depth mining of the person as an interior space. This private identity of the modern individual, which provides the necessary counterpoint to his/her civic role, is the subject not only of modern autobiographies and diaries (see Chakrabarty 1992b), but also of modern psychological discourse (see Taylor 1989). Such a subject increasingly imagines healing as the exploration and eventual expression of his or her true inner self. The movement toward a more "humanistic" medicine acknowledges the need to involve this inner self—with all of its motives, fears, dreams, and ambivalence—in the treatment of illness. Therefore it is not surprising that after the first day or two I felt intrusive in Dr. Upadhyay's office only during the visits of North American, European, or Australian patients. Inevitably I felt compelled to ask these patients for permission to be present during their examinations and consultations. Even after they consented to my presence, sometimes protesting their openness, I felt and imagined a mutual embarrassment. The psychological problems of these patients, unlike those of the Indian patients, rarely opened out into social and moral dilemmas. A North American woman confided that as a child she had been left to eat only cold food out of the refrigerator. She volunteered that as an adult she experienced chronic anxiety. An Australian man revealed that his physical problems began with a relationship breakup. He also disclosed that he was subject to emotional suppression, occasionally erupting in violent fits of anger. Psychological problems were smoothly traced to social sources but nonetheless interpreted as inner states often following the hydraulic processes of contents under pressure (Lutz 1988).

Dr. Upadhyay is in the business of convincing Indians that they need the systemic medicine for which consumers in European-based societies are beginning to clamor. At the same time, however, he is in the position of denying "Westerners" the prefabricated doṣic identity they seem to crave. A European man with a handful of chronic complaints visited Dr. Upadhyay from a nearby ashram. Later the same day, when advising an Indian patient to spend more time in quiet contemplation, the doctor mentioned the European. He threw out a comment to the effect that foreigners in India practice meditation, yet ironically Indians themselves do not. Then he added that actually *saṃnyās* (the ascetic's vow to relinquish worldly ties) "is easier." It is more difficult to be a householder, care for your family, "face the music." In the international market Ayurveda may seem to advertise a pre-integrated identity, just as ashrams may seem to advertise a retreat from society. But for Dr. Upadhyay, Ayurveda, like meditation, is less an item to be purchased than an ethic to be practiced.

Ironically "Westerners" already seem to have the "faith" that he must continually test in Indians. Yet that faith in Ayurveda is also an expectation that Ayurveda will confirm their individuality. Dr. Upadhyay promotes Ayurveda in terms that resemble European and North American holism, and yet he practices Ayurveda in terms that defy that holism. For holistic medicine is marketed toward those who imagine that the road to health is at the same time a road to individuation. For such individuals medicine is entangled in self-description, self-reification, and self-enframing. As Arney and Bergen have pointed out, the fashion in holism and "humanistic" medicine disciplines patients to be true to "their own nature." (1984, 138).[10] When it is part of a psychological self-help program, holistic treatment easily becomes a medicalization of life choices and trajectories. Dr. Upadhyay's treatment, however, is better understood as a moralization of medical trajectories. If there is a "nature" to which his patients must be true, it is transpersonal, unencompassed, detached from personal position and interests. In fact, it is less a "nature" than a complex of choices, a moral direction.

During one conversation Dr. Upadhyay commented that one of his "worries" about my research was what he described as my "fascination" with Ayurveda and perhaps with India more generally. He was reluctant to say more for fear of being misunderstood. Perhaps, however, it is fair to free-associate my "fascination" with the eager self-diagnosis of the North American patient of "pure" pitta prakṛti. The danger from foreign consumers of Ayurveda, whether seekers of a health that is conflated to identity or sympathetic social researchers, is our readiness to interpret Ayurveda as a new commodity to satisfy our own cultural hungers.

Subverting Modernity

Since the early part of this century the proponents of Ayurveda have defended it from the encroachments of biomedicine on many platforms. On one platform they defend it as an embodiment of certain eternal truths. On another they defend it as a symbol of national identity. On another they defend it as a useful addendum to biomedicine. On yet another they defend it as a solution to the atomistic excesses of modern science.[11] Each of these tactical responses to biomedical power is evident, alone or in mosaic, in the three medical practices considered here. All three doctors, to a greater or lesser degree, engage in a dialogue with modernity, not only in their conversations with me, but also in their medical practices. Vd. Sharma, both imagining and perceiving my complicity with empiricism and with diagrammatic models of medical treatment, preached the importance of absolute principles and diachronic narratives of medical treatment. Dr. Karnik, imagining and perceiving my complicity with a modern desire for the counterbalance of tradition, insisted on the evaluation and development of Ayurveda along strictly scientific lines. Dr. Upadhyay, imagining and perceiving my and his non-Indian patients' complicity with holistic fashions and touristic romanticism, offered an Ayurvedic cure that required not consumption but commitment. These practitioners undermined my three assumptions—that medical phenomena can be mapped onto the person, that local medical knowledge can be isolated and defined, and that illness is a private matter—sometimes unwittingly, but sometimes quite deliberately. In a sense they offered me no basis on which to make the typological comparisons I was originally trying to make: with Vd. Sharma I failed to compare concepts of person; with Dr. Karnik I failed to compare ethnomedical paradigms; and with Dr. Upadhyay I failed to compare brands of holistic humanism.

These practitioners' statements to me were not transparent expressions of their conceptions of medical phenomenology but political gestures. They spoke not only to their patients and to the anthropologist, but also to allopathic doctors, to government agencies (who are responsible both for valorizing Ayurveda as Indian and for prioritizing allopathy over Ayurveda), to their Ayurvedic colleagues, and to European or North American consumers of imagined Asian wholeness. All these interlocutors had their ghostly presence in our conversations and in patient consultations. These Ayurvedic physicians address themselves to such wide-ranging forces and discourses as biomedical science, national identity, and neo-orientalism. What is at stake in their discourse and practice is not so much that Ayurveda might be lost as a cultural form. The very construction of Ayurveda as a cultural form fits rather well into a project of biomedical dominance, as does the construction of Ayurveda as a local version of the interior gaze. The first allows biomedicine to bracket Ayurveda as a merely cultural practice; the second allows it to absorb Ayurveda as a subordinate medicine, a source of a few drugs and a few insights. What is at stake, rather, is Ayurveda's subjection to the domination of enframing epistemologies.

It is not that there is no trace of the modern interiorization of the person in the practices of these three physicians. The files of Vd. Sharma's patients hold X ray films of their chest cavities. For Dr. Karnik the instruments that survey the interior of the body are the final diagnostic arbiters. Dr. Upadhyay discusses illness as readily in terms of physiological dysfunction as in terms of doṣa imbalance. Nor is there a total disregard for the notion of privacy. Vd. Sharma is careful to tell me that he *can* close the screen between his consultation alcove and the rest of the room, even though he rarely does. Dr. Karnik's and Dr. Upadhyay's waiting rooms and examination rooms are definitively separate. Yet within these seemingly private spaces the discourse often has a distinctly public character—social, moral, and political—in its references to the contest between allopathy and Ayurveda. The anatomo-clinical method, the positivist representation of an objectivized reality, the dualism of inside and outside, are not rejected, but rather subjected to a variety of sometimes calculated, sometimes casual maneuvers that subvert, invert, divert, and otherwise play with a modern episteme. For these practitioners the interiorization of persons and the enframing of medicine are epistemological moves that remain partial and ambivalent. Even if they allow the modern exhibitionary gaze to focus to some extent on Ayurvedic patients and illnesses, they are reluctant to allow it to focus squarely on Ayurveda itself. Ayurveda as cultural difference will not be diagrammed by Vd. Sharma, defined by Dr. Karnik, or packaged for a North American market by Dr. Upadhyay. Ayurveda is not so easily reduced to exoticized ethnomedicine or the latest brand of commodified holism. The idea of "true" Ayurveda is a deftly maneuvered political tool. Its meanings may alter with historical circumstances as long as the control over its meanings remains in Ayurvedic hands and not in the hands of allopathic doctors, government agencies, or passing anthropologists.

three Healing National Culture

How did practitioners come to alternately invite and evade the enframing of Ayurveda as a culturally defined system of medicine? The strategies of the practitioners discussed in chapter 2, whether to prevent the marginalization of Ayurveda as merely culture or to take advantage of the healing powers of cultural imaginaries, resonate with nearly a century of discourse over Ayurveda as a sign and a healing force of national culture. Vd. Sharma's implicit references to Ayurveda as a cultural term, no less than Dr. Karnik's explicit resistance to Ayurveda as a cultural term and Dr. Upadhyay's creative use of Ayurveda as a cultural term, all refer back to the work of earlier generations of practitioners to define Ayurveda as culturally distinctive. During my stay in India, when I was not observing in Ayurvedic teaching hospitals or private practices, I sat in Ayurvedic college libraries, perusing broken-spined books with crumbling pages and antiquated typography that were published by the indigenous printing industry established at the end of the nineteenth century. Around me Ayurvedic students would be talking noisily, keeping an eye on the hallway for their professor. If he or she was seen walking down to the classroom for a lecture, the students in that class would get up from their tables and follow. At times I went along; at other times I stayed, poring over the old books as if they could help me understand the uneven bursts of activity in contemporary Ayurvedic education.

In this chapter I turn to these books and to the fragments of a genealogy of Ayurveda as culture that can be found in them. For in these texts, written at the turn of the century, there begins to be a shift in focus from concern over the loss of physical health to concern over the loss of cultural health. Social malaise begins to be attributed not simply to moral lapse, but also to the compulsive mimicry of European ways of life. Ayurveda accordingly begins to be understood as a remedy not only for bodily illness, but also for the power imbalance of colonial rule. In these texts, as I will show, the problem of specious healing moves from a concern with the incompetence and incomplete knowledge of certain vaidyas to a concern with the imitation of European approaches to health. The category of legitimate healer itself shifts to delineate an explicit binary between authentic and fake, in place of the hierarchy of *vaidyak* (related to vaidyas) qualities found in earlier texts.

In these texts, then, a modern notion of cultural authenticity begins to emerge, an idea of an original and true Indian medicine that would allow practitioners to call upon their countrymen and women to be true to themselves and to their science. The genesis of the modern sense of authenticity is hinted at in the etymology of the word: when "authentic" entered English in the fourteenth century, it was synonymous with "authoritative"; in the fifteenth century it took on the sense of "reliable" and "actual, not imaginary." It was not until the eighteenth century, however, that it began to mean "genuine, not counterfeit" (Hoad 1986, 28). At first, then, the truth inherent in the authentic depended on its authorship by those in particular social positions; then that truth began to depend on the separation of the authentic from the merely imagined; finally that truth depends on the difference between the authentic and a copy that poses as itself. The modern sense of authenticity thereby conceals its link to social authority and carries a sense of that which is not only real, as opposed to imaginary, but also primary as opposed to mimetic. The authentic is both that which is original and that which is not simply concocted. As such, the authentic is imagined to be perfectly self-present, a final referent that has no need to refer elsewhere for meaning and yet paradoxically is unthinkable except through a relation to the false or imitative.

Such a notion of authenticity arose alongside historicism, a modern arrangement of events in time that, to paraphrase Chakrabarty (1992b, 1992c), involves a sense of anachronism (and therefore of progress), laws of cause and effect, and a split between the secular and the sacred. It is not surprising, therefore, that in the Ayurvedic texts with which I am concerned here, there is also a tension between historical and ahistorical temporalities. In these texts, currents of the "homogeneous empty time" of the modern nation (Anderson 1991; Benjamin 1968) compete with currents of a more textured heterogeneous time that does not depend on causal relations, a sense of anachronism, or a secular-sacred split. These works therefore set a precedent for a particular Ayurvedic historiography, discussed in the final section of this chapter, that is not fully assimilated to European ideas of history. For while this historiography makes use of the linearity of a modern historicism, it reverses its order, so that Ayurveda is not so much evolving as devolving from its divine origins as a perfect science. This refusal of a historicist repression of the mythic reinforces the ideological power of Ayurvedic histories.

Temporalities in a Healing Text

Śivanātha Sāgar, published in 1912, is a vernacular compilation of aphorisms and recipes gleaned from Sanskrit ancient and medieval Ayurvedic texts, along with other healing lore gathered by the author, Śivanāth Singh. Singh begins the introduction to his book by writing the following:

> These days, because of British rule, there has been progress in the mechanical arts; so many printing presses have started up, and many scholarly treatises and practical books have been printed and have become well known. As a result, many of the local people have become proficient in various skills and knowledge. This has been happening everywhere, but in our own Rajasthan, in the Jodhpur dialect, many books of social benefit have become celebrated. Among these, the books of vaidyak knowledge are often less famous because in this region, for a long time now, the tradition of vaidya śāstras has been lost, and false ascetics and other such people have become vaidyas and have set up practice. It is difficult to find any knowledgeable, trained ascetics in this group (1912, 1).[1]

Singh goes on to more closely define the problem of incompetence. He notes that lower-caste boys are being apprenticed by irresponsible vaidyas. After learning three or four recipes, they take the name of some great guru, and "swindling the poor, simpleminded householder," they ruin many lives with their *aśuddh* (incorrect, impure, or perhaps unpurified) medicines (1912, 1). "These people are ascetics in name, but in the accumulation of wealth they are even greedier than householders. From their false and inadequate medicines not only do patients fail to become well, but they fall sick from new diseases and die" (1912, 1). As a result, Singh observes, there are scarcely three or four men in the Rajasthani region who live to be a hundred years old; most die at the early ages of sixty or seventy.[2] Due to the improper medicines of ignorant vaidyas, Rajasthani bodies have become weak and unable to sustain life. The physical well-being of the Rajasthani people has decreased because of the treatment by ignorant practitioners over such a long period (1912, 2).

Singh goes on to say that there is no tradition of teaching and studying vaidyak knowledge in the regional vernacular. Generally, the practitioners in this region use only five or ten medicinal substances because the śāstras have not been disseminated as much as in other places. Poets here have written countless poems, verses, and songs of every variety eulogizing the king. "Yet of all types of well-being, physical well-being is the highest. Although the means of attaining a state of physical well-being is described in Ayurveda, no poets have given it any attention" (1912, 2). Since the knowledge of healing remains "unsung" or "unstudied" (in the copy I was reading most of this word had been chopped off in the final trimming of the book), people suffer from disease. After observing this sad state of affairs for several years, in 1886 the author resolved to "write a book on Ayurveda for the people of my own country in which the complete method of diagnosis, treatment, *bhasma* [medicinal ash], extracts, *rasāyana* [rejuvenation therapies], techniques, and all other topics would be explained" (1912, 2). Later on in the introduction Singh relates to us certain biographical information. He was born in 1851 in a village near Jodhpur. Always clever, he practiced healing in his home from the age of ten, relying only on donations.

Singh lists the Sanskrit texts from which he has drawn, including major ancient and medieval works on Ayurveda, many of which are still cited by Ayurvedic scholars today. He tells us that there are more than eleven hundred topics in his book and many other subsidiary topics. The task of distributing the book and of bringing health to the people of the region depends on the people themselves. Because no such book has previously been written in the Jodhpur dialect, he is hopeful that great men will offer their patronage to assure that the book is distributed in their areas. He writes, "It is useless to give this work any special praise. It is said that . . . the fragrance of *kastūrī* [the substance found in the navels of deer, valued for its healing properties and known for its fragrance] cannot be experienced by swearing oaths about it but only by holding it in your hand" (1912, 2). He goes on to enumerate the various verse forms he has used in the text.

This text is noteworthy for several elements that separate it both from the ancient and medieval works that it cites and from the books on healing that will flood the bookstalls in the coming century. First of all, the introduction is different from earlier texts in that it links the book to the current state of affairs in the society. This introduction is written in a continuous expository prose that assumes the "homogeneous empty time" of the nation (and of modern history) that can be inscribed with any variety of contemporaneous information (Anderson 1991), the author's biography, the spread of illness in Rajasthan, the metrical forms to be found in the text, and so on. By situating himself in a sociological landscape, the author connects the world in the text with the world outside the text (Anderson 1991, 30). Observing with dismay the ignorance of vaidyas in the Rajasthani communities around him, he determines to remedy the situation by writing this book. His narrative, sprinkled with sociological plurals such as ignorant vaidyas, threatening illnesses, feeble people, and negligent poets, is marked not by a grandiose uniqueness of events but by their typicality, comparability, and representativeness (Anderson 1991, 30).

Following this historically situated introduction, however, *Śivanātha Sāgar,* though an original work and not simply a translation of earlier works, is composed in poetry. In fact, the verse forms, whether conceived aesthetically or as mnemonic devices or (probably) both, are mentioned in the introduction as one of the assets of the book, not incidental but integral to its value. In these verse forms, the social realism of the introduction gives way to a mythic grandeur that has no ground in historical time. The words in the metrical structures of *Śivanātha Sāgar* move through a different temporal medium than the words of its introduction. Here time is not an empty medium across which contemporaneous events can be traced, but rather a richly grained time where eternal truths unfold in musical rhythms.[3] The relatively modern introduction places *Śivanātha Sāgar* in the genre of works created by the new printing industry and intended to be read, while the stanzas on healing place it in a genre of works intended to be, if not sung, then at least recited aloud. To this day in Ayurvedic colleges, while the prose of contemporary textbooks is silently perused for its content, with no regard at all for its language, the Sanskrit *ślokas* (verses) of ancient texts are recited aloud by professors who have commended a few of them to memory. The syllables are thought to embody wisdom in a way that is completely unfamiliar in modern technical works. As a whole, then, despite its mass production, *Śivanātha Sāgar* does not fully conform to the standards of a nationalist print media, in which technical information would be conveyed in expository prose without poetry or hyperbole. There is, in this work, a certain creative tension between the historical preoccupations of the introduction and the timelessness of the rest of the text, the first serving almost to enframe the sacredness of the second.

There is a tension here also between a modern comprehensiveness and an *a*modern open-endedness. While on the one hand the author proudly claims to have covered eleven hundred topics, on the other hand each topic seems to serve as a starting point, rather than end point, for study and contemplation, a polyvalent stanza to turn over in the mind, rather than a totalizing statement. A passage entitled "Characteristics [*lakṣaṇ*] of the Heart," for example, reads as follows:

> That is the heart's place that has an opening that is low and slightly open like a lotus bud. In that place consciousness and the bliss of ātmā reside, and *oj* [the seventh of the dhātu, understood as semen or reproductive fluid and associated with strength, immunity, and an overall glow of health], which is the splendor of all the dhātus, also resides in its shelter. You should know this. It is called the place of the veins and arteries that nourish the body. The veins and arteries radiate out from the center [*nābhi,* literally navel], spreading throughout the body. Day and night they mix with vāyu [the doṣa associated with air and movement] and deliver the *ras* [food essence, the first of the dhātu] to all the dhātus throughout the body, thereby nourishing them [Singh 1912, 32].

It is noteworthy that in this passage, the idea that this information has been received from others and is being conveyed now to the readers is highlighted rather than elided. The importance of the heart to the veins and arteries is attributed not to empirical fact, but to linguistic act: the heart is "called" the place of the veins and arteries. Here the social creation of information is not masked in empiricism.

Furthermore, this stanza refers far beyond itself, invoking several different narratives of the heart: the seat of the soul, the key to the body's strength, a center point for physical nourishment. These narratives of the heart speak intertextually with other narratives—of diet, doṣa, and dhātu. The passage therefore opens up rather than sums up the significance of the heart to life processes. The significance of the heart, like the trajectory of the veins and arteries, radiates outward in possibilities of spirito-physical sustenance and bliss. Moreover, there is an element here not only of elucidation, but also of delight. Oj, also known as *ojas,* is not simply the seventh dhātu but the "splendor" of all the dhātu; it is not simply located in the heart but sheltered there. In *Śivanātha Sāgar* neither the organs nor the dhātu, neither disease nor patients themselves, are simply passive, neutral objects of a scientific gaze. The morally charged meanings of bodily processes are reinforced by the etchings accompanying the texts, in which fevers are personified, a drawing of lungs is placed next to a drawing of the author worshipping the god of Ayurveda, and messengers of death distinguish between virtuous patients and sinful ones (figures 2, 3, 4, and 5).[4]

Except for its historically focused introduction, *Śivanātha Sāgar* is more similar to ancient Ayurvedic texts dating from approximately 1000 B.C. (as well as to texts of the intervening centuries) than it is to the texts that were to appear in the coming decades. Consider, for example, this translation of a series of verses on the heart in *Caraka Saṃhitā:*

> The six parts of the body, the intellect, senses, five kinds of sense objects, the ātmā along with its qualities, the mind along with its objects are joined together in the heart. The heart specialists regard the heart as the resting point of these entities, similar to the central girder of the beams in a house. . . . It is the seat of the excellent ojas and the receptacle of consciousness. From the heart as from a root, ten great vessels carrying ojas pulsate throughout the body (P. V. Sharma 1981, 1:237).[5]

The next three lines go on to extol the virtues of ojas, without which no creatures can live; the essence of the embryo and that which sustains the embryo, the "cream" of the fluids that nourish the body; the fruit of the ten vessels that produce many fruits and are therefore called *mahāphala* (great fruit) (P. V. Sharma 1981, 1:237). How different this language is from that of the modern textbooks I will discuss in chapter 5. In this

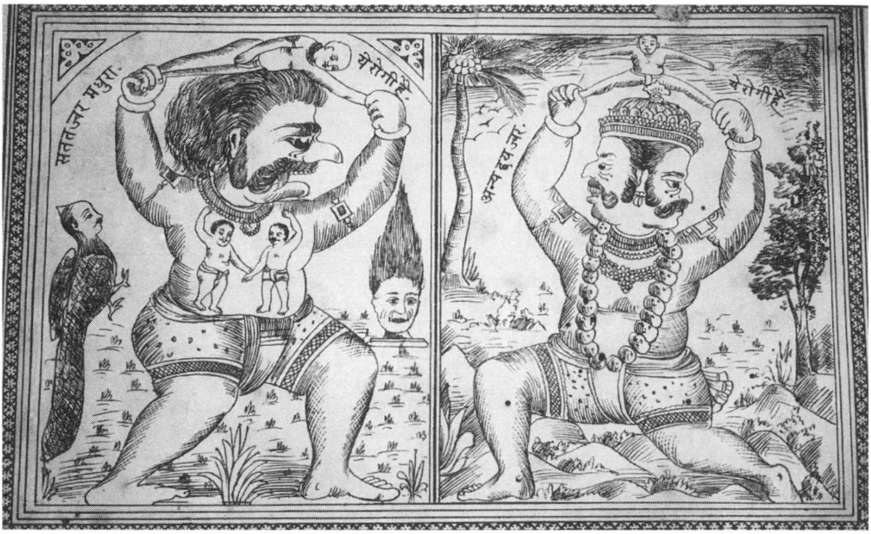

Figure 2. Personified Fevers. *Satat jwar,* remittent fever, taking hold of the ill person (left). *Anyadway jwar,* fever that recurs every twenty-four hours, seizing the ill person (right) (Ś. Singh 1912, 3).

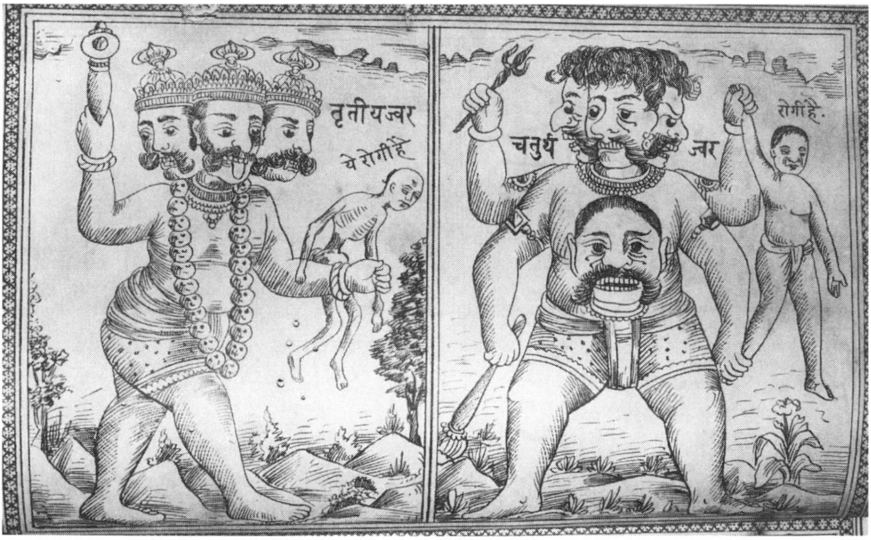

Figure 3. More Personified Fevers. *Tṛtīy jwar,* the fever that recurs every second day (left) and *caturth jwar,* the fever that recurs after an interval of two days (right) (Ś. Singh 1912, 4).

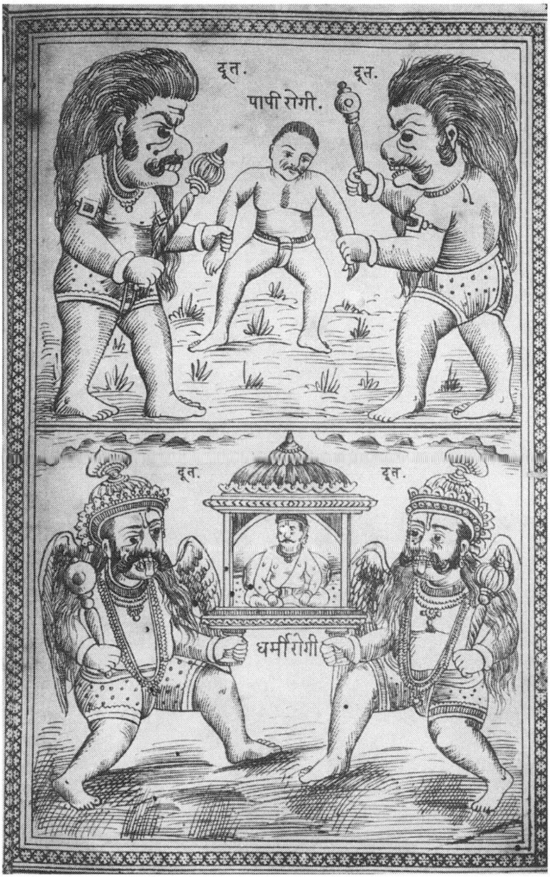

Figure 4. Sinful and Dharmic Patients. *Dūt* (messengers) with a sinful patient (top) and with a *dharmī* (dutiful, virtuous) patient (bottom). This is probably a depiction of the messengers of death who come for a dying patient. These messengers are said to carry meritorious persons away with great respect and to drag sinful persons away by their extremities (Ś. Singh 1912, 5).

poetic work, as in *Śivanātha Sāgar,* meaning is less delimited than compounded, and description is an aspect of praise.

If the poetry of *Śivanātha Sāgar* does not assume a "homogeneous empty time," the introductory prose, despite its historical consciousness, does not quite imagine an Indian nation, referring only to the local problems of the author's own region. Singh even goes so far as to say that the

Figure 5. God and Lungs. Dhavantari, the *vaidya mahārāj,* being worshipped by author Śivanāth Singh, *vaidya rāj* (top). An unborn child in the womb (bottom left). Lungs (bottom right) (Ś. Singh 1912, 1).

vaidya śāstras have been much more neglected in Rajasthan than elsewhere. Similarly the introduction lacks any negative assessment of the impact of foreign rule on indigenous medicine. Rather, the author mentions the British only in order to credit them with the introduction of the printing technology that permits the expansion of knowledge. Clearly this author, who was around age sixty at the time of publication, conceives Ayurveda as a route to good health but not yet as a sign of Indian nationhood. Accordingly *Śivanātha Sāgar* does not identify the crisis of health as a crisis of the imitation of foreign ways.

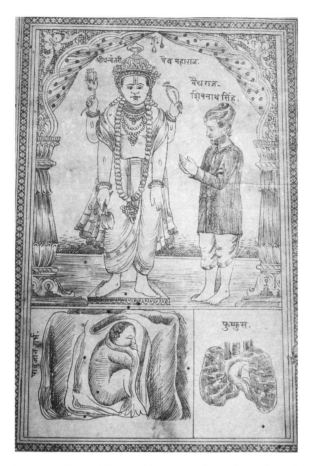

For Singh, then, *cultural* inauthenticity is not an issue. What is an issue is another sort of falseness: pretension to competence. In *Śivanātha Sāgar* the problem of imitation is the problem of ignorant vaidyas parading themselves as knowledgeable vaidyas. The passage on incompetent Ayurvedic practitioners or quacks is worth a closer look because of what it may reveal about the incremental development of a modern sense of authenticity. Singh discusses several criteria for incompetence in this passage. First, the ignorant vaidyas do not belong to a lineage—that is, they are not successors to particular lines of respected healing practitioners. Second, their knowledge is slight, limited to three or four medicines. Third, some of their medicines are actually harmful—whether from being improperly prepared or through being simply incorrect, it is not clear. Fourth, though ascetics in name, they are mercenaries in practical effect. In some ways this characterization of incompetent practitioners is closer to that of Ayurvedic texts compiled around three thousand years earlier than it is to that of the present day. A comparison of this discussion of malpractice with that in the *Caraka Saṃhitā* allows us to see more clearly the notion of authenticity that has, however faintly, begun to emerge, a notion that is the ground for contemporary understandings of culture, selfhood, institutional integrity, and scientific proficiency. For in the ancient text by Caraka, false Ayurveda appears as an especially incompetent healing practice, while in Singh's work, false Ayurveda begins to appear as imitative practice that simultaneously posits and displaces an originary practice.

The first reference to incompetent physicians in the *Caraka Saṃhitā* appears in chapter 1 of the first section of the work, "Sūtrasthānam." Here the reader is warned against practitioners who believe themselves clever but are ignorant of the proper use of medicines. Accepting medicine from such vaidyas, who wear only the garment of knowledge, is more dangerous, the text says, than being struck by lightning, bitten by a poisonous snake, or swallowing red-hot iron. The verse ends by advising that the one who aspires to be a physician should endeavor to develop good qualities so that he may give life to others. Practitioners endowed with good qualities can, moreover, be recognized by their successful cures (P. V. Sharma 1981, 1:13–14). In the chapter summary the word used for the ignorant vaidya discussed in the previous lines is *vaidyapavāda*, or one who passes himself off as a vaidya.

There is further reference to incompetent practitioners in chapter 9 of "Sūtrasthānam," which deals with the quadruplet of healer, medicine, attendant, and patient. Here the ignorant physician is described as one who proceeds with too much fear and too little confidence and may cure one person with a long life span by chance while sending hundreds with an uncertain life span to an early death (ibid.). By contrast, life-giving practitioners are those who are dedicated to sacred texts, comprehension of meanings (*arthavijñān*), application (of principles) (*pravṛtti*), and practical philosophy. The best of these practitioners are the ones who are knowledgeable about the causes, signs (*liṅga*), cures, and prevention of illness (ibid.). Therefore physicians should purify their intelligence (*prājñā*). In the next few lines the text states that even *one* of the qualities of learning—wisdom, practical insight, experience, accomplishment (*siddhi*), or popularity—is enough to justify the title of vaidya, but all of these qualities together earn the title of a vaidya who bestows happiness on living creatures (ibid.). Another verse in *Caraka Saṃhitā* refers to practitioners with mercenary motives, avowing that those who sell cures for a livelihood are devoted to a pile of dust while disregarding a cache of gold (P. V. Sharma 1981, 1:34). There is, however, no overt association in this verse of greed with ignorance.

A more extensive characterization of incompetent practitioners appears in a chapter avowedly concerned with the vital breath but veering quickly into a lengthy comparison of practitioners who promote vital breath and those who destroy it. The former are recognized by their high birth; scriptural and practical knowledge; cleanliness; self-control; friendliness to all; and the complete grasp of a long list of specific information, including everything from the "thirty-two ointments" to the "six hundred evacuatives" and from embryology to blood disorders (P. V. Sharma 1981, 1:233–234). The latter are characterized by their vaidya's garb; self-praise; flattery and entertainment of clients; avoidance of scholarly congresses; irrelevant recitation of aphorisms; terror of questions; and lack of preceptors, disciples, or colleagues (P. V. Sharma 1981, 1:235). "The wise patient," one translation reads, "should avoid these great fools, full of physician's conceit, who are like serpents saturated with air" (P. V. Sharma 1981, 1:236). There are, then, many criteria of incompetence suggested in these ancient pages: ignorance of medicinal substances, lack of confidence, pretension, insufficient knowledge of Ayurvedic texts, inadequate grasp and application of principles, deceptive appearance, and so on. The most repeated criterion would seem to be simply the failure to embody the qualities of an accomplished practitioner.

The most succinct statement about incompetent healers in *Caraka Saṃhitā* appears in a section on the three types of physicians, which is included in a chapter addressing seven other triadic aspects of Ayurveda: the three desires, the three pillars of bodily support, the three kinds of strength, the three causes of disorders, the three types of diseases, the three types of therapy, and the three ways of vitiating the three doṣa. Here the three types of physicians (*bhiṣak*) are enumerated as follows: those who pretend to be healers (*chadmacara*), those who have learned healing by experience rather than by study (*siddhasādhita*), and those who embody the qualities of a vaidya. The pretenders are defined as those who take the title of physician on the strength of appearance, a few containers of medicine, and random talk. These practitioners are called *pratirūpaka,* a word that Monier Monier-Williams alternately defines as "image, picture," "forgery," "having the appearance of something," and "charlatan" (1993 [1899], 663). The experiential healers are defined as those who practice in the name of physicians who possess wealth, fame, and knowledge. In the interpretation of one twentieth-century Ayurvedic scholar, they are "those that become physicians by heredity" (and not by training) (Mukharjee and Narayanarow 1954, 307). The practitioners who embody the qualities of physicians are defined as those who are accomplished in healing techniques (*prayog,* which the translator renders as "rational administration" but which is susceptible to a broader interpretation), knowledge (*jñān*), and specialized or worldly knowledge (*vijñān*) and who promote happiness and life in their patients (P. V. Sharma 1981, 2:78–79).

What is interesting from a contemporary standpoint is that we do not find in this passage a binary division between fake vaidyas and authentic vaidyas, but rather a ternary division between superficial vaidyas, experiential vaidyas, and highly accomplished vaidyas. In this classification, healing based on experience or inheritance rather than textual knowledge may indicate a lesser order of skill but is not to be equated with fraudulence. The second group of practitioners have learned Ayurveda (perhaps even under the competent vaidya in whose name they practice) but have not (perhaps *not yet*) themselves embodied the qualities of a vaidya. Even if we understand the accomplished vaidyas as "true" vaidyas and the vaidyas in appearance only as "false" vaidyas, their inclusion on a list with inadequate or not fully developed vaidyas has the strange effect, for a modern reader, of turning reality into a matter of gradation. It is difficult to assimilate this list to a modern duality of original and copy, authentic practitioner and imitator. One possible way of understanding this list is as an enumeration of more or less effective kinds of mimesis. Mimesis was at that time, and for many centuries following, an essential practice of Ayurvedic scholarship, from the mnemonic repetition of ślokas to the imitation of the guru by the *śiṣya* (disciple). If we interpret the list according to a criterion of mimetic efficacy instead of genuineness, then the competent practitioners are those who successfully imitate all the qualities of vaidyas so completely as to imbibe them, the less competent are those who imitate only the practical and not the intellectual qualities of vaidyas, and the pratirūpaka are those who imitate only the surface qualities of vaidyas.

While healing malpractice is a concern in both *Caraka Saṃhitā* and *Śivanātha Sāgar*, the context of malpractice differs from one text to the other. In *Caraka Saṃhitā* this context is one of enduring categories arranged in numerological constellations of threes or fours or sevens. Here the "plurals" of the various kinds of vaidyas are not part of a historical narrative but rather of an apparently timeless typology. In the narrative parts of *Caraka Saṃhitā* plurals are replaced by particular epic figures, the mytho-historical gods and sages who expound Ayurveda in guru-śiṣya dialogues and symposia. In the introduction to *Śivanātha Sāgar* the context of malpractice is one of social-historical conditions in which vaidyak knowledge has been lost and is being restored. How far the imagination of this context depends on the introductory prose form (and vice versa) is suggested by another text, probably also published around the turn of the century, that proceeds directly from a prayer to Ganeśa (the elephant-headed son of Śiva, often invoked at the beginning of an undertaking) to the body of the text, without recourse to a prose introduction. Here the passage on qualified practitioners and less than qualified practitioners, like that in *Caraka Saṃhitā,* is a list of the qualities of each. Vaidyas are described as speaking the truth; having learned from a guru; knowing the proper terminology, diagnostic method, and treatment; having complete knowledge of a vaidya; having hands like nectar; being praised wherever they cure; fully competent to prescribe medicines; patient; without greed; compassionate; pure; without lethargy; and honest. Proscribed (*niṣiddh*) vaidyas, on the other hand, wear torn and dirty clothes; have an angry temperament and behavior; practice fraud; are excessively arrogant; live in small, insignificant villages; and come without being called. Here also there is a third category of vaidya, which is defined as "foolish" (S. P. Singh c. 1900, 17).

In Caraka's typology, one who is a vaidya in appearance only is still one of the three types of vaidyas. This is a matter of identification, not historical crisis. In the situation described by Śivanāth Singh, on the other hand, those who are vaidyas in appearance only are replacing the accomplished vaidyas. The notion of an authentic Ayurveda is beginning to emerge as a superior healing knowledge that is not simply coexistent with an inferior healing knowledge but displaced by a spurious healing knowledge. The possibility of such a displacement is essential to a modern idea of the authentic, which appears as the longed for original behind the insufficient copy. Yet the discussion of incompetent practice in these two texts is also alike in at least one important respect. In neither text do the discussions of Ayurvedic incompetence emphasize the unhealthy consequences of the loss of indigenous knowledge or the imitation of foreigners. The problem of healing incompetence has not yet begun to blur into the problem of *cultural* inauthenticity.

The Problem of Copying Europe

In *Arogyaśikśa* (Health instruction), published in 1908, Muralidhar Śarma also laments the rise of disease but this time with definite gestures toward an Indian nation. "First," he begins, "we must thank Bhagavān [the Lord], but then we must consider how much disease has been increasing in Bhāratakhaṇḍ [the Indian land]. Who can fail to notice that today there is not even one-tenth, not even one-hundredth of the health there was fifty years ago?" Ninety out of a hundred people are sick. New diseases are appearing every day. Everyone is terrified of becoming ill. Fifty years ago, although there was less concern for hygiene and fewer medicines, there was more contentment. Today all the towns and villages and even the forests are clean; there are dispensaries in every lane of every village. Even people who have no *roṭī* (bread) in their stomachs and no clothes on their backs have two or three bottles of medicine in their huts. But what is the result? Death is rising as quickly as the number of medicines. In these words the author asks his readers to envision the world around them, a world where new and terrifying illnesses have appeared even though the landscape is clean and the villages overmedicalized. It cannot be hygiene, then, or lack of medical supplies that is the problem. "Dear brother," he goes on, "why are we in this predicament?" The main reasons are adharma and improper conduct (*anācār*). "When you hear that the main reasons are adharma and anācār, don't be alarmed; simply understand that diet and lifestyle are the cause of every disease." Dharma, he continues, is vanishing from Bhārat. If people now were as virtuous as people had been previously, then health and happiness would spread throughout the land.

Then he adds, "Besides improper diet and lifestyle, worry and poverty are also powerful causes of disease. These are on the rise in Bhārat today." If you put on new-fangled spectacles, he writes, you see progress (*unnati*). But the amount of inflation and the current obsession to fill one's home with new commodities lead to worry:

> With all this worry how can physical health be sustained? A person beset by worries is not strong but weak. A weak person cannot endure any slight change in diet, heat, cold, or sunlight. It is my firm belief that as long as we continue to see all these shiny new things in our neighborhoods and in the homes of our friends and in the market, then the reduction of expense, of weakness, and of disease will be not only difficult but impossible. . . . The weak have a particular need for a health regimen. Everyone knows this but doesn't attend to it. *They think only of copying the Europeans,* without considering that [the Europeans] come from a cold country, are robust, possess a strong digestive fire, and can digest food eaten five times a day. While we are from a hot country, our digestive fire is not strong, and we ourselves are weak. If we eat more than twice a day, we won't be able to digest our food. Eating five times a day suits the Europeans, and hot and cold are both agreeable to their nature. But for us these are harmful. We form the habit of eating hot and cold foods like an addiction to intoxicating drink (Muralidhar Śarma 1908, 4–5; emphasis added).

In this passage Śarma decries the notion of a consumption-oriented progress that leads to poverty and weakness. He faults his countrymen and women for imitating European lifestyles. He then makes a clear demarcation between the indigenous and the foreign and urges allegiance to the former. Yet it is notable that there is not, for him, any loss of national face in the admission that Bhārati *log* (people) are weak, incapable of digesting excessive foods in hot and cold combinations. At this historical moment what is at stake in the copying of Europeans is not quite cultural pride but rather health itself. He goes on to argue that the medicinal substances found in each country are those that are suitable for its inhabitants. Indian plants yield the medicines appropriate to Indian constitutions. The problem of copying Europe is a problem not of inauthenticity but of inappropriateness. Furthermore, in understanding the imitation of Europeans as an instance of adharma, the author invokes a grander cosmic and moral order than colonial politics.

In the next passage, Śarma speaks not simply within modern historical time but even against it, criticizing the obsession with progress. First, he cautions against the dangers of fast-acting medicines whose ingredients are antagonistic to the bodily elements:

> Doctors, vaidyas, and hakīms [Unani practitioners] are handing out medicines for terrifying diseases that need to be systematically uprooted by medicines acting over many months. . . . The doctors these days . . . are advertising medicines that can cure diseases like leprosy, diabetes, and so on in just two days, and the price of medicine for any persistent disease is inflated four- or eightfold. This is the way the country is going. And why wouldn't things come to this, with people promising speedy recoveries, when by railway a journey that used to take six months takes only one day and news that used to arrive in a month arrives in four hours and work that once took years is now finished by a machine in a few hours? If all these things are speeded up, why should it take any time to get cured of disease? But people fail to realize that the dharma of life and the dharma of inanimate things are not the same (Muralidhar Śarma 1908, 6).

Śarma here suggests that the dharma of life, and therefore of healing, moves at a different pace than modern industrial progress. The attempt to force this modern timing onto matters of health results in the harmful imitation not only of European lifestyle, but also of European medical treatment.

This idea is echoed in the introduction to a vernacular translation of a medieval Sanskrit text, *Vṛndavaidyak,* published under the sponsorship of a still ruling maharaja. The author of the introduction, named Maheśamanda Śarma, writes:

> There can be no doubt that in modern times, because of the rule of ignorant *devī* [literally, goddesses], Indians' descendants have forgotten the grandeur of their own fundamental śāstras, have no energy left to grasp their essence; having become senselessly infatuated with the impure/false foreign medicines only, they are prepared to destroy their own prosperity. It is this that is at the root of their destruction. There is no doubt that it is the medicines originating in this very country that are appropriate to the nature of the people raised in this country. But as the kingdoms began to change, many śāstras and much knowledge began to disappear, among them the books of medicine, until a mere two or three books were considered sufficient. So Ayurvedic knowledge nearly vanished but was not quite able to disappear because of two events: a great number of books began to be published, and, because of this, there began to be hopeful signs of the entire spirit of Ayurvedic knowledge rising again (Maheśamanda Śarma 1910, 9).

Again the central problem is the imitation of European medical treatment, along with a loss of śāstric knowledge traced to the erosion of the princely dominions. Yet there is a shift in attention in this work. While Muralidhar Śarma was concerned simply with the decline of health, which he attributed to the imitation of European lifestyle or medicine, Maheśamanda Śarma is concerned with the decline of indigenous medical knowledge per se.[6] The spread of physical disease is coupled with the disregard for the presumably primordial glory of Ayurveda, the "grandeur" of the śāstras. In this text the concern of *Śivanātha Sāgar* with the loss of vaidyak knowledge returns, but with a new significance. While Śivanāth Singh blamed the loss of knowledge on certain local social problems, the author of this text blames the loss of knowledge on the erosion of the power of the Indian princes. The unmistakable subtextual theme is the decline of Ayurveda due to foreign rule. Yet the text refers not to

British rule but rather to the rule of ignorant devī, thus still casting the problem in terms of divine rather than colonial order.

The theme of foreign influence becomes more pronounced in the introduction to another vernacular translation, published nearly a decade later, of another medieval work, *Bhāvaprakāś*. The author of the introduction, named Śaligrama Vaiśya, elaborates not only on the deleterious adoption of European medicine, but also on the ancient glory of Ayurveda. He begins by invoking the glory of Bhārat, which has been an inspiration to other countries. In the time of the Hindu *rājā,* he reminds us, when pure Ayurvedic treatment (*śuddh Āyurvedīy cikitsā*) was more common, "the distress of disease was almost totally absent" (Vaiśya 1919, unnumbered pages of introduction). When people did fall ill, their illness took a less "terrifying form." "At that time," he declares, "this earth seemed like heaven." There was an Ayurvedic school in every region. The local doctors were possessed of full knowledge and skills. With Ayurvedic treatment "all the diseases vanished."[7] By following the lifestyle (*niyam*) recommended by Ayurveda, people became strong. "Because of the effectiveness of Ayurvedic medicine, Indian vaidyas were greatly praised throughout the world: residents of Europe, Persia, Arabia, Romania, and many other countries came here for medical training. These same foreign doctors, with the changing times, call us idiots today" (ibid.). Remedies produced here were once exported to places such as Persia, Arabia, Romania, Russia, Kabul, Germany, England, Asia, Africa, Italy, Portugal, Sweden, France, and so on. Even today they are exported. So what use do the people of Bhārat have for the remedies of other lands? "We have the testimony of many European doctors on the antiquity and excellence of Ayurveda."

"But," the author continues, "it is a matter of great sorrow that . . . such an inauspicious day has come to Bhārat." All the many branches of the śāstras, including Ayurveda, have become ruined. The Mogul rulers burned and tossed in the Yamuna River books that scholars had produced through years of effort. Finally only those medicines that had never been written down but were simply remembered were still in use by vaidyas. Once these vaidyas themselves died, their successors became complete fools. When the primary texts had been burned, how was reading and writing possible? Eventually even the names of Sanskrit medical books vanished from the world, and all the lesser books, *vaidyaraṭna, amṛtasāgar* (books composed primarily of medicinal formulae), and so on, began to be considered great:

> Whoever remembered even one powder considered himself a full-fledged vaidya. Thus vaidyas took great pride in very minor works until they were drowned in negligence to such an extent that they forgot how to read and write and recalled only twenty or twenty-five medicines such as myrobalan and its fruit, amla, dry ginger, pepper, pipal, ajwain, asafoetida, coriander, and so on. Only the names of Caraka, Suśruta, and Vāgbhat [authors of the earliest Ayurvedic texts] remained, while the subjects of their books or the vast number of ślokas written in them were no longer of any concern. . . . In this way the entire medical knowledge of Bhārat was reduced to zero. Doctors and Unani hakīms began to gain in prestige. They opened dispensaries here and there, and the words quinine and sodawater began to pour out of everyone's mouth. . . . People respected doctors instead of Dhanvantari [the name of a god and preceptor of Ayurveda, used also as a title for Ayurvedic practitioners]. Everyone thoroughly believed that Ayurvedic medicine was not very effective compared to European medicine. Any vaidyas who knew how to make medicines stopped making them because no one was asking for them any more (Vaiśya 1919, unnumbered pages of introduction).

Gradually, the author reports, "Bhagavān had pity on us." Through the compassion of our benevolent rulers a wide range of Ayurvedic books began to be published and distributed, of which this edition is one.

In this text the crisis of physical disease begins to be conflated with the crisis of cultural disease. The shift is subtle but momentous. The salient issue now is less that health has been threatened by adharma than that indigenous medical knowledge has been threatened by foreign invasion. Vaiśya's concern here vacillates between loss of health and loss of face. The precolonial paradise he imagines is one in which Bhāratīy log were not only physically strong, but also nationally and culturally proud. Indian medicine was praised and imitated across the globe. In this text it is the foreign destruction of indigenous knowledge that is responsible for the current social, moral, and intellectual degradation of Indian people in general and Ayurvedic practitioners in particular. Here Ayurveda begins to be associated with a Hindu national-cultural essence to be restored after centuries of colonialism. This colonialism is, moreover, a curious conflation of British and Mogul rule, in which both Europeans and South Asian Muslims are framed as foreigners. When Muralidhar Śarma lamented the sad state of medical knowledge practice he implicated doctors, hakīms, and vaidyas all in the same breath. Vaiśya, on the other hand, has singled out doctors and hakīms as foreign agents who "gain in prestige" at the expense of vaidyas. Even as he clearly articulates a problem of European dominance, he also articulates an antagonism between Hinduism and Islam that prefigures the modern ethnic categories of the nation.

In these last three texts the imitation of Europe is understood as a problem, whether at the level of health regimen (the imitation of European habits) or at the level of cure (the imitation of European medical treatment). In these works ignorant vaidyas are neither simply one of the varieties of vaidyas, as in *Caraka Saṃhitā,* nor the result of certain regional social troubles, as in *Śivanātha Sāgar,* but rather the effect of British (and, in the last text, Mogul) rule. Quackery as a problem begins to be situated in relation to colonial medicine and power. These texts suggest both that quacks are those who imitate European medicine and that those who practice Ayurveda are wrongly considered quacks. Tellingly, however, at this historical moment and in these vernacular texts, the imitation of Europeans is still a problem not because it is inauthentic or fake, but because it is geographically unsuitable. That is, there is no invocation of genuine medicine, whether European or Ayurvedic; rather there is an invocation of medicine suitable to places and groups of people. The problem is not imitation itself, but a wrongly chosen object of imitation. With the rise of Ayurveda as an emblem of national culture, however, the crisis of imitation was to shift. Little by little imitation became a problem in and of itself. Attention shifted from the loss of physical health and śāstric knowledge to the loss of cultural authenticity, a loss that is intelligible only within a modern frame of meaning.

Notice that even with the nascent nationalist sentiments and sociological space of their introductions, these works do not quite assume a progressive, secular history. For aside from the introductions, the bodies of these texts are concerned not with current medical practice, nor even a course of medical progress, but rather an omnitemporal and sacred medicine, descended from the gods, practiced in a heavenly yug by ṛṣi of great wisdom, and only recently ruined by the adharma or inappropriate mimesis of the modern age.[8] Even in the introductions, the primary narrative conflict in these works is more focused on the struggle between dharma and adharma than on the struggle for political power that would come to characterize a nationalist history (Chatterjee 1993, 85, 91). Despite their gestures toward modern historicism, then, these texts remain poised just outside the time of a nationalist history.

Ayurveda as a Sign of the Nation

In the mid-1800s, Ayurvedic literary works were copied by hand and passed from teacher to student. It is not surprising, therefore, that the introductions to the turn-of-the-century texts considered above nearly all expend at least a few words on extolling the print media. The author of the introduction to the *Vṛndavaidya* begins with effusive thanks to a certain maharaja "by whose grace a great number of books are being published, along with translations, for the benefit of humankind" (Maheśamanda Śarma 1910, 9). He goes on to praise the maharaja for undertaking the vernacular translation and publication of ten or twenty rare books from his Ayurvedic library in order that every Indian might both know "the glory of ancient vaidyak knowledge" and receive the benefits of that knowledge in the form of strength and a long life. The author of the introduction to *Bhāvaprakāś* concludes by thanking God for the recent spate of Ayurvedic publications in the vernacular. Such comments remind us of the importance of the rise of print capitalism, in its transcription of vernacular speech, to the development of national-cultural identity (Anderson 1991). In the introductions to some of these texts the authors make an initial gesture toward the imagination of an Indian nation by contrasting a primordial Ayurveda reflecting the glory of ancient civilization with a contemporary Ayurveda reflecting the sad decline of that civilization. This narrative, which was to become increasingly salient in Ayurvedic works of the coming decades, dovetails in part with a British orientalist scholarship that valorized Aryan antiquity over medieval or contemporary India. This scholarship, which furthered British agendas by both supporting the idea of a classical origin of modern nations and justifying colonial interference in Mogul rule, shaped British Indological studies of many subjects, including Ayurveda.

Colonial scholars of the early nineteenth century understood the problem of imitation rather differently than the Ayurvedic scholars cited above. For the Ayurvedic scholars, the imitation of Europeans was harmful not because it was inauthentic, but because it was inappropriate. For the colonial scholars, on the other hand, imitation of any kind was harmful in and of itself. Merely to say something was an imitation was enough to invalidate it. In his lengthy study of Indian medicine Thomas Wise listed the replacement of ancient medical works with imperfect copies as one of the problems facing Ayurveda. The ignorance of the śāstras, he wrote, has led to "the substitution of superstition and quackery." As an example of this superstition, Wise notes "the system of *bhūtavidya* [knowledge of ghosts], which included the offering up of certain prayers, and incantations" (1986 [1845], v). He apparently missed the passages in the *Caraka Saṃhitā* that discuss the practice of prayers and incantations to drive out not only *bhūt* (ghosts), but also certain fevers and other disorders (P. V. Sharma 1981, 2:170, 83). The spiritual or "superstitious" references in the "classical" texts were elided by British scholars in order to facilitate the construction of ancient Ayurveda as empirical as opposed to magical. In orientalist discourse, quackery was conflated with magic or religiosity.

In the defenses of Ayurveda dating from the early twentieth century, Ayurvedic scholars themselves also valorized ancient texts over current practices.[9] At the founding ceremony of Benares Hindu University in 1916, Gananath Sen emphasized that Ayurveda had served humanity even from "under the weight of ruins." He went on to say that works such as *Caraka Saṃhitā* are only remnants of a vast Ayurvedic literature that existed a thousand years before. Then he cautioned, "I do not here propose to discuss or defend some effete material that has crept into mutilated Ayurvedic literature. . . . Such effete material is nothing but interpolation and is like the chaff that must be eliminated if the nutritious grains are wanted" (Sen 1916, 23). Referring to the "crying need for reform," he said, "We must not be timorous to admit that the present methods by which so-called Kavirajas [synonymous with vaidyas at that time] are manufactured out of idle pupils or compounders in many cases are fit to be mercilessly condemned" (Sen 1916, 26). In fixing their gaze on ancient texts, such Ayurvedic revivalists tended to overlook intervening centuries of Ayurvedic practice, with all its regional variations, innovations, and fruitful exchanges with Unani and other healing practices.[10] Even today the trend of associating Ayurvedic knowledge almost exclusively with early texts, especially the *Caraka Saṃhitā* and *Suśruta Saṃhitā*, rather than with the practices of vaidyas that have been passed and altered from generation to generation is very strong.[11] The discourse of revival therefore had the effect of detaching Ayurvedic knowledge from immediate practical contexts and locating it within remote texts. Revivalist discourse also delineated Ayurveda as the exclusive province of a group of high-caste, Sanskrit-literate pundits. Separating the wheat from the chaff was also a matter of separating the elite from the riffraff. One aim of "revival" was to wrest the name of Ayurveda away from the myriad "compounders" who did not fit a middle-class image of professionalism.

What is crucial to my argument here is that the revivalist ideology evokes the idea of imitation no longer simply as the copying of climatically improper regimens and remedies, but rather as the contamination of authentic Indian culture. It is no longer that a mimetic learning style is simply focusing on a wrong and foreign object. Rather, as in the Wise text, it is mimesis itself that is suspect as a displacement of the real. Quackery now begins to take on a more fully historical dimension: fake doctors are a consequence of the decay of ancient Ayurveda. The authenticity invoked here takes its force as a sign not from concepts of geographical unsuitableness, but from socio-temporal ideas of adulteration and counterfeit. The authentic cultural object is distinguished from an object that is a corrupted version (grain mixed with chaff) or a mere copy. Revivalism goes beyond orientalism in endeavoring not only to scholastically preserve knowledge of the "classical" era, but also to revive it. Ayurveda is not to be simply a museological object but a national medicine. As Sen told his listeners in 1916, "We have taken the vow, not merely to lament the bygones but diligently to dig up the diamond fields which were there, are yet there, though covered with ruins. We shall not cease in our efforts till we get back our treasures and leave them to posterity repolished and replenished for the benefit of the whole world" (1916, 2).

In order to be commensurate with other national medicines, Ayurveda would have to be framed as both secular and scientific. Revivalism thus adopted the orientalist narrative of an ancient scientism, followed by a medieval process of "sacrilization," to be corrected by a project of "secularization" (Leslie 1976a). Sen was one of many twentieth-century theorists engaged in an effort (examined more closely in chapter 5) to demonstrate that ancient Ayurveda anticipated and encompassed European science.[12] This effort involved a reinterpretation of certain topics such as bhūtavidya, one of the eight specialties of Ayurveda. Thus in a 1954 Ayurvedic textbook, in a section entitled "Reference to Bacteriology," bhūt are defined as "particular groups of minute beings which do harm to men," or, in other words, microorganisms (Mukharjee and Narayanarow 1954, 266). Similarly in a contemporary introduction to the *Caraka Saṃhitā,* bhūtavidya is translated as "pertaining to micro-organisms or spirits" (Sharma 1981, 1:v). One urban practitioner I met, Dr. Pathi, told a group of industrial scientists that bhūt, *piśāca,* and *rākṣasa* (ghosts, spirits of the dead, and demons) should be understood as "nothing but bacteria, fungi, and viruses." Alternatively, a 1959 government report on the status of Indian medicine (usually referred to as the Udupa Report after the practitioner who headed the committee responsible for preparing the report) glossed bhūtavidya as psychotherapy (Government of India 1959, 1).[13] In the narrative of decline, ancient Ayurvedic knowledge is comprehensive and rational, while contemporary Ayurvedic knowledge is fragmented and riddled with irrationality.

Yet despite this rationalization there is an ambivalence in twentieth-century Ayurveda on the matter of spirit. Zimmermann (1978:100) has traced the ambivalence to a conflict between rationality and ritual in classical Ayurveda itself. I suggest, however, that the ambivalence is rather the splitting effect of a modern understanding in which something called spirit is isolated in order that it may be alternately marginalized and harnessed to political use. For even as Ayurveda began to be framed as national medicine and therefore science, it also began to be framed as an aspect of Indian "spirituality." We cannot assume that this "spirituality" is a preexistent entity that nationalism gathers into its embrace.[14] In both the ancient and the turn-of-the-century vernacular texts cited above, the mingling of precepts that we, as moderns, might categorize as spiritual with those we would categorize as scientific is both unproblematic and unself-conscious. In *Śivanātha Sāgar,* for example, the signs/features (lakṣaṇ) and treatments of various fevers are interspersed (without any clear categorical distinction) with the signs/features and treatments of possession or seizure (*grahaṇ*) by ghosts (bhūt), demons (rākṣasa), and celestial musicians (*gandharva*). Here the realm of nonhuman agents works not as a separate category of spirit but as part of the etiological landscape.

In later works, however—particularly those written in English and therefore addressed to a more Anglicized (and to some extent English) audience—the framing of Ayurveda as "spiritual" becomes not only overt, but also elaborately justified. In one of the testimonies on the state of Ayurveda delivered to the Madras government in 1923, for example, an elegant argument is made against medical materialism, quoting British writers to draw connections between the "supernatural" elements of Ayurveda with such aspects of European society as Christian Science, saintly miracles, and hypnotism (G. Srinivasa Murti, Government of Madras 1923, appendix 1:70–72). Here the "spiritual" (or parapsychological) is invoked not as part of a thorough inventory of the world, but as an aspect of national-cultural rhetoric that excludes all those ghosts, gandharvas, and mad sadhus who might exceed its modern grasp.[15]

The tension between Ayurveda as national medicine and Ayurveda as "spiritual culture" is startlingly illustrated in this passage of a 1923 letter of advice on the revival of Ayurveda to the secretary of the Ayurvedic Committee of the School of Tropical Medicine in Calcutta:

> It will come to you as a surprise that many Ayurvedic physicians now use quinine in malaria but though they do not admit it, we should not be astonished to find in some tantras or puranas later on, the properties of the drug described in the form of a dialogue between Śiva and Parvati. It would be done so, not to cheat the public, but to create a faith in the minds of the patients: and we know that similar devices had been adopted in recent times by Europeans, when, in order to stimulate faith in vaccination, some Sanskrit poems were composed to show that vaccination was sanctioned by the religious books of the Hindus (cited in Mukhopadhyaya 1994 [1922–1929], 2:33–34).

Here the Ayurvedic imitation of European medicine is mingled with the imitation of ancient scriptural poetry in order to be effective. This mimetic tactic is, moreover, itself imitative of British tactics to promote European medicine. Such a colonial display of mimesis and countermimesis—

mimesis in support of mimesis — will be useful to keep in mind when in chapter 6 I introduce Dr. Mistry, a master of the simultaneous imitation of both scientific and religious authority. Meanwhile, the semiparadoxical work of Ayurveda as a sacred sign of the nation is nowhere more clearly inscribed than in the mythic structures of Ayurvedic histories.

Mythic Histories

The surprising temporal cadences of modern Ayurvedic historiography were impressed on me in an Ayurvedic college one afternoon during a lecture on the history of Ayurveda. I sat with the students on hard wooden benches, sweating in the monsoon heat. The previous history lecture had been about medieval treatises on the use of metals in medicine. I was listening only haphazardly this afternoon, lulled by the rain pouring down outside the open windows, trusting my tape recorder to register what I missed. Suddenly I was startled into alertness by the mention of Mahatma Gandhi. The lecturer was recounting the accomplishments of a man who had written volumes of interpretation of the ancient seminal texts of Ayurveda, the *Caraka Saṃhitā* and the *Suśruta Saṃhitā*. His mention that this man had studied with Mahatma Gandhi in college alerted me to the fact that from the last lecture to this we had been catapulted from the sixteenth century to the twentieth. He went on to talk about the establishment of modern Ayurvedic colleges. It was as if the history of Ayurveda evaporated between medieval times and the twentieth century. Some days later I had the opportunity to question the history professor about this curious gap. He told me that ever since Caraka's time, Ayurveda has been in decline. Literary works became more concise, consisting sometimes of only a few recipes, until finally they became completely negligible. There was, therefore, virtually nothing to report about Ayurveda during the seventeenth, eighteenth, and nineteenth centuries. Fortunately the *Caraka Saṃhitā* was preserved and, in the present era, could be reinterpreted.

The history professor's answer is indicative of a perspective on Ayurvedic history that I encountered from many Ayurvedic professionals in diverse settings. From this perspective, the history of Ayurveda is one of increasing deterioration, beginning with its divine origins, its development in the satyayug, and its increasing decay in the kāliyug. This history differs from Puranic histories in its revivalist subtext and from orientalist histories in its religiosity. Despite their packaging in nationalist institutions, such as textbook prose and college curricula, contemporary Ayurvedic histories do not assume a "homogenous empty time," but instead imagine a parabolic time in which the problems of contemporary Ayurveda constellate with the possibilities of Ayurveda in a golden age.

The main thrust of Ayurvedic histories is therefore not the development of medical knowledge over time but rather its devolution. Where this devolution diverges most sharply from orientalism is in its conflation of the classical past with a closeness to the divine. The separation between sacred and secular time on which a modern notion of history depends (Chakrabarty 1992b) is absent in these contemporary temporalizations of Ayurvedic knowledge. Three volumes of what was to have been a six-volume work, *History of Indian Medicine: Containing Notices, Biographical and Bibliographical, of the Ayurvedic Physicians and Their Works on Medicine from the Earliest Ages to the Present Time,* were published between 1922 and 1929. In the introduction to the first volume the author, Girindranath Mukhopadhyaya, writes that he has followed the design of a medical history in which "every chapter might have as its heading the name of a great surgeon or physician, who as pioneer has determined and guided progress" (1994 [1922–1929], 1:9). Because his third volume took him only as far in his account as the first century B.C., it is not possible to determine whether the author believed that progress in Ayurveda extended into medieval times.

Despite the introductory comment, Mukhopadhyaya's history resembles a European chronicle more than a history since it traces a sequence without offering narrative significance or closure (White 1990, 17). On the other hand, Mukhopadhyaya certainly gestures toward "the discourse of the real" that characterizes history (White 1990, 20). The word "legend" appears frequently in the biographies of ancient physician-gods. In the third volume, European scholars are occasionally cited on the question of the mythic or historic status of a particular person. Nonetheless, there seems to be a certain ambivalence in this work toward the break between myth and history in its very organization, structured around a lineage that crosses unproblematically from the divine to the human. In the first chapter, after writing, "Brahma is said to be the originator of medical science," Mukhopadhyaya cites the assertions of several nineteenth-century European doctors and scholars to the effect that all medicine descends from God and then ends the section with several healing formulae attributed to Brahma (1994 [1922–1929], 1:4–17). When considered as a modern work, this early modern history seems to hover between genres, the accounts of the life of Rama suggesting a history of literature or legend and the many passages attempting to date a certain scholar suggesting a history of persons or events. Contemporary textbook histories of Ayurveda also begin by saying that Ayurveda originated with Brahma, was transmitted from Brahma to the Aświn twins (who are associated with medicine), then to Indra, and finally, through his compassion, to human sages (e.g., Mukharjee and Narayanorow 1954; Śukla and Tripāthī 1993). In the Ayurvedic legacy the lineage of guru and disciple moves smoothly back from clearly historical authors such as Bhāvamiśra to more ambiguous authors such as Caraka, whose singularity or plurality is still in question, and then ultimately to members of the divine pantheon. In these histories, there is seldom any modern caveat to the effect that Ayurveda's origin story is merely a parable or a metaphor.

As often as it is argued by Ayurvedic scholars today that Caraka's and Suśruta's works were grounded in the strictest and most thorough empiricism, it is also argued that their works were rooted in divine omniscience and the singular meditative powers of ancient savants. This idea appears in a testimony to an official report on the state of Ayurveda to the government of Madras in 1923. One pundit wrote that whereas modern scientists seek to overcome the limits of the senses through instruments such as the microscope and cardiograph, ancient sages "sought to effect the same results, not by providing their sense with external aids, but by improving their own *internal* organs of sense, so that their range of perception may be extended to any desired degree." He went on:

> It is possible for master-minds to perfect their "sense" (in which term, they include the mind also—"the sixth sense" as it was sometimes called) to so great a degree as to include, within their range, everything from the most microscopic to the most macroscopic. . . . Hindu tradition asserts the original propounders [in Indian philosophy] of such theories as that of the Evolution of the Atoms were persons endowed with the immense ranges of vision of which I have spoken; it is claimed, for instance, that when they taught about the structure of Atom, they

> did not merely speculate in the matter, but described what they really saw; . . . herein lies the difficulty of the Hindu method; because, the perfecting of the senses to the desired degree can be achieved, if at all, by only exceptional individuals of our generation; and therefore the satisfaction of direct observation is not possible to the great majority of us. Herein also lies the immense value of the external aids which Western Science provides us with (Murti, quoted in Government of Madras 1923, appendix 1:21).

In confirmation of this view, another vaidya testifies in the same report, "The ancient Hindu yogis knew the scientific truth by their meditation and worked wonders through their mental force" (Menon, quoted in Government of Madras 1923, part 2:94). Many contemporary practitioners agree. One professor and researcher in an Ayurvedic teaching hospital commented that it is amazing that one person commanded all the knowledge in *Caraka Saṃhitā*. The ancient vaidyas, he said, must have had some *divyadṛṣṭi*, divine vision. Another college-educated practitioner told me that whereas certain modern researchers of Ayurveda analyze plants in the laboratory to determine their medicinal properties, the ancient ṛṣi simply meditated in front of a plant, intuiting its medicinal properties by a kind of mental osmosis. A student in an Ayurvedic college told me that one of his teachers had told him of one book by a ṛṣi that told of a particular medicinal plant for bone fractures that, when touched, gave the vaidya a vision of the bone. "This dramatic thing we don't have in Ayurveda now. "Therefore," he went on, "we have to use X rays instead." For many Ayurvedic practitioners and educators, then, the superiority of ancient science was due not so much to secularism as to advanced yogic skills.

Correspondingly, the quasi-magical "folk medical" practices that the British orientalists framed as "superstition" and magic are more likely to be framed by contemporary Ayurvedic scholars as fraudulence and trickery. It is not a serious engagement with spiritual realms that makes such medical practices suspect, but rather a mock engagement with spiritual realms, a false posturing of religiosity. One day I was discussing with an Ayurvedic professor the questionable claim of a local doctor that he could detect how many miscarriages a woman had had from her pulse. After declaring the impossibility of such a diagnosis, the professor added that then again, perhaps the doctor had a gift from god. Unlike for the orientalists, for Ayurvedic scholars a sincere religiosity does not in itself signal quackery, but rather tends to preclude it.

In Ayurvedic history, then, science and religion are joined.[16] The closer we come to divine knowledge — i.e., the further back in mytho-history we go — the closer we come to a perfect science. One day I was sitting in the office of the principal of an Ayurvedic college listening in on an energetic conversation between one of the professors and the principal about a particular Ayurvedic precept. Suddenly the principal turned to me and began to explain that Ayurvedic science was eternal, whereas modern science was constantly changing. At some point, he said, some scientist decided that the smallest unit of matter was an atom. Now an atom is no longer recognized as the smallest unit of matter. Ayurveda, he concluded, is a "perfect science," not like, he seemed to imply, the imperfect European science that keeps changing its mind. Shiv Sharma, a vaidya who, for reasons I discuss in the next chapter, is credited by some with "saving" Ayurveda in the twentieth century, answered those orientalists who argued that Ayurveda had stagnated with these words: "an unstable science groping in the dark, is not necessarily progressive, nor a stable science based on true and unchanging principles stagnant. Progress means a move in the right direction and it ends when the destination is reached. The conflicting and unfounded theories of the Western medicine cropping up in large numbers lead nowhere" (Sharma 1929, 276). A similar observation was made at around the same time by a group of seventeen vaidyas responding to a questionnaire sent out during preparation of the Madras Report on Ayurveda. This group of practitioners first noted that the questionnaire implicitly discounted the third means of knowledge recognized in Ayurveda, scriptural authority — the first two being direct observation (*pratyakṣa*) and inference (*anumān*). They then went on to criticize modern science as follows: "They are changing their ground almost every year by refuting the old theories, and experimenting, each according to his own whims, upon poor creatures, without any proportionate gain to anybody. Is it this that deserves the name of science? Our idea of science is that it should be a storehouse of incontrovertible, universal knowledge which holds good for all times — past, present and future" (Sharma et al., quoted in Government of Madras 1923, part 2:76). In the same report another vaidya testified that while Ayurveda employs theories and formulae proven over time, the "allopathic system is changing and has not yet come to any definite form. What is truth in one generation is falsified in another and reappears in a third; hence it is in a more or less experimental stage." He went on to state that the neglect of Ayurveda had led to a failure to make certain necessary changes due to "changed conditions of habits, foods, etcetera" (Anjaria, quoted in Government of Madras 1923, part 2:80). Although Ayurvedic practice needs to be adjusted to fit the times, Ayurvedic theory, he suggested, was already perfect. Histories of Ayurveda invariably emphasize its influence on other ancient healing practices, and thereby ultimately on European medicine, through its exchanges with other empires of the ancient world such as Greece, Mesopotamia, and Egypt. In the lecture following the one mentioned above, the history lecturer spoke extensively of the evidence that travelers from other continents had studied ancient Ayurveda and transported its concepts back to their native lands. In the assertion that Ayurveda was the source of these other healing traditions lies the suggestion that it can still compete in the international arena. This era in Ayurveda's past is therefore invoked to restore its potency in the current century. These histories of Ayurveda are charged with the nationalist purpose of the present time.

Moreover, this nationalist purpose carries within it an implicit communalist impulse. In evoking eternal knowledge belonging to a golden age, Ayurvedic histories tacitly make Ayurveda available to Hindu fundamentalist imagery of Ram Raja, a Hindu golden age. One obvious effect of a history that skips from the sixteenth to the nineteenth century is to erase much of the Mogul era and to enforce the Hinduness of Ayurveda, erasing centuries of exchange between vaidyas and hakīms. This has the effect, in turn, of enforcing the Hinduness of the national culture to which Ayurveda contributes.[17] It is true that most of the government reports published over the twentieth century discussed the modernization of Unani medicine and other indigenous medicines alongside Ayurveda. During the early 1990s there was at least one modern-style institution in India that was billed as a college of both Ayurveda and Unani. The Ayurvedic practitioners I know are neither militantly Hindu nor exclusionary in their practice. Nonetheless, when a narrative of spiritual community, such as that evoked by these Ayurvedic histories, dovetails with the narrative of modern nationhood, it tends to be articulated in state violence against communities or community violence in service of imagined communal states.

In the early twentieth century Ayurvedic professionals faced the danger that indigenous medicine would be excluded from the invented Indian (and largely Hindu) culture around which nationhood was organized. In meeting this danger, these professionals expanded the purpose of Ayurveda from the healing of people to the healing of an exclusionary culture. The same Dr. Pathi who said that bhūt should be understood as bacteria made the point in more than one lecture that Ayurveda had, for the last few centuries, been transmitted by technicians and not by scientists. The scientists, he said, were "massacred by the Muslims and the British," and the technicians began to "imagine they were scientists." To explain why bhūt are not presently understood as bacteria he said,

> Unfortunately, our entire Ayurveda was in the hands of some quacks [until recently]. But those quacks were very, very useful to us, like tape recorders. They recorded our entire science, without knowing it, and we don't mind. They transported it, without disturbing a single word or sentence, to us, and the scientific part of Ayurveda was destroyed by foreigners; especially [in the] Mogul era, it was destroyed. And the technicians only, or these so-called quacks, I say, those who were not knowing the meaning of it, they had this Ayurveda. And then this Ayurveda, what they were knowing [of] it, it was all perverted science.

Here Dr. Pathi shows how thoroughly a modern sense of inauthenticity is intertwined with an idea of rigid and antagonistic cultural boundaries.

In referring to quacks as tape recorders he also calls attention to the connection between the notion of authenticity and modern possibilities of mechanical reproduction. He evokes the mechanical mimesis of a modern age, in which words can be accurately reproduced without comprehension. In other conversations, however, he worked with a different sense of mimesis, an imitation that, he said, is the basis of all learning. Those students who wish to learn Ayurveda well, he told me, should spend two or three years after college with a practitioner like himself, simply observing and imitating. The imitation of these students, like the mimesis praised in the *Caraka Saṃhitā,* amounts to an embodiment of the qualities of a vaidya. For Dr. Pathi, while the mimesis of apprenticeship carries a connotation of fully absorbed knowledge, the mechanistic mimesis carries a connotation of superficial knowledge. In the next chapter I turn to the development of that more mechanistic mimesis within the standardized structure of modern Ayurvedic education.

four The Effect of Externality

I was sitting in the office of the director of an Ayurvedic teaching hospital in an Indian city, describing my research project in carefully chosen phrases. When I told him that the project was entitled "Sansthānik Āyurveda mẽ Rog kā Vicār" (The concept of disease in institutional Āyurveda), he asked brusquely, "Matlab kyā hai?" (What does that mean?). As I stumbled to explain, invoking the difference between Ayurveda within a guru-śiṣya *parampara* (guru–disciple lineage) and Ayurveda within *adhunik sansthān* (modern institutions), he interrupted to say irritably that whatever the "means" (using the English word) of education, the concept of disease as defined in the śāstras remains unchanged. He seemed to be arguing that the content of Ayurvedic knowledge could and must be distinguished from the form in which that knowledge was packaged and transmitted. His reasoning rested on the presumably commonsensical assumption that an institutional structure is a form that contains and represents a particular content or function. Once, a professor at the same institution told me that the only difference between his practice and his grandfather's was the "uniform," the "packaging." His grandfather, he said, wore a lungi, while he wears Western clothes. Both these college professionals seemed to take for granted, or at least invite me to take for granted, that Ayurvedic teaching hospitals are structures that unproblematically contain and represent Ayurvedic knowledge, a static and discrete body of ideas.

An understanding of the relationship between institutional form and institutional content or function is possible only through the exercise of the knowledge practice Mitchell has termed enframing.[1] While the idea of enframing owes much to Foucault's discussion of disciplinary power, it goes a step further in recognizing that even as power is diffused through everyday practices of surveillance, it is projected as residing in external frameworks. It is due to the resultant externality (and internality) effect that institutional form can be considered separate from institutional function. In the case of biomedicine, for instance, control of the body is exercised through daily practices of examination, isolation, and reification by means of diagnostic tools such as stethoscopes and sonograms. Yet medical control is largely perceived by patients and others to originate in such institutions as hospitals and professional associations of physicians. This projection of control onto external frameworks makes possible a split between politically motivated agencies of institutional power and (supposedly) politically neutral exercises of medical truth. Medical knowledge can be understood as being pure content, separable from and not contingent on the institutional forms through which it is enacted. It is crucial to understand that the success of the externality effect rests on its naturalization. That is, the pervasiveness of modern discipline is accompanied not only by the effect of externality, but also by the masking of the artificiality of that effect. The recognition that the effect is (merely) an effect would inevitably put its efficacy at risk.

In this chapter I investigate the disturbance of the relationship between form and function or form and content within contemporary Ayurvedic teaching hospitals, where the curriculum and the degrees granted routinely *mis*represent the educational and knowledge practices of the classrooms and wards. During the above conversation with the director of the hospital I seemed to offend him still further with a request to follow the daily activities of the college in the company of a student with a sincere interest in Ayurveda. Ayurvedic doctors had repeatedly warned me that most students in Ayurvedic medical colleges had less interest in Ayurveda than in the degree, which would allow them to practice a freestyle, pharmaceutically directed medicine. The director replied gruffly that all the students had a sincere interest in Ayurveda. A few months later I heard from both an Ayurvedic undergraduate examiner and another institutionally affiliated Ayurvedic doctor that the director's daughter had received her Bachelor of Ayurvedic Medical Science despite very poor answers on her final exam and that she was now about to receive an Ayurvedic M.D. despite her failure to conduct independent research as nominally required. The case was presented to me by both doctors not as atypical, but rather as exemplifying the corrupt state of contemporary Ayurvedic education.

A historical understanding of the development of Ayurvedic institutions within the colonial and postcolonial eras suggests that widespread corruption and other slippages between form and function resulted in part from the introduction of European institutional models into the Ayurvedic practice of the late nineteenth and early twentieth centuries. These institutional models, originally introduced by British colonialists as part of European medicine, were reproduced by Ayurvedic practitioners who were persuaded that the only way to compete with European medicine was to develop Ayurveda as its institutional parallel and equal. Once practitioners began to reconceive Ayurveda as a sign of the nation, they were faced with the task of packaging it for the nationalist movement and later the Indian state as a standardized national medicine commensurate with biomedicine. Increasingly, then, they addressed a disequilibrium not just in the physical body or the social body, but also in the body politic, specifically the part of the body politic that governed medicine itself.[2]

In this chapter I suggest that while the effect of an external framework was indeed created through the establishment of Ayurvedic institutions, this effect was never fully naturalized. Slippages between institutional form and function were exaggerated to the point that contemporary Ayurvedic institutions are frequently described in disgusted tones (even—perhaps especially—by Ayurvedic professionals) as mere empty formality without meaningful function. In this chapter I explore the possibility that such open acknowledgment and often tacit acceptance of the failure of Ayurvedic teaching hospitals to properly contain and represent Ayurvedic knowledge may signal a recognition of the artificiality of an external framework that has little relationship to the actual workings of the institution. For modern Ayurvedic institutions were established not so much to better transmit Ayurvedic knowledge as to balance the scales with European medicine.

Despite his irritation with my research topic, the hospital director gave me permission to observe activities in the Ayurvedic college. One day a couple of months before final examinations, I was talking with a few of the professors in the faculty lounge while I waited for a lecture I had planned to attend. In recent weeks I had noticed that the lectures on the class schedule seemed to start late or not at all. When I questioned students and professors on this matter, they gave me different explanations at different times: the students might say that a particular professor was very busy, while the professors might say that the students were engrossed in "self-study." Except for me, no one seemed to find the discrepancy between schedule and actual classroom practice disconcerting. The students simply read in the library or sat talking and studying in the narrow wooden desks jammed together in the classroom. The professors, meanwhile, gathered in the lounge. That day as I prepared to leave the lounge for the lecture I wanted to attend, I realized that the lecturer was still sitting there talking to a colleague. "Are you not lecturing this period?" I asked. His colleague countered, "There are no students in the classroom, are there?" I said, "There are a few, but most are waiting in the library." "Yes," she said, as if we had settled the question of the students' attendance, "the library is the common room." Then she added, in contradiction (I thought) to the previous exchange, that these days the students all go home after the first two periods.

This incident was emblematic for me of a frustrating thinness I experienced in my ethnographic visits to this and other colleges. Despite the hours spent in observation and conversation with students and faculty, I seemed to be only skimming the surface, recording haphazard scraps of instruction, without penetrating to the depths that must surely lie behind. My frustration betrays the particular expectations and conditioned longings of an anthropological hermeneutics. For I continuously had the feeling that I was failing in the Geertzian ideal of layered interpretation, thick description (Geertz 1973). Margaret Trawick (1992, 89–90) has recommended that we stop thinking of the anthropological project as a stripping of the surface to reveal the depth. She suggests that we acknowledge that there is only the turbulence of a confrontation that includes ourselves, the participant-observers. My visits to Ayurvedic colleges make the most sense to me when perceived as aspects of such confrontational turbulence, involving not only my own epistemically situated presence and those of the students and staff, but also certain absences or spectral presences, such as those of British colonialists, ancient pundits, Indian politicians, allopathic doctors, and Ayurvedic quacks. I think now that in sifting the daily activities of Ayurvedic colleges for deeper layers of meaning, I was seeking complexity in the wrong place — that is, in place at all — in densities of experience within an institutional space, rather than in intricate narratives of political necessity. Modern Ayurvedic education became comprehensible to me when I was able to view it no longer as a disassembled or dissembling text, but as an improvisation, not as an empty or corrupted form, but as an "ab-use," to borrow Spivak's (1992) phrase, of an Enlightenment language of form and content, a rearrangement of a modern institutional syntax.

From Guruparampara *to Curriculum*

At first, after Macaulay's *Minute* and the momentous cannon blast discussed in chapter 1, Ayurvedic training persisted in the form it had probably mostly taken for hundreds of years, the guru-śiṣya parampara, or teacher-student lineage.[3] Since the time of the compositions of the oldest extant texts there had also been a few renowned centers of the healing arts at certain periods. From the fifth to the twelfth centuries, for example, many of the healing practices now encompassed in the name of Ayurveda were taught at Nalanda, a center of scholarship spanning half of a square mile, boasting three hundred lecture halls, fifteen hundred teachers, and ten thousand students (S. Kumar et al. 1985, 2). "Vaidyaka" was one of seventy-two subjects of study at Nalanda, which admitted students from all over Asia (P. V. Sharma 1972, 6; Jaggi 1981, 83). Admission standards were apparently stiff, but those who became students were offered not only free instruction, but free food and clothing as well, thanks to the generous endowments of wealthy and royal families. The healing arts were also taught at Taxila (located in what is now Pakistan), an important center of learning dating from the sixth century B.C. that also attracted foreign students. There is also supposed to have been a center of the vaidya arts in the city of Kashi (Benares or now, officially, Varanasi) that specialized in surgery (S. Kumar et al. 1985, 2).

In addition to these large centers of learning, there were small *gurukulas,* rural residential centers led by one or two gurus. Both Wise (1986 [1845]) in his scholarly work on indigenous medicine and William Adams (mentioned in Leslie 1973, 221–223) in his work on indigenous education describe the gurukulas or *tols* of the mid- to late nineteenth century. A handful of students lived in the home of an experienced vaidya, studying the śāstras and participating in the preparation of medicines and the treatment of patients for five to seven years. Some version of this guru-śiṣya practice dates at least from the time of Caraka, who describes the initiation ceremony for a vaidya novitiate, as well as the responsibilities of both guru and student (P. V. Sharma 1981, 1:350–355). *Gurutols* continued to exist into the twentieth century, even after the advent of modern Ayurvedic education. According to the Udupa Report of the late 1950s, three-quarters of the vaidyas then practicing had been "traditionally trained" (Government of India 1959, 153). The authors of the Madras Report on indigenous medicine identified two methods of instruction, "tol" and "syllabus." In the first, study is centered on particular ancient or medieval texts and practical training is guided by an experienced vaidya, while in the second, identified as the "Western model," study is not centered on particular texts and practical training is conducted in hospitals and clinics. They went on:

> Each method has its own advantages; but at a time when, due to various causes, there has been an arrest in the progress of Indian Medicine, the confining of teaching to ancient text-books alone may tend to crystallization unless the professors keep themselves in active and intimate touch with all that is happening around them, so that they may be able to include in their teaching the newer conception of things, either by way of commentaries, explanations or in any other manner that may appeal to them (Government of Madras 1923, part 1:30–31).

A few pages later the authors offered an example of how the ancient texts were to be updated by advocating that the electron theory of matter be grafted on to the numerically based Indian philosophy of Sāṃkhya. (More such proposals to synthesize Ayurveda with European science are considered in chapter 5.) The concern of these authors to update the gurukula methods in part reflects the fact that by then the popularity and viability of the tols were being severely undermined by colonial policies. After Macaulay's *Minute* the British encouraged defection from indigenous medicine by distributing free European medical books and supplies and by offering scholarships to modern medical colleges. More and more Indians, including sons of vaidyas, were attracted to the well-equipped colleges of European medicine. The loss of British support at this stage was all the more critical since British rule had been steadily eroding the royalty on which Ayurvedic practitioners had previously relied for support.

By the end of the nineteenth century prominent Ayurvedic physicians were concerned that because of the establishment of colleges of European medicine in Indian cities, the diminishing patronage of Ayurveda, and the increasingly coercive tactics by the colonialists to impose European medicine, the Ayurvedic profession was falling into disregard. In organizing professional associations, pharmaceutical companies, and medical colleges to defend and preserve their profession, they began to frame Ayurveda as a medical system that would be comparable with other medical systems. In September 1890 a group of such vaidyas in Bombay formed the first modern Ayurvedic association, the Mumbai Vaidya Sabhā (Bombay Vaidya Society; hereafter Sabhā) for the promotion and development of Ayurveda. Following British organizational models, the Sabhā elected a chairman and two secretaries. Partly with the aid of the Sabhā, similar groups were formed in Gujarat and other places. While at first the Sabhā engaged in social activities such as the maintenance of a library and dispensary, very soon it began to engage in political activities on behalf of the Ayurvedic profession. When the British issued a ban on the production of an alcoholic substance used in Ayurvedic medicines, an allopathic doctor who was the son of a vaidya and sympathetic to the Ayurvedic cause initiated a successful lawsuit on behalf of the Sabhā to reverse the ban. In 1907 the members of the Sabhā were instrumental in founding the Akhila Āyurvedīy Mahāsammelan (All-India Ayurvedic Congress; hereafter Mahāsammelan), which is still the most influential Ayurvedic association at the national level.

According to a recent history of the Sabhā written by a few of its oldest members, the vaidya community of Bombay came to the realization early in the twentieth century that "Ayurvedic study should be *structured in a way that was appropriate to the time,* in order to turn out skilled doctors who would be able to both promote Ayurveda and serve the public" (Mumbai Vaidya Sabhā 1990, 9; emphasis added). To this end two separate educational institutions were established, the Aryan Medical School and the Mumbai Āyurvedīy Pāṭhaśāla (Bombay Ayurvedic School). In 1907 the latter organized the curriculum of the Nikila Bhāratiy Āyurvedīy Vidyāpīṭh (All-India Ayurvedic Vidyāpīṭh, or center of scholarship), which in 1908 established a system of uniform examination for Ayurvedic pupils studying in gurukulas or under senior vaidyas. The Vidyāpīṭh offered three levels of examination: one for the title of bhiṣak (physician), the second for the title of *viśarāda* (one who is well versed), and the third for the title of *ācāryā* (preceptor). The bhiṣak exam was administered in vernacular languages, the viśarāda exam in rudimentary Sanskrit, and the ācāryā exam in high literary Sanskrit. In addition to their practical apprenticeships under experienced vaidyas or doctors, the pupils studied ancient and medieval Ayurvedic texts. Vd. Shukla, who was active in the still-thriving Sabhā when I first met him in 1992, told me that it was the lack of regard for Ayurveda among the nationalists that prompted the Sabhā to undertake the structuring of Ayurvedic education. Ayurvedic practitioners had perceived an opportunity to promote Ayurveda on a nationalist platform by arguing its unique connection to Indian cultural identity. The members of the Sabhā became convinced, however, that Ayurveda could be promoted as one of the contents of national culture only if it were packaged in a standard institutional form.

Yet in this early structuring of Ayurveda education the form adopted was only partially parallel to the disciplinary form of European medical education. The gesture toward standardization implied by the use of uniform examinations was counterbalanced by the persistence of training specific to the lineage of particular gurus. As described in one account, the Vidyāpīṭh "regularized the Guru-Shisya tradition of education of Ayurveda with a goal to organize regular education by examinations throughout India" (Kumar et al. 1985, 3). The Udupa Report stated, "The Vidyapeeth has laid down standard syllabus for their studies and examinations giving every importance to the subjects and not so much to the old textbooks" (Government of India 1959, 33). The accounts of gurukulas given to me by various elderly vaidyas, however, suggest that the gurukulas of that era, whether connected to the Vidyāpīṭh or not, were still organized to some extent around the old Ayurvedic texts.

Vd. Shastri, a North Indian small-town vaidya in his eighties at the time of our conversations in 1994, told me that Ayurveda had been practiced in his family for four generations. His father had learned through parampara. He himself, however, like every other older practitioner with whom I spoke who was raised in an Ayurvedic family, had studied not under his own father, but in a gurukula. Vd. Shastri attended a gurukula in Haridwar for five years during the 1930s, along with one hundred other students. He told me that the students first learned about *jaḍī-būtī* (medicinal herbs) and *divya* vijñān. When I expressed confusion at this second term, which literally means divine knowledge or knowledge of the divine, he defined it as *padārth* vijñān, a subject in the contemporary Ayurvedic curriculum that is discussed at length in the next chapter but can be glossed here as a cosmo-epistemology in which ideas about the world and about knowledge of the world are intricately interwoven. After this they studied *śarīr kriya,* a recently coined term for physiology denoting the activities of doṣa, dhātu, mala (understood as the products of bodily elimination), and agni (literally fire and often understood as digestion but not just of food). Then they studied *nidān* (usually translated as diagnosis or etiology), which is concerned with the causes and progressions of illness, and finally cikitsā, or treatment. During their third year of study his class also dissected cadavers. At this time in this particular gurukula, then, the outlines of a modern division of subjects had just begun to take shape. At home Vd. Shastri learned about jaḍī-būtī by accompanying his father into the forest to gather plants for medicinal preparations. In the guru-śiṣya paramparā, Vd. Shastri told me, the guru and student used to regularly gather plants together. They would examine them, grind them, give them to a patient, and observe their effects. In the gurukula at Haridwar, however, the gurus and students went into the forests together only very occasionally, maybe a few days a month. Later even that practice was ended.

Dr. Pathi, introduced in chapter 3, also attended the gurukula in Haridwar nearly three decades later but still before the imposition of a uniform, nationally enforced Ayurvedic curriculum. He had already obtained Master's degrees in biochemistry and medicine when he relocated to Haridwar expressly for the purpose of attending a gurukula rather than a *miśra* (mixed—i.e., with allopathy) Ayurvedic course. He wanted an education in the "Indian style," which, he said, involved not teaching but rather learning by observation and imitation. He gave me a more detailed account of the gurukula, which clarified the textual emphasis in the course of study. He explained that in the morning the students studied theory and the preparation of medicines. Then they accompanied the guru who headed the gurukula while he examined and consulted with patients. Later they attended lectures followed by questions and answers with the guru and other teachers working below him. After studying herbal horticulture in the afternoon, they attended more discussions in the evening. During the first two years the literary study concentrated on several branches of Indian philosophy (which Vd. Shastri had generalized as divya vijñān); in the third year it concentrated on the seminal Ayurvedic texts such as the *Caraka* and *Suśruta Saṃhitās.* The students saw their guru once or twice a day. At the gurukula vaidyas were trained to three levels: *śreṣṭh* (best, most honored), *madya* (medium), and *kaniṣṭha* (junior). The śreṣṭh students learned *nāḍī* vijñān, the knowledge of pulse, as well as the use of the most dangerous bhasmas or medicinal ashes. The guru would tell each student which of the three types of vaidyas he should be, based on his talent. The Haridwar gurukula was apparently never connected to the Vidyāpīṭh. Both Vd. Shastri and Dr. Pathi agreed that the gurukula had been completely ruined by the introduction of the standard modern curriculum in the 1970s.

Until he graduated from secondary school in 1932, Vd. Shukla had no idea that he was going to be a vaidya. Despite the fact that his father was an Ayurvedic practitioner, he felt no calling to the profession. He was, however, drawn to the nationalist movement, which was made up of professionals such as lawyers, professors, and biomedical doctors. He thought that he might become a professor. By the time he graduated, however, his father was very ill, and he himself had married at the urging of his grandfather. Since he was forced to take up an occupation quickly, he studied in a gurukula with ten or fifteen other students under several Ayurvedic pundits, passing the bhiṣak exam in 1933 and the viśarāda exam in 1936. His knowledge of Sanskrit was not extensive enough to pass the ācāryā exam. The course of study focused on the poetic texts—medieval texts such as *Bhāvaprakāś* for the bhiṣak exam and ancient texts such as *Caraka Saṃhitā* for the viśarāda exam. Alongside the textual study, the students studied *dravyaguṇa,* or the properties of (medicinal) substances. During this period Vd. Shukla also worked as an assistant at an allopathic clinic run by a friend of his father. He told me frankly that while at the same time his "theory was Ayurvedic," his practice, based on his clinical experience, was allopathic. Like other vaidyas of the era, he dispensed aspirin and quinine. He did not yet feel the political pressure to make his Ayurvedic practice represent a distinctive cultural tradition.

When we discussed the shift from guruparampara to modern education, Vd. Shastri, the small-town vaidya, told me:

> The difference between the previous manner of study and today's is that the student used to learn according to the ancient pattern in which scholarship was full of affection [*sneha*] between the guru and the disciple. This was the ancient "system" [English word] in which there

> was a close bond [*yog*] between the guru and the disciple. These days instruction follows the modern method, which is a business transaction [*hisāb*] in which the student has less faith [*śraddhā,* also connoting reverence] in the guru and so is not able to grasp the knowledge in its true form. In ancient times knowledge was acquired through absorption [*tanmay*] in the guru. The pupil who received the blessings of the guru was very successful. These days it is not like that.

For Vd. Shastri, then, the capitalist concept of an approved educational package available for purchase by generic consumers does not address the need for reverence, subtle rapport, and even love between teachers and students, which alone seem to assure that knowledge will be assimilated. This affection is not easily transposed into modern institutional relationships, where kinship-style bonds of imitation and sympathy between people understood to have divinely ordained roles are replaced by the rights and duties of abstract individuals understood to be equal. The absorption in the guru of which Vd. Shastri speaks can be thought of as that aspect of mimesis that, as we learned from Dr. Pathi, permits knowledge to be passed on not just as a mechanically reproduced set of words and concepts, but also as a substance to be shared and embodied.

Vd. Shastri and Dr. Pathi are not alone in their concern over the institutional interruptions of guruparampara. A Bengali vaidya who was the founder of one of the first modern Ayurvedic colleges and president and examiner for the Vidyāpīṭh testified in the Madras Report that he had lived and studied first in a gurukula headed by his own father and later with another guru "as his own son." He goes on:

> It is difficult to exaggerate the immense value of such a holy atmosphere of study and learning. I recognize that at the present day it is not practicable to revive the beautiful institution of our ancient Gurugriha nivas [residence in the guru's home]. Nevertheless something of its ancient glory may be preserved if we could found residential Ayurvedic colleges standing in their own grounds, where reside not only the pupils but as many professors as possible, so that the students may as far as possible live and study in the immediate and inspiring presence of their preceptors. If even this is not possible, we may so arrange our curriculum that for at least a couple of years every student lives with at least one of his professors. It is only thus that the

> pupils learn many invaluable things, without feeling or knowing that they are being taught. . . . Especially for the student of medicine, it is highly essential that, in the plastic period of his life, he should learn to build up into his life that high sense of duty and honour, as also that spirit of service and self-sacrifice, which is best fostered under a system of Gurugriha nivas, provided, of course, the Gurus are not of the mercenary type that is unfortunately becoming increasingly common at the present day (K. J. B. Roy in Government of Madras 1923, part 2:15).

Again, there is the conflict between the kinlike relationships of residential gurukulas and the transactional relationships of modern colleges. Here, moreover, there is also the hint of a possible risk in the attempt to graft a kinlike relationship onto the public, business relationship between abstract individuals. For what if the self-interest expected in the second kind of relationship betrays or—even worse—masquerades itself as the trust and care expected in the first kind of relationship? This is a question that, in various phrasings, continues to haunt modern Ayurvedic institutions and the rest of this chapter.

Institutionalizing Purity

In 1930 during the noncooperation movement the Bombay Sabhā helped to establish a clinic to assist activists who had been wounded by the *lathis* (billyclubs) of the colonial police force. The Indian National Congress had given nominal support to indigenous medicine as early as 1920, resolving that "having regard to the widely prevalent and generally accepted utility of the Ayurvedic and Unani Systems of Medicine in India, earnest and definite efforts should be made by the people of this country to further popularise Schools, Colleges and Hospitals for instruction and treatment in accordance with Indigenous Systems" (Indian National Congress, cited in Government of India 1948, 5). It is noteworthy, however, that this resolution, which was reconfirmed in 1938, advocates Ayurveda and Unani not because of their truth but because of their popularity and practical application, recognizing them, in a sense, as culture rather than as science. Moreover, the resolution emphasizes the necessity of enframing Ayurveda and Unani in schools, colleges, and hospitals that undoubtedly are to be organized along modern lines. Vd. Shukla, who lived through the nationalist battles of the 1920s, 1930s, and 1940s, claims that the majority of nationalist politicians consulted allopathic doctors and not vaidyas. Even Gandhi, he told me, used to consult the head of an allopathic hospital in Bombay. Paradoxically, even as the Congress was campaigning for the recognition of Ayurveda as national culture, the educated elite that was its leadership was steadily losing faith in Ayurveda as a healing practice (see Frankenburg 1981).

In 1938, just a year after Congress rule had been established in several provinces and two years after Vd. Shukla had passed his viśarāda exam, the Medical Practitioners Act was passed in Bombay Presidency to regulate the registration and education of vaidyas. Other provincial governments soon followed suit. Similar legislation, excluding indigenous practitioners and even making it illegal for registered doctors to use indigenous medicines, had already been passed for biomedical doctors between 1912 and 1917 (Patterson 1987, 128). It is not surprising, therefore, that the authors of the 1959 Udupa Report to evaluate the state of Ayurveda praised the liberality of the 1938 act in bestowing on registered Ayurvedic practitioners many of the privileges enjoyed by biomedical practitioners. They wrote, "We can very well imagine the healthy effects of this Act on the practicing Ayurvedic physicians of the Bombay State" (cited in Government of India 1959, 150). The members of the Sabhā, however, viewed the act very differently: on the one hand, the act extended to vaidyas medical rights similar to those of doctors, but on the other hand, "Ayurvedic study through guruparampara and *vanśa* parampara [family lineage] was abolished" (Mumbai Vaidya Sabhā 1990, 13). The effect of the act, Vd. Shukla told me, was to officially recognize only those Ayurvedic courses of study that were mixed with European medical subjects. It was at this time, he said, that the terms miśra Ayurveda and śuddh Ayurveda came into existence. The Sabhā historians concur: the Act led to a sharp split among vaidyas throughout the subcontinent that eventually solidified into the division between the advocates of śuddh and miśra Ayurveda. Nearly sixty years later, in an impassioned interview he would not allow me to tape-record because of what he still experienced as the political volatility of the topic, Vd. Shukla said vehemently, "No government has the right to stop any science." He said that those who were educated in the miśra courses became contemptuous of vaidyas who were educated in other ways. They were, he said bitterly, "full of vanity and egoism and took themselves as better physicians [even] than medical doctors."

Vd. Shukla insisted that the harmful impact of the miśra course was not the use of allopathic medicines or medical knowledge, but rather the erosion of Ayurvedic principles. Even today, he said, some allopathic medicines are useful for offering quick relief in the short term. Nonetheless, he stopped prescribing biomedical injections and tablets in the early 1950s. When I asked why, he said that when he became involved in the Sabhā, he felt the need to align his medical practice with his political stance. This allegiance to śuddh or presumably pure Ayurveda, a loyalty motivated by politics rather than healing efficacy, markedly proclaims the historical shift from Ayurveda as a set of eclectic and ever-changing knowledge and healing practices to Ayurveda as a medical system and a sign of Indian national culture. By the 1980s the assimilation of Ayurveda into the Indian national identity was so complete that a history of Indian medicine could easily state, "After the first independence revolution of 1857 the Indians realized an urgent need of preservation of their national socio-cultural heritage including Ayurveda" (Kumar et al. 1985, 3). Ayurveda is perceived to carry that aura of "primordialness" that overdetermines its place in the national agenda (Anderson 1991). The contest over its inclusion in this agenda is, therefore, all too easily elided.

The proponents of miśra Ayurveda wanted to subsume biomedical practices and concepts (such as laboratory analysis or viruses) within an overarching Ayurvedic theory to develop one system of medicine. The proponents of śuddh Ayurveda, as the writings of the Sabhā attest, wanted to build counterparts to biomedical institutions to develop a parallel Ayurvedic system of medicine. It is evident that in Vd. Shukla's mind śuddh Ayurveda is identified with gurukulas while miśra Ayurveda is identified with colleges. This view is corroborated in an early modern textbook of Ayurveda, published in the mid-twentieth century, that contrasts gurukulas with colleges as follows:

> 1. The Real Indian Method, viz., the Individual system, i.e., The Gurukula system (tols) is the one in which a Guru or teacher undertakes the complete responsibility of the physical, intellectual and social growth of the students admitted by him for education. . . . Trained

under such environments, the students of Ayurveda developed as custodians of National Health and Missionaries of Humanity. 2. The Modern Method of Mass Education where all classes of students (intelligent, moderate, indifferent) are classed together and taught by paid teachers in urban surroundings as in present day Colleges and Schools. . . . They, however, produced a large number of the so-called Ayurvedic practitioners who are not only not proud of their own science but who are satisfied to occupy a subordinate rank as imitators of the Western Medical Practitioners (Mukharjee and Narayanarow 1954, 344–345).

This identification of śuddh Ayurveda with gurutols was not to hold, however. The two camps were united from the first in their concern to sustain Ayurvedic practices against the hegemony and economic power of biomedicine and in their identification of Ayurveda as an important symbol of national identity. Increasingly, they were also united in their support, to varying degrees at various times, of the introduction of modern institutions and methodologies (Brass 1972; Leslie 1976a). Despite the apparent ideological polarity, the difference between these two positions has largely been one of strategy in the face of competition from biomedicine. Both śuddh and miśra Ayurveda are national signs, the first relying on the ideological seductiveness of cultural authenticity and the second on the ideological seductiveness of modernity. Since cultural authenticity and modernity are equally essential to a national imaginary, however, the eventual, if nominal, victory of the śuddh camp (to be discussed below) is probably better attributed to the lesser threat it seemed to pose to the biomedical profession than to its ideological emphasis.

Shortly after the enactment of the Medical Practitioners Act of 1938 in Bombay, Shiv Sharma was elected the chairman of the Mahāsammelan. Over the next several decades he became the leading proponent of śuddh Ayurveda, campaigning forcefully against the miśra curriculum. Sharma, the son of the vaidya of a powerful maharaja and a cosmopolitan Brahmin, was a man who had equal facility with English jokes and Sanskrit śloks (Leslie 1992, 182). He expanded his base of support through appeals to noninstitutionally trained vaidyas who were threatened by the new graduates of the miśra course. His advocacy of the complete purging of modern subjects and technologies from Ayurvedic education appealed not only to conservative vaidyas, but also to government ministers of health who subscribed to the superiority of European medicine and were wary of hybrid practitioners. Leslie (1973, 238) has suggested that the actual purpose of śuddh institutionalization was the strangulation of Ayurvedic colleges. Nonetheless, every Ayurvedic physician in Bombay with whom I spoke about Shiv Sharma credited him with a major role in saving Ayurveda from absorption into biomedicine. The historians of the Sabhā write of his "exceptional brilliance, vigorous voice and irrefutable logic" (Mumbai Vaidya Sabhā 1990, 13). As a consequence largely of Shiv Sharma's forceful campaigning, many of the provincial governments shifted their support to śuddh Ayurveda.

The śuddh-miśra controversy can be traced through the reports of several government commissions established in the years after independence to make recommendations on the future development of Indian medicine. In 1948 the Chopra Committee recommended that Ayurvedic education be integrated with allopathic education. A synthesis of the two medicines was expected to combine Western diagnostic tools, surgery, physiology, and pathology with Ayurvedic philosophical principles. The writers of the report argued that this would eliminate rivalry between two separate medical professions and provide for adequate health services in rural areas. The Chopra Report was in some measure conceived as a corrective to the 1946 Bhore Report of the colonial administration, which ignored indigenous medicine altogether.

Nonetheless, the proposals of the Chopra Report were opposed by the Mahāsammelan and other proponents of a śuddh curriculum. In 1950 an editorial in the official periodical of the Mahāsammelan vehemently objected to a proposal by the health ministry that was in line with the recommendations of the Chopra Committee. The main thrust of the criticism was that the inclusion of physics and chemistry in the admissions requirements for Ayurvedic colleges would undermine Ayurvedic theory. These subjects, the editorial contended, were "necessary to understand the physical world but not to understand Ayurveda. For Ayurveda it is the study of Sanskrit and philosophy that are most essential" (Āyurveda Mahāsammelan 1950, 532). The editorial went on to assert that "without a proper understanding of Sanskrit and śāstric philosophy, the students will have difficulty understanding the benefit and brilliance of Ayurveda" (1950, 533). The editorial also objected to the stipulation that anatomy, physics, and certain other subjects were to be "taught according to modern medical knowledge" and at a level to be decided by the biomedically dominated Indian Medical Council, while other subjects were to be taught according to both modern and indigenous knowledge (1950, 533). The editorial noted that this policy imposed on the Ayurvedic student a double burden of study in addition to a need for advanced competence in English in order to read biomedical textbooks. Finally, the editorial strongly opposed the jurisdiction of the Indian Medical Council over Ayurvedic education, noting that the council had to date been "violently opposed to Ayurveda" (1950, 534). The editorial concluded, "If the state governments adopt the proposal of this congress then there will definitely be fewer students of Ayurveda and those few will be vaidyas in name only. The result will be that in twenty years the country will be deprived of the services of Ayurvedic science" (1950, 534). Ironically, as becomes obvious below, most of the aspects of the miśra curriculum opposed by the Mahāsammelan were later incorporated into the śuddh curriculum.

In 1954 the Sabhā and its allies in the provincial government at last succeeded in persuading the government of the Bombay presidency to adopt a śuddh policy. The Sabhā historians write, "When this demand of the vaidyas was met a wave of joy swept through the vaidya world" (Mumbai Vaidya Sabhā 1990, 19). As the Udupa Report explained the event, "Many people felt that the original way of teaching Ayurveda on the traditional Guru-Parampara method was the only thing that could save it from extinction. Therefore they met together and drafted a Shuddha Ayurveda course under the patronage of Bombay government in 1952" (Government of India 1959, 32). Tellingly, however, Vd. Shukla admitted to me that "even in that [new curriculum] some modern knowledge was being imparted," including biomedical anatomy. Part of the reason for this was that in Bombay, as in many other parts of India, there was increasing student demand for modern subject positions and subject matter. Paul Brass (1972) reports that between 1958 and 1964 there were are least fifty-five student strikes or demonstrations at Ayurvedic colleges, most of which put forward demands for equal status with allopathic students and the modernization of college facilities and curricula. At the gurukula in Haridwar that Dr. Pathi attended in the 1960s, the students had rebelled, like students elsewhere, against śuddh Ayurveda. They compared themselves, he said, to students in biomedical colleges; they wanted, like them, to wear "pants and shirts," study modern medical subjects, and earn a Bachelor's or other acronymic degree rather than a title such as bhiṣak or ācāryā. In the fight against the degradation of the Ayurvedic profession the strategy of the turn-of-the-century Ayurvedic authors had been to campaign *against* the imitation of European medical practice. The seemingly opposite yet perhaps complementary strategy of mid-twentieth-century Ayurvedic students was to campaign *for* the imitation of European institutional practice. These students believed that vaidyas could compete with doctors only if they received a commensurate training and certification.

Following the Chopra Report, several other committees produced reports on the appropriate direction of indigenous medicine. In 1959 the Udupa Committee again pleaded for the integration of Ayurveda and modern medicine up to the postgraduate level. One key recommendation in this report was that while the principles of Ayurveda could be taught in lecture, "modern medicine" should be taught in hospitals (Government of India 1959, 54). Of śuddh and miśra Ayurveda the Udupa Report had this to say:

> A general impression has been created by previous reports that the integrated system of education has been a failure. This unsatisfactory and one-sided decision led to the so-called "Shudha Ayurveda" movement, which in turn created confusion in some of the important Ayurvedic institutions in the country. It left nothing but frustration in the mind of students who naturally rebelled. The strikes in the various colleges and the closing down of the institutions for long periods are too well known to be repeated or gone into here. The fact remains, however, that the "Shudha Ayurveda" movement has turned the hands of the clock backward to a considerable extent. . . . It is felt that the new syllabus chalked out by the "Shudha Ayurveda" people is only a rehash of the old integrated system of medicine and that even the pure Ayurvedic institutions have included in their syllabus modern science subjects (Government of India 1959, 8).

In 1962 the Vyas Committee was assigned to draft a curriculum for śuddh Ayurveda. By this time there was widespread belief that the graduates of miśra programs were proficient in neither Ayurveda nor biomedicine. Yet while the resolution that prompted the formation of the

Vyas Committee stated that "Subjects of Modern Medicine in any form or language should not be included in the course," the final report of the committee stated, much more equivocally, that "some knowledge of comparative medicine and, particularly, its fundamentals in their relationship to Ayurveda, must be made available to students" (quoted in Brass 1972, 360–361). Not only was the inclusion of biomedical subject matter left open, but also the practice of guruparampara was declared no longer practical and the study of anatomy by dissection was declared to be essential. In 1970 the Ministry of Health established the Central Council for Indian Medicine (CCIM) for the purpose of regulating education and practice and cultivating research programs for Ayurveda, Unani, and Siddha. Then in 1977 the government ordered the Ayurvedic curriculum prepared by the CCIM to be adopted by all Ayurvedic institutions.

Even as the commitment to śuddh Ayurveda solidified, then, the meaning of śuddh Ayurveda seemed to have subtly changed. There was no attempt to recreate guruparampara. Over time the Vidyāpīṭh syllabus had come to concentrate more and more on subjects and less on seminal texts. Shiv Sharma himself in a 1957 address had stated that the śuddh curriculum he advocated differed from the miśra curriculum in only two particulars: that the number of Ayurvedic subjects vis-à-vis biomedical subjects was increased, and that the biomedical subjects were placed at the end of the course "to enable the Ayurvedic student to grasp the tenets of Ayurveda on a clean and unconfused mind before any additional subject was taught to him" (quoted in Government of India 1959, 39). In contemporary education, as will be apparent below, this "clean and unconfused mind" is considerably compromised by being steeped in modern scientific concepts during secondary school instruction. In the separate Ayurvedic educational structure that has evolved over the 1980s and 1990s, many of the demands of the militant students and many of the proposals of the government reports advocating miśra education have been implemented. The standardized curriculum is organized primarily around a modern division of subjects (including modern anatomy and pathology) rather than around particular Ayurvedic texts or pundits. The syllabus has expanded beyond the ancient and medieval Ayurvedic classics to dozens of textbooks organized on modern lines and written in an expository style. The students admitted have pursued a science track in middle school and have little or no background in śāstric philosophy or

Sanskrit, while their professors are largely, though not exclusively, graduates of the widely disparaged miśra courses. Ayurvedic subjects are taught primarily in the classroom, while biomedical subjects are taught primarily in the laboratories and hospital wards. The degree system has been brought into parallel with the degree system of biomedicine. In addition, a huge percentage of Ayurvedic graduates (anywhere from 80 to 90 percent, according to the practitioners with whom I spoke) have continued, like the graduates of integrated courses, to practice an eclectically mixed medicine. This shift in the institutional organization of knowledge, the implications of which I consider more fully below, could not have been accomplished without a corresponding shift in the textual organization of knowledge. Not only schools, but also books had to become the preformatted containers for a modernized Ayurveda.

Poetic Logic and Textbook Exposition

Several of the government reports mentioned above spoke of the need for modern Ayurvedic textbooks. The ancient and medieval texts studied in the gurukulas were compendia of recipes and scholarly colloquia, interspersed with poetically phrased aphorisms about health and illness. The Chopra Report complained of the "confusion" of these texts, stating, "Information about one topic is not found in any single chapter, and frequently the author seems to digress from the main topic into less relevant ones" (Government of India 1948, 106). The Udupa Report noted the lack of standard "subject-wise textbooks [that] can be easily followed by a novice" (Government of India 1959, 56–57). This need had begun to be identified several decades earlier. The Madras Report of 1923 noted that the Ayurvedic texts were "aphoristic" and required elucidation by "competent gurus," who unfortunately were becoming increasingly rare (Government of Madras 1923). In 1919 Nagendra Nath Sen Gupta, a vaidya with an extensive list of modern credentials (including membership in the Society of Chemical Industry in London and Examiner in Hindu Medicine at a Delhi Sanskrit institute) published a defense of Ayurveda in which he addressed the discrepancy between the organization of knowledge in the Ayurvedic texts and the organization of knowledge in European science. Of the aphoristic character of the Ayurvedic texts, he noted, "The truth is, these aphorisms constitute only heads of discourses. They are for the use of the preceptor in the lecture hall. The learning and experience of the preceptor enable him to dwell largely on them for assisting the comprehension of the pupils" (N. Gupta 1919, ii). On the next page he wrote the following of the *Caraka Saṃhitā:*

> The topics may not be closely connected with one another or even directly connected with Medical Science as it is now understood. But then it is the method of the Rishis. . . . The fact is the Rishis were opposed to system building before the collection of facts. They thought that the first step in building science consists in the collection of materials. They, therefore, set down their experiences of facts and the results of their reasoning without much attention to rigid principles of classification (Gupta 1919, iii).

Gupta's clearly defensive praise for the method of the ṛṣi was, however, merely by way of an introduction to his own book, a prose exposition of Ayurveda in English. He asserted that it was the first book of its kind, comparable to Wise's work on Hindu medicine but more comprehensive. On the one hand, then, he insisted on the value of the aphoristic style of the ṛṣi. Mere prose exposition cannot substitute for the knowledge exchanged between guru and śiṣya, much of which is exchanged through practical demonstration. On the other hand, however, he was pioneering a new type of Ayurvedic text that seemed to offer modern-style explanation as a substitute for the teacher-student rapport of the guruparampara.

Gupta's reference to the "rigid principles of classification" that are not found in the *Caraka Saṃhitā,* or indeed in almost any Sanskrit or vernacular text prior to the twentieth century, may be taken to refer to a modern ordering of phenomena that draws definite distinctions between reality and representations and arranges things in hierarchies of type (Foucault 1970). The organization of topics not only in *Caraka Saṃhitā,* but also in the turn-of-the-century texts examined in the previous chapter partly resembles, from a modern perspective, that classification of animals in Jorge Luis Borges's imaginary Chinese encyclopedia, which prompted Foucault (1970, xv) first to laugh out loud and then to assiduously analyze the episteme that makes such a classification impossible in modern Europe. In *Śivanātha Sāgar,* the section on the lakṣaṇ of the heart, which describes the heart as the seat of consciousness, ojas, and the bliss of ātmā, is immediately followed by sections on the function of *prāṇa* (breath/life, one of the five types of vāyu), the lakṣaṇ of life and death, and "that which is called" the creation of the world, the protection of the body by four substances, and the creation of the world.[4] A section on the twenty-four *tattvas* of creation (translatable as elements / constituents) is immediately followed by sections on the movement of "the ego [*ahaṃkāra*] and so on," the movement of food, "that which is called" the condition of food, and the lakṣaṇ of the seven prakṛti (constitutional types). This, in turn, is immediately followed by sections on the natures of two prakṛti, the lakṣaṇ of remorse and lethargy, and the lakṣaṇ of yawning, sneezing, and burping; these are closely followed by sections on the lakṣaṇ of ill persons and the lakṣaṇ of medical treatment. Later in the book a section on the god of the pulse and the gods of each of the three doṣa is immediately followed by sections on the location and movement of the pulse, the motion of the pulse, the pulse of two-doṣa fever, the pulse of happiness, the pulse examination for sensory awareness, and the examination of urine.

While this arrangement of medical topics may be somewhat more acceptable to a modern mind than the arrangement of animals in Borges's imaginary encyclopedia, it still displays a certain incongruity, betraying a lack of differentiation between mind and matter, cosmology and physiology, the apparently real and the apparently fabulous. What is the basis, for example, of juxtaposing the movement of the ego and the movement of food, or the characteristics of remorse and the characteristics of burping? How can a verse on gods, if it is to appear at all in a healing manual, be tucked among verses on seemingly empirical phenomena? What can it mean for topics that are mediated by their representations—for example "that which is called the creation of the world" or "that which is called the condition of food"—to be mentioned alongside topics that are not so mediated? The taxonomy seems not only more loosely associative than hierarchical, but also riddled with gaps and overlaps. Why should there be, for example, a verse on two-doṣa fever pulse juxtaposed with a verse on happiness pulse, yet no verse on one-doṣa fever or three-doṣa fever and no verse on the pulses of sadness or anger or fear? What might be the motive for the apparent redundancy and disregard for orderly series wherein pulse movement appears in one stanza as a subtopic and in the very next stanza as a topic?

In 1814 a British surgeon struggled to translate two separate Indian healing texts. After giving up the effort, he noted the impossibility of translating Indian texts because of their "poetical style," characterized by "similes, metaphors, and all kinds of figures" and adding up to "a banquet of absurdity sufficient to satisfy the most voracious guest" (Benjamin Heyne, quoted in Arnold 1993, 50). Zimmermann has referred to the knowledge practice of the ancient Ayurvedic texts as "logico-poetic." That is, there exist in these texts taxonomies of climates, tastes, vegetable and animal remedies, illnesses, somatic types, and so on that are ordered in part according to a literary aesthetic. Contrasting the Ayurveda of these texts with modern science, he writes, "There could have been no zoology in the minds of the Indian scholars, no osteology, or physiology. Instead, based on a Sanskrit image, there are endless 'garlands of names' (nāma-mālā). Onto these name lists are grafted an amazing combinative system of 'savors' (rasa) and 'qualities' (guṇa)" (1987, 98). The logic of these texts is not causal and linear but rather combinative, based on a vast network of resemblances. Zimmermann concludes, "No examination, no research, no enquiry or attempt to find a reason for the data: that is what I meant when saying the model of natural history was alien to India. Its place is filled by the collection, recitation and combination of the formulas consecrated by Tradition" (1987, 158). Here he seems to accept the Enlightenment paradigm that opposes the empirical knowledge of modernity to the received knowledge of tradition and privileges the former over the latter.

We can understand the poetic logic of Ayurvedic texts in another way if we investigate why we find them poetic. In literary language, according to Hartman, "words stand out as words (even as sounds) rather than being, at once, assimilable meanings," and their "quality of reference may be complex, disturbed, unclear" (Geoffrey, cited in Mitchell 1988, 143). In expository language, on the other hand, words do not possess a plenitude in and of themselves, but rather a capacity to represent something outside of themselves. This dichotomy between poetic and expository language is, however, peculiarly modern. Mitchell reminds us that it was not until the late 1800s that language in Europe began to be conceived as a system of arbitrary codes standing in for supposedly real objects. He quotes the revelation of a French professor of grammar heralding the new conception: "Words are signs. They have no other existence than the signals of the wireless telegraph" (1988, 140). In the ancient, medieval, and pre-twentieth-century Ayurvedic texts, on the other hand, words have multiple and layered evocations. They work not through denotation of discrete concepts, but rather through reverberation in one another's polysemic sounds and senses, proliferating meanings through the text in a way that we today consider poetic or literary. Like texts of medieval Europe, the early Ayurvedic texts abound in long, rambling lists as knowledge piles up on itself through a process of association.

In the list of topics of *Śivanātha Sāgar* noted above, the intermixing of things that are prefaced by the phrase "what is called" with things that are not suggests also that there is no hard distinction between what is said and what is known. It is not simply that the oldest Ayurvedic texts were based on received knowledge, but also that they unproblematically interspersed received knowledge and empirical knowledge. In recounting what was known about healing, the authors seem to have had no reason to separate what was observed in the world from what was learned from other healers There is no assumption here that reality can be any more directly apprehended through sensory observations than through oral lore. The authors drew from a continuum of language, whether it was the language of the world, the properties of plants and animals, or the language of the poets, the phrasings of human insight. The physical signs of land, waterways, and winds required interpretation just as much as the words left by previous generations. To gather all the knowledge about health and illness meant to gather both what was written in the landscape and what was written in books.[5] If, in these texts, words are physical objects with the same substance and potency as other objects, similarly so-called natural objects are themselves signs, indicating other sign objects along an endless progression of echoing resemblance.[6]

Moreover, like the language of the world, the language of these texts is not a transparent medium through which the meaning is immediately evident. Verse acts as a mnemonic and organizing vehicle carrying the sound-substance of medical wisdom into the mind of the reciter and listener, writer and reader. The rhythms of poetic texts were evidently designed to enhance memorization, recital, and even comprehension. In *Caraka* it is said that the Ayurvedic student "sitting comfortably on even and clean ground should recite the aphorisms in order with clear voice attentively repeating it [*sic*] again and again. At the same time, entering deeply into the ideas he should understand them well in order to get rid of his own defects and to know others' defects. In this way, he should continue the study without wasting time in midday, afternoon and night. This is the method of study" (P. V. Sharma 1981, 1:351–352). Repetition is intended as a device for simultaneous memorization and contemplation. The knowledge in a sūtra exists in a latent form that unfolds its interpretations and practical uses over time and repetition, contemplation and experience, elucidation and discussion. This is perhaps the reason that one vaidya testified in the Madras Report, "The Modern method of teaching followed in colleges enables the students to acquire more knowledge, *albeit less deep,* in a shorter time than is or was possible in tols" (Government of Madras 1923, part 2:29; emphasis added). If the expository texts of allopathy (and modern Ayurveda) allow the student to amass vast amounts of knowledge, the poetic texts of Ayurveda challenged the student to unfold deeper levels of knowledge. In these texts, words do not so much invoke preexistent meanings as produce contextual meanings through active practices of writing and reading. One Ayurvedic professor put it to me as follows:

> Everything is clear in allopathy. When you take the book and open the page, then you will have all the clear, clear things there. While in Ayurveda everything is not clear. That you have to get yourself with *manana* [reflection, careful study], or you have to think over it one hundred times, and then you will know what that is. Not for everything, one hundred times, but some things are there that you have to learn by heart. . . . See what happens, our science is in śāstra; sūtras are there, one line is given, and in that one line the meaning is so hard that you have to take out the meaning, so implementation of that line is very, very difficult, and everyone has to think over it.

If modern textbooks convey the effect of an enclosed and exhaustive knowledge, the poetic texts of Ayurveda convey rather the effect of a knowledge that is neither enclosed nor exhaustive. Francis Ellis of the Madras civil service noted that memorized verses were like a "tap root" that a pundit could draw upon to expound certain principles. As Nagendra Gupta observed, the cryptic poetics of the earlier texts were starting points for scholarly discussion and exegesis, rather than comprehensive expositions in themselves. One contemporary Ayurvedic practitioner told a group of foreign students that he was always finding new things in *Caraka.* "You don't just have to read between the lines," he said; "you have to read between the words." He went on to recount how he had realized that the whole explanation of hemoplasia was contained in two lines of *Caraka.* One young practitioner went even further in his interpretation of the importance of the old texts, claiming that over time exposure to the Sanskrit śloks enhances the "sattvic [pure, virtuous] qualities of mind" so that the capacity to understand Ayurveda gradually increases. The Sanskrit words, he told me, "massage the nervous system."

Unlike Ellis, most colonialist scholars had not been able or interested to read between the lines of Sanskrit poetry or to notice that anyone else might be doing so. One orientalist scholar noted in 1823 that great attention was paid to proper pronunciation of "poetical" language but not to the "meaning" of that language (cited in Cohn 1985, 323). William Adams, commissioned to write reports on vernacular education in Bengal and Bihar, found the education in indigenous schools to be "superficial and defective" (Cohn 1985, 324). He argued that while the students could chant long passages of the Vedas, they showed no understanding of the meaning (Cohn 1985, 323). In his final report he suggested that the gurukulas be employed to improve medical training. To this end he recommended that textbooks be prepared to combine modern science and local practice, "European theory and Indian experience" (Leslie 1973, 222). These books would be distributed without charge to indigenous teachers as preparations for public examinations, and gurus would be paid endowments for successful students. While this proposal was never implemented, a century and a half later such textbooks have become keystones of contemporary Ayurvedic education.

The Slippage of Frames

The purpose of modern textbooks was not only to comprehensively cover Ayurvedic knowledge, but, equally important, to map it out in a modern division of subjects. The modern Ayurvedic curriculum for a Bachelor of Ayurvedic Medical Science degree established by the CCIM is divided into three "years" actually spanning about a year and a half each, for a total of five and a half years, including school breaks. The sequence of courses as of 1994 is listed in table 1. *Swasthavṛtt* refers to the regimens of preventive health outlined in Ayurvedic texts. As an academic subject, nidān is translated as pathology or etiology, while *śarīr racana* refers to

Table 1. Curriculum for Bachelor of Ayurvedic Medical Science Degree.

First Year	*Second Year*	*Third Year*
Sanskrit	Swasthavṛtt	Kāyacikitsā
Padārth Vijñān	Caraka Part 1	Caraka Part 2
Śarīr Racana	Nidan	Śalya
Śarīr Kriya	Dravyaguṇa	Śālākya
Itihas	Rasaśāstra	Kaumābhṛtya
Aṣṭānga Saṃgraha	Agadatantra	Prasautī-Strīrog

anatomy. *Śalya* is surgery, *śālākya* is a specialization related to illnesses affecting the head and neck that is understood as a parallel to the biomedical specialization of ears, nose, and throat. These two along with *kāyacikitsā* (treatment), *agadatantra* (toxicology), and *kaumabhṛtya* (pediatrics) are included among the eight parts of Ayurveda identified in ancient texts. The other three parts of Ayurveda (which are not taught as separate subjects in Ayurvedic colleges) are rejuvenation therapy (rasāyana), the healing of illnesses caused by spirit beings (bhūtavidya), and *vājikaraṇa* (aphrodisiacs). Dravyaguṇa is understood as botany of medicinal plants, while *rasaśāstra* is translated as pharmacology, and *prasautī-strīrog* refers to obstetrics and gynecology. *Aṣṭāṅga Saṁgraha* is an ancient text that is often grouped with the *Caraka* and *Suśruta Saṃhitā* as one of the most revered texts of Ayurveda. *Itihās* is translated as history.

For each of the topical subjects listed in the curriculum the CCIM has provided a long list of acceptable textbooks in various vernaculars, any of which may be studied by the students. In addition, the students attend lectures in each class during designated periods. The scheduling of activities cannot be taken in and of itself as a manifestation of modern disciplinarity. Timetables were probably also followed to some extent in gurukulas. There is, however, an important distinction to be drawn between the more monastic discipline of the gurukulas, in which the rhythm of activities was directed by the authority of teachers and texts to perfect the student's mind, and a modern discipline, in which time is regulated according to a rational hierarchy of grade levels to subject the student's body. It is this modern temporal discipline of "docile" bodies that has been implemented in Ayurvedic colleges. Yet, as hinted above, there are curious lapses in this corporeal discipline. Not only do students and professors show up only haphazardly and at odd times for classes, but during a particularly monotonous lecture students sometimes also speak freely and noisily with each other without any reprimand from the professor. Foucault suggests that in the imposition of disciplinary space, "One must eliminate the effects of imprecise distributions, the uncontrolled disappearance of individuals, their diffuse circulation, their unusable and dangerous coagulation" (1979, 143). Yet all these were manifestly not eliminated in the Ayurvedic college I most often visited.

The supervision of student bodies as they are moved from classroom to classroom or of patients' bodies as they are lined up in numbered beds on hospital wards occurs in what Foucault (1979) has referred to as the "techno-political" register of modern bodily discipline (Figure 6). The analysis of bodies within the modern Ayurvedic curriculum, on the other hand, exemplifies what he calls the "anatomo-metaphysical" register of bodily discipline. These two registers are part of one technology of rational distribution, deployed, on the one hand, in institutional space and time, and on the other hand, in scholarly operations. European disciplines were instituted in Ayurvedic colleges not only through timetables and arrangements of space, but also through the tabulated analysis of human organisms.[7] Gridlike arrangements are useful in both registers of discipline, that of supervising the body and that of surveying it.

In the surveillance of the body, the most dramatic reorganization of ancient Ayurvedic knowledge occurs in the two subjects identified in the curriculum as śarīr kriya and śarīr racana. These two subjects bear the least resemblance to any topics identified in the ancient and medieval texts. The isolation of Ayurvedic physiology from Ayurvedic anatomy is a concession made to a modern understanding of how medical knowledge should be organized. Here, enframing is implemented at the somatic level, for anatomy refers to structures and physiology to the functions of these structures. In Ayurvedic colleges, anatomy is almost exclusively taught according to biomedicine, with the marginal inclusion of a few Ayurvedic subjects such as the ātmā and the *marmas* (particular points on the body sensitive to injury and also, according to some, susceptible of healing stimulation). In the meantime, doṣa, agni, and other bodily processes are taught in śarīr kriya but are never mentioned in śarīr racana. In śarīr racana labs, the organs are handled and named, usually in at least three languages, while in śarīr kriya labs, doṣa are examined via lakṣaṇ in the patient but never discovered in a cadaver. There is no pretense that the

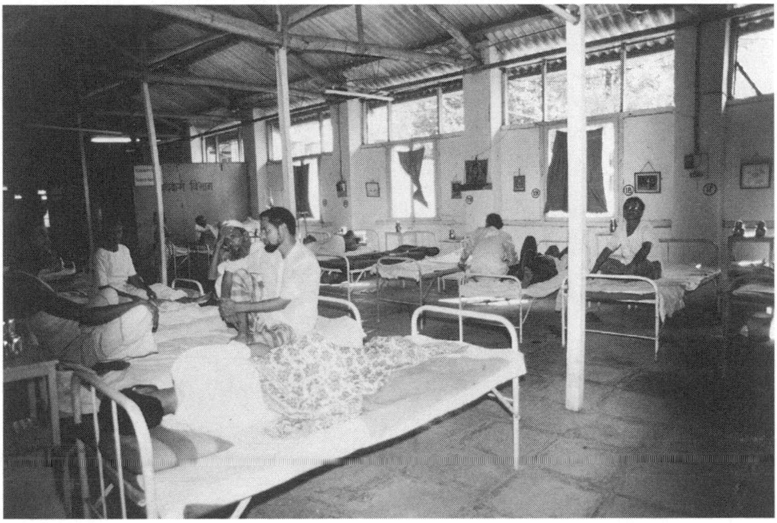

Figure 6. Ayurvedic Hospital Ward. Patients lined up in numbered beds.

names and corresponding body parts of anatomy class can enframe or limit the doṣa. In Ayurvedic pathology, insofar as it is based on the notion of doṣa, simply to "open up a few corpses," as European doctors were advised to do at the dawn of biomedicine, does not make the disease process visible (Foucault 1973, 146). It is the doṣa of the physiology lectures that, moving freely and invisibly among the organs, are responsible for all the processes of the body. When I asked students how they cope with the conflict between anatomy and śarīr kriya, they explained that they understood each topic exclusively in its own terms. The contemporary Ayurvedic curriculum therefore renders onto biomedicine the (anatomical) *things* (that belong to biomedicine) while apparently reserving for Ayurveda the *processes* that belong to Ayurveda: the flow of the doṣa, the workings of agni, or the conversion of the dhātus from one to the other.

In the modern Ayurvedic curriculum, even if doṣa cannot be found in corpses and charted on anatomical diagrams, they can at least be quantified. There has been a determined effort to standardize doṣa and other Ayurvedic phenomena. In the first-year śarīr kriya class there are examination forms for doṣa, mental and physical prakṛti, agni, dhātu, and mala. These forms are composed of tables in which a given body part or process is written in the left-hand column while various lakṣaṇ that act as signs for particular somatic states are written in a series of columns on the right. As one professor told me, "In this department we teach how to calculate the percentage of vāta, pitta, and kapha. . . . In vāta prakṛti there are ten symptoms [the usual translation of lakṣaṇ]; in pitta there are ten as well; in kapha there are ten. . . . It means that for these thirty symptoms the student has a chart; he goes to the Ayurvedic ward, he asks the patient, he watches the patient, and he ticks [it off]. After ticking, he calculates the percentage of vāta, pitta, and kapha." Such examination forms are techniques for turning a chain of signs connected in narratives of life or illness into a tabular order. Signs of illness or health are now separated from narrative accounts, translated into quantities, and arranged in discrete doṣic columns that enable calculation within columns. The tables theoretically allow the precise classification and thereby treatment of a patient according to Ayurvedic concepts. The six-page examination form for physical prakṛti, for example, lists dozens of lakṣaṇ, ranging from "soft body hair" to "idle chatter" to "loose joints." The students calculate the person's prakṛti by counting the number of positive lakṣaṇ related to each doṣa and then calculating the percentages of vāta, pitta, and kapha.

One day a group of students and I were waiting for a lab session for a class in śarīr kriya. Other students also loitered in the same room, waiting for a śarīr racana lab, drilling one another about hemoglobin, blood viscosity, temperature, oxygen, plasma, and so on. I asked one of the students if the kriya lab was about to start. "I think so," she said, "if he shows up." Soon the professor did show up, and the students began to practice examining the state of the dhātu in one another, filling out the dhātu *parikśan* (examination) forms in their lab books. The lab books contained lists of lakṣaṇ or features that indicated the state of a particular dhātu. If there were ten possible lakṣaṇ for well-developed *asthi* dhātu or bone tissue (such as strong joints or nails or teeth), then each lakṣaṇ was worth ten points. If the student observed four of these lakṣaṇ in her lab partner, then she gave him a score of 40 percent for asthi dhātu. All the dhātu were scored in this way. Privately the students confessed to me that they could not identify many of the lakṣaṇ in the journal since they have Sanskrit names. In their opinion, the professor for this lab was not very good, but at least he translated the words so that they did not have to look them all up in the dictionary. I knew what they meant since I had spent many hours leafing through my Monier-Williams for terms on the prakṛti parikśan form such as "cloud-like sound," "ocean-like sound," "*mṛdaṅg* (a two-headed Indian drum)-like sound," and "lion-like sound" for the voice qualities of kapha prakṛti patients, or "lotus-like" and "like durba grass" for the complexion of kapha prakṛti patients, or "poison arrows" and "lightning flashes" for the dreams of pitta prakṛti patients.

A few months after observing this lab, I found myself discussing dhātu parikśan with an Ayurvedic practitioner who had graduated from college five years earlier. In his particular college the students rated each dhātu with a series of from one to three pluses. It was, he said, a "totally absurd situation. It is not even right to record it like that. What am I going to get from it?" "To be frank," he added, he and his fellow students used to first peruse a patient's diagnosis as recorded on the case forms and then assign dhātu values that accorded with the illness. If a patient were arthritic, for instance, they would assign a low number to his asthi dhātu. The dhātu exam, when transformed into an "absurd" quantifying exercise, ceases to be a *tool* of Ayurvedic diagnosis and becomes instead the *product* of a (frequently) biomedical diagnosis. Medical signification is thrown into reverse. The dhātu score that is supposed to signify a particular disease is instead itself signified by the disease name. The secret duplicity of any signification, as noted by Derrida (1976), is exposed here: the signified never truly precedes the sign, and every signified, however cleverly masquerading as a self-present object, is on closer scrutiny itself a sign. Diagnosis is taught as an empirical process of correct identification, correct matching of sign and object. Yet it is openly acknowledged here that this identification is less a matter of apprehending reality than of arranging and rearranging signs. Diagnosis as practiced in modern Ayurvedic teaching hospitals is recognized as more of an assignation than a discovery. The tables, in a sense, have been turned.

Everyone with whom I spoke who was attending or had attended an Ayurvedic college spoke about the disparity between classroom and clinical instruction. Just as recommended in the Udupa Report, Ayurvedic concepts tend to be confined to the classroom, while biomedical concepts tend to dominate the clinical instruction. While in the classroom students cram Ayurvedic theory, on the hospital wards they learn primarily which Ayurvedic drugs to prescribe for which biomedical disease categories. Ayurvedic graduates therefore almost universally agree that their undergraduate education leaves them with no idea of how to actually apply

Ayurvedic concepts to a clinical situation. This is partly due to the fact that in the routine of a modern hospital there is little time to carry out a full diagnosis, including an assessment of prakṛti, doṣa, dhātu, agni, and mala. It is also due to the fact that few of the professors in the colleges, often graduates of miśra courses, are themselves accomplished clinicians. While diagnostic methods are taught in the classroom, pathology is taught in a lab according to biomedical laboratory techniques. Moreover, at least in the two institutions where I conducted the closest observations, the examinations learned in śarīr kriya labs for doṣa and dhātu are practiced only during the first year, when their relationship to diagnosis is purely hypothetical, and not during the third year, when their relationship to diagnosis would be necessarily clinical. In the part of their lab book that final-year students use to record the results of outpatient exams for their class on kāyācikitsā, there are no forms for dhātu or agni parikśan. There are a few lines allotted for the signs of disease, half a line for aggravated doṣa, and no mention at all of prakṛti. In the part of this lab book designated for inpatients, there are shortened forms for prakṛti parikśan and a form for mala parikśan, but no forms for doṣa, dhātu, or agni examinations. It would be tempting to suppose that by the third year the examinations of prakṛti and doṣa have become second nature to the students and so do not have to be disciplined by blank forms. The students work on their lab books, however, while accompanying senior doctors in crowded outpatient departments (OPDs) or on hurried hospital rounds, when there are rarely more than a few minutes to spend with each patient. In the dozens of hours I spent in these two settings there was seldom any consideration of prakṛti and only occasionally any consideration of doṣa. If Ayurvedic anatomy concedes the body parts to biomedicine, then Ayurvedic physiology, at least as presented to undergraduates, concedes the tabulation of Ayurvedic doṣa and prakṛti largely to nonclinical, theoretical contexts.

As I pointed out in chapter 2, such a restriction could have the effect of either marginalizing these phenomena or privileging them as beyond tabulation. Within clinical if not classroom discourse, prakṛti is kept at a remove from quantifying constructions, as if it does not belong to medical science but to an older, Sanskritic knowledge. As one of the professors explained, the examinations students perform in the third-year kāyacikitsā lab are oriented toward treating the "disease." A third-year student confirmed this, telling me the main concern at his level was to identify the disease, often in biomedical terms. A young practitioner remembered that in her education basic Ayurvedic concepts had been studied only via the texts, while clinical experience was focused on which drug to prescribe for which disease. Students therefore receive much more practice in a quasibiomedical diagnosis than in Ayurvedic diagnosis. Most BAMS (Bachelor of Ayurvedic Medical Science) graduates have a clear sense of how to apply the evaluation of doṣa to a prescription, noting, for example, that a person of primarily vāta constitution should not be given a vāta-inducing drug. Few, however, have any sense at all of how to apply doṣa to the understanding of pathological process.

Dr. Pathi has been an examiner for the subject of śarīr kriya for more than fifteen years. On this exam, he told me, there are no questions linking doṣa to clinical cases. He continued, "Dhātus they can understand; mala they can understand because they touch it. But doṣas they cannot understand. And then throughout the curriculum they just blindly accept what the teacher has told them without understanding it. And then the real concept of Ayurveda they don't understand at all. And they try to forget about these doṣas throughout their career." In another conversation he reiterated this, saying, "Doṣa, dhātu, mala—first year they have passed [it]. Then they forget it." The study of doṣa, dhātu, and mala, he said, ought to be continued through all the years of the curriculum. The author of an article on teaching methods in Ayurvedic education voiced a similar opinion, writing that doṣa, dhātu, and mala should not be confined to the classroom but "explained in relation to clinical examination and application" (V. R. Mehta 1989, 481). First-year Ayurvedic students assured me that they did not consider doṣa to be substances, but rather, in the words of one student, "active factors": pitta, they said, is called bile, but it is not totally bile, while kapha is called mucus but is not totally mucus. This knowledge remains vaguely hypothetical, however, as long as they are not clinically alert to how these active factors manifest. At a conference on Ayurvedic research in the early 1990s Dr. Upadhyay commented that the graduates he had taught had clearly been trained to see doṣa as something like substances. The concepts of vāta, pitta, and kapha, he said, need to be taught "from day one right in front of patients." Dr. Pathi told me that when he was on the state board of Ayurvedic education, he suggested that academicians teach the academic side and practitioners teach the clinical side. The academicians protested that they were fully capable of teaching the clinical side also. He told me that he replied, "I also am capable of teaching the academic side, but if I do, my students will fail their exams, and if you teach the clinical side, they will fail in their clinical practice." As one analyst of Ayurvedic education, P. Himasagara Chandra Murthy, writes, "It may not be improper to say that the whole process of Ayurvedic education has become disoriented and dysfunctional producing a number of young men and women who are preferring more to jobs [*sic*] instead of serving the community on their own. Though the financial constraint is also a reason for this situation, the lack of strong practical and clinical orientation at the undergraduate and postgraduate levels is no less a cause" (1990:46). Therefore, the letters BAMS, seen on the shingles of numerous medical shops across India, generally signify a quasibiomedical practice, including perhaps a few Ayurvedic remedies but rarely based on diagnoses of the state of the doṣa, dhātu, and so on. It is tacit knowledge that this particular sign rarely is linked to its supposed referent.

The director of the hospital had been insulted when I implied that some of the students might be less than sincere. Yet students are quite frank about the weakness of their commitment to Ayurveda. Most of them are attending Ayurvedic college only because they did not receive high enough exam scores (or exercise enough influence in high places) to enter biomedical colleges. Only a small percentage of students have chosen Ayurveda of their own free will, usually because their parents are Ayurvedic practitioners. Until starting college, few of the students had any knowledge of Ayurveda. Fewer still have any background in the Indian philosophies, such as Saṃkhya, that inform the Ayurvedic śāstras or sufficient knowledge of Sanskrit to read the older Ayurvedic texts with any degree of comprehension. Instead they have the background in biology, chemistry, and physics that is required of any medical career track. Many students feel more at home in their comparatively biomedical anatomy or pathology classes than in other Ayurvedic subjects. When I asked one student shortly before exams which subject she and her friends were studying the most, she replied, "Anatomy, because it is easiest for us to understand." "When we study doṣa, we have to think about dhātu," she explained, "but when we study the brain, we do not have to think about the stomach." Because of their background in European science many students feel that much of what they are taught in Ayurvedic college is nonsense. Two students explained to me that in the class on padārth vijñān (the subject that deals most explicitly with philosophy), they were told that when the mind is thinking, it is located in the brain, and when the mind is feeling, it is located in the heart. "We don't know what sense it makes," one of the students said. They were also told that modern physics identified speed and velocity, but Ayurveda discovered "direction." "What is this?" the student said. "It's nonsense really. . . . It's funny. . . . We don't know what it all means." In an article on Ayurvedic teaching methods V. R. Mehta notes, "A student going for medical study whether in modern medicine or Ayurveda has a background of modern Physics, Chemistry and Biology as taught in the science stream of Higher Secondary Education. He will be confronted with the Panchabhoota theory of matter [the idea that all matter is composed of five elements, as described in chapter 2]. The confusion arises in mind as to the modern conception of matter and properties which he has learnt and another concept of Mahabhoota which he has to face" (1989:481). As one young practitioner recalled to me, arriving at an Ayurvedic college can be like arriving on an "alien planet." It is only later, in the more clinically oriented classes, when they are able to match Ayurvedic drugs to biomedical diseases, that most students feel at home.

Many of these students freely admit that they intend to practice a blend of Ayurveda and allopathy after graduation. They realize that very few of them will be admitted to the Ayurvedic M.D. programs, which offer more concentrated clinical experience, study, and research, and qualify graduates for faculty positions in teaching hospitals. In addition, these students largely believe that social pressures make it impossible to exclusively practice Ayurveda in private clinics. Some of the students with whom I spoke were actually surprised to learn from me that there are many successful private practitioners who diagnose and treat according to doṣa, dhātu, and mala. When I asked one student whether he agreed with the common belief that the use of allopathic medicines would produce side effects that would then lead to further illnesses, a friend of his interjected impatiently, "Yes, yes, we understand all this, but the point is not to help the patients; the point is to earn money; his parents have spent one lākh rupee on his education." In other words, they will expect him to start earning money right away. Professors may actually reinforce students' feelings that it is impractical to practice Ayurveda. Once a professor of Ayurvedic history commented to me, in the presence of two students, that because of the lack of public interest in Ayurveda, these students would have no choice but to practice allopathy as well. Their families, he said, want them to be "doctors." The students feel that the perception of Ayurvedic practitioners by the general population is far from favorable. One young woman mentioned that she had recently passed a tent on the sidewalk sporting a banner that read "*Davakhāna*" (dispensary; literally, medicine-food) and advertising Ayurvedic medicines. This, she protested, is what Ayurveda has come to. (Ironically it might be argued that it is also what Ayurveda has come *from*. *Caraka* actually means itinerant or ascetic and may signify less the name of a person than the description of a kind of practitioner.)[8] When the students discuss Ayurvedic notions with their families or friends, they are met with laughter and cries of "nonsense." As P. H. C. Murthy concludes,

> The emergence of Modern Medicine into the Indian culture has a definite influence on the teaching and learning of Ayurveda. . . . The curriculum planning has given much importance to modern medicine. This is reflected in the nomenclature division and allotment of the subjects and the diagnostic approaches, and study of Sarira Racana and Sarira Kriya. This way, it is possible to get only rudimentary or half knowledge in both the systems and ultimately a graduate is, rather bent to take up Modern Medicine in his practice which earns him a fast-luck (1990, 46).

With this rhyming pun he sums up the particular way that the promise of fast money or opportunity can make an Ayurvedic graduate into an allopath.

Institutionalizing Corruption

Just as it is widely acknowledged that Ayurvedic colleges do not, mostly, produce Ayurvedic clinicians, so it is also widely acknowledged that Ayurvedic education is pervaded by "corruption." Stories of corruption abound, particularly in the conversations of private practitioners who are associated with, yet independent of, Ayurvedic teaching hospitals. Dr. Pathi estimated that fully 50 percent of the research theses required to obtain an Ayurvedic M.D. are purchased from professors for a price of around fifty thousand rupees. In his role as an examiner in Ayurvedic colleges, he has read six or seven M.D. theses that were simply copied from books. "To tell you frankly," he said, "the Ayurvedic M.D.s don't know ABC of that subject." Examiners in both biomedical and Ayurvedic education are susceptible to bribery. While the identities of the students are coded, the codes can still be leaked. Dr. Pathi discovered that another examiner had been accepting bribes in his name when the parents of a student arrived with a box of sweets to thank him for their son's passing grade. Disgusted, he asked the other examiner to refund the family's money, saying "This is a useless thing on my name." On another occasion he examined a first-year student who was not able to answer any of the questions. When Dr. Pathi asked how he had been admitted to college, the student said that his father had bribed the principal. Dr. Pathi failed him but recommended that his parents pay for private tutoring. Many years later the young man was able to open his own practice. Dr. Pathi was also one of the examiners for the daughter of the hospital director mentioned toward the beginning of this chapter. After he gave her twenty marks out of a hundred, her paper was returned to him for reevaluation. When he then gave her three marks out of a hundred, someone approached him and asked, "Do you realize whose paper this is?" The order for reevaluation had come from a high official. The case went to court. Even though all the examiners had given the paper low marks, the young woman was ultimately given a passing grade. Later this woman's father asked another practitioner I know to supply his daughter with one of his research papers for an M.D. dissertation topic. The practitioner refused but said to me, "She will get the M.D. I know it." The very next day he informed me that she had.

Akhil Gupta (1995) has pointed out that the definition of corruption changes according to sociohistorical circumstances. He points out that an action such as accepting a sum of money for making entries in a register of land records, which might not have been considered "corrupt" under colonial rule, is necessarily considered corrupt by the rules of a democratic nation-state. In nationalist regimes, as opposed to colonial ones, he notes, there is a new discourse of accountability, according to which government employees are answerable to the populace. Nationalism has created new subject positions, unknown in colonial India, of accountable public employees and citizens with inalienable rights. These new discourses and subject positions, Gupta suggests, are indispensable to contemporary perceptions of corruption in Indian society. In the case of Ayurveda there has been a swift transition over several decades from training sponsored by patrons to education legislated by the state. In a patronage arrangement the salient subject positions are those of kinfolk, patrons, and friends, not public employees and citizens; among such subject positions gifts and favors are expected to flow freely. In such a community the concept of bribery is meaningless. As long as there is no ideology of identical subjects equal before the law, the notion of favoritism and selective gift giving has no pejorative sense. Many of the problems in Ayurvedic education may be interpreted in part as the result of a misalignment between the standard institutions of nationalism and local practices. What is labeled as corruption is one manifestation of this misalignment.

One Ayurvedic practitioner, Dr. Mishra, told me of the following conflict between himself, trained in modern institutional settings, and his father, trained in a gurukula. Behind his back, his father arranged to have his daughter-in-law registered as a vaidya, even though she had neither education nor experience. When Dr. Mishra discovered that this had been done, he was exceedingly angry. The father reasoned that his son might some day have need of his wife's assistance in his practice. In that event he could teach her himself whatever she needed to know. As Dr. Mishra told me the story, he said that he suddenly felt he understood why, on his graduation, his father had wanted him to assist in his clinic rather than to study for an M.D. From his father's point of view, medicine was actually learned through observing and assisting senior practitioners rather than from institutional study. According to his father's logic, the license was a mere formality, without any necessary relation to the competence of the practitioner. Dr. Mishra went on to draw a distinction between the historical circumstances thirty years ago and those today. He said that thirty years ago, it was justifiable to issue degrees and licenses, through the Vidyāpīṭh, to large numbers of unqualified practitioners in order to strengthen the Ayurvedic ranks. This use (or "ab-use") of modern institutional structures was necessary, he continued, because by modern standards, guruparampara training could never be recognized as comparable to modern medical education. Now, he said, such discrepancy between structure and practice is no longer necessary and so no longer condonable.

It is probable that the individualized guru-disciple training simply did not yield the kind of standardized knowledge that could be tested by one uniform exam. Ironically, sheer pragmatism may have dictated that the examination had to be rigged in order to be fair. Today, that corrupt examination system, having contributed to the disintegration of the distinctive knowledges of particular gurus, also compromises the standardized knowledge that has displaced them. Not surprisingly, some contemporary practitioners question the assumption that the generic knowledge that is guaranteed by a supposedly uniform (but corrupt) educational system is of a higher standard than the knowledge guaranteed by the authority of a particular guru and the monastic discipline of his gurukula. At the Ayurvedic research conference mentioned above, Dr. Karnik (who was introduced in chapter 2) commented that in the guru-śiṣya parampara a certain standard was maintained within the guru's lineage. In "institutionalized" Ayurveda, on the other hand, there is no standard at all. "There should be something common," he said.

The practices of contemporary Ayurvedic education jeopardize not only the generic knowledge they are supposed to produce, but also the generic subject positions they are supposed to protect. First-year Ayurvedic students worried to me that because they would be examined by an outside board rather than by their own teachers, they had no idea what the examiners would expect. The examination by an outside board is supposed to solve the problem of the "partiality" of the teachers toward particular students (even though it is clear that partiality can be bought). "Partiality" here takes its negative valence from a modern liberalism that assumes abstract human subjects with equal rights to equal treatment. In the gurukulas of the nineteenth century, the concept of partiality would have been meaningless or at least quite different in meaning. When an affective bond between student and teacher is expected, partiality is not an issue but a matter of course. One practitioner recounted to me the *im*partialities of his examination experiences in one Ayurvedic college. The professors were often upset with his mother, the college principal, because she transferred them to new departments every few years. The examiners vented their frustration with this policy on him. In a rasaśāstra exam, for example, he was asked to tell the examiners the chemical composition of Surf, a popular laundry detergent. He asked what this had to do with rasaśāstra. The examiner replied that he should know about everything. The student got up and left the room, saying, "Okay, see you next year." (A student who fails an exam has the option of studying the subject further and retaking the exam the following year.) Later he spread a rumor that he was going to have people removed from the examiners' list through his mother's influence. Although his mother was actually unwilling to interfere, the rumor itself was effective: the examiners stopped harassing him, and he was able to graduate. In the interstices of modern educational equality, then, particular affiliations and affective ties continue to have authority, but outside of the avowed gurukula ethos of affection and respect.

In the conversation with Dr. Mishra about the shifting appropriateness of corrupt behaviors I was reminded of Cohn's (1987b) work on the introduction of courts of law to an Indian village. I briefly synopsized Cohn's thesis: because lawsuits, unlike earlier ways of settling disputes, were an impossible means through which to reach compromise or allow everyone to vent his/her feelings, they were perceived merely as a means through which to attack one's enemies. Similarly, I wondered whether Ayurvedic institutions might be an inappropriate, if not impossible, means through which to transmit the locally specific healing practices of fifty years back. If so, then perhaps these institutions were originally perceived merely as a means by which to obtain professional status. Dr. Mishra quickly agreed and commented that close to 90 percent of the cases in contemporary Indian courts are intended simply to delay an outcome. He asked me then if I had been following the Khairnar story in the national media. G. R. Khairnar was a Bombay municipal employee in charge of demolishing illegal buildings constructed by underworld figures. He was suspended from his job when he accused the chief minister of Maharashtra of links with organized crime. Although Khairnar could not immediately substantiate the charges, his peasant upbringing and reputation for honesty, combined with the popular belief that corruption was rampant among government bureaucrats, made him an instant hero. The Khairnar story had been front page news in both the English and vernacular press for about two weeks running. The story inspired such headlines as "The Myth of the One-Man Demolition Squad" (T. Singh 1994), "Striking Back at the Empire" (Seshu 1994), and "Khairnar's Crusade" (Rahman 1994).

Dr. Mishra referred to a recent editorial in one of the English dailies written by Nani Palkhivala, one of India's foremost jurists. Palkhivala had begun by noting Khairnar's heroism: "This simple man, personifying the rustic simplicity and the basic integrity of the ordinary villager, has succeeded in proving that to the soul of India sacrifice appeals more than success. He risked more than his job—he jeopardized his life itself and multitudes rallied round him. The 'illiterate intelligence' of our masses still has what I would call 'ethical ethos'" (1994, 1). The jurist then went on to distill what he felt were the main issues of the case: "Khairnar's case presents two issues, which are totally separate and distinct. One is the legal aspect of the matter—is the action taken against Khairnar sustainable in law? The other is the great moral issue involved in the whole episode. The legal aspect is almost insignificant compared to the ethical questions, which Khairnar's case has thrown up." Palkhivala argued that Khairnar should not protest his suspension in court, partly because he was by law guilty of breach of discipline under the Municipal Servants' Conduct and Discipline Rules, but even more importantly because he would then be restricted from speaking to the public while the case was sub judice. The jurist asked,

> Is it worth stifling the public response and silencing the agitated public mind, for the sake of a legal indication which, even if it materialises, would be a negligible gain compared to the vastness of the moral stakes involved? The real issue is light-years apart from the legal question. Khairnar's case proves that the law and morality do not coincide. What is legally wrong is, sometimes, morally the only right thing to do. When Mahatma Gandhi was charged with violating the law and was tried before a British judge, he pleaded guilty and requested the judge to pass on him the maximum sentence. . . . He [Khairnar] would deserve to be remembered in history if he has awakened us to the fact that we have so far been content to run a third-class democracy under a first-class constitution (1994, 1).

While the supervisor responsible for the suspension may have been legally right, Khairnar was morally right. Like Gandhi, Palkhivala advised, he should bow to the law but continue to publicly advance his moral position. The point to which Dr. Mishra particularly wanted to call my attention was that such a renowned jurist would draw a distinction between law and morality, and would concede by implication that the courts are ineffective to enforce the social ethic.

About the same time, while visiting Vd. Shukla's wife, I happened to watch part of a Hindi movie on television that bore some resemblances to the Khairnar story. The plot involved the relationship between two brothers whose poverty motivated one of them to become a doctor and forced the other into banditry. Both brothers were heroes, valiantly protecting a personal ethic. The bandit held an ethic of vigilante justice, while the doctor held a professional ethic, and both brothers (and their mother as well) held an ethic of family loyalty. At one point the doctor protected a patient who was his brother's enemy with the proud words, "I am a doctor." The bandit ultimately died rescuing his brother from jail, where he had been confined for aiding banditry by treating his brother's wound. Meanwhile, this "ethical ethos" was championed against bureaucrats and law enforcement officials, who were portrayed as villainous, wantonly violent, and devoid of ethics. The film dramatized the opposition between law and morality, noted by Palkhivala, that complicates the imagination of Indian citizenship and occupational integrity. Some weeks later I heard, not surprisingly, that one of the Bombay film companies was considering turning Khairnar's story into a screenplay.

Both Khairnar's story and the Hindi movie about the two brothers seem to convey that the modern state in its various branches cannot enframe and enclose the social ethos. Similarly, many practitioners seem to feel that modern Ayurvedic institutions cannot enframe and enclose the practices by which Ayurvedic knowledge is actually transmitted. The Ayurvedic graduates who manage to develop the most commitment to and competence in Ayurvedic diagnosis and treatment are those who assist and observe in the Ayurvedic practices of either their parents or other experienced practitioners after completing their degrees. One graduate who had a sincere interest in Ayurveda but no idea how to practice it has been working with Dr. Upadhyay for several years. She now feels confident to diagnose and treat patients on her own. Several graduates, including one of his own daughters, have worked with Dr. Pathi for one or two years. In a paper submitted to the Ayurvedic research conference one practitioner recommended that elements of the gurukula practice be introduced into modern education: "It should be made clear to the student that the possession of a degree certificate at the end of the stipulated five and one half years of study does not give him/her the license to play with people's lives. The student will have to pursue his studies rigorously with some expert master until such a time when the master deems him/her fit to undertake the responsibility of looking after the community health problems" (Kutty 1994, 3). Unfortunately, however, it seems that even gurukulas, when inserted into a modern paradigm of form and content, can become empty forms. I heard from a couple of sources that the same hospital director who had sought a ready-made M.D. thesis for his daughter was leading a project to establish gurukulas for post-M.D. study. When I mentioned this to Dr. Mishra, he said that the project was a sham: one person is designated a guru and paid three or four thousand rupees; another person with an M.D. is designated a śiṣya. And then? I asked. Then nothing, he replied, with a gesture of disgust. The student is given a title that is supposed to signify a higher status than an M.D. On the one hand, he said, the hospital director participates in the national administration of institutional Ayurveda, and on the other, he keeps his name associated with guru-śiṣya parampara, thereby trying to "control" both.

While there are slippages between form and content in modern institutions everywhere, in modern Ayurvedic institutions the illusion of an alignment between form and content seems to be less fiercely sustained than it would be, for instance, in the United States. In the Ayurvedic community, as in other sectors of Indian society, corruption is continuously noted and censured as if it were as inevitable and ubiquitous as drought (though perhaps more predictable). The people I knew spoke of corruption with bitterness or irony but without hope of recourse. In the United States, on the other hand, each instance of corruption that is brought to light is treated, at least in the media, as singular and outrageous, raw material for a legal battle. Could the difference be partly that in modern India the dualism of form and content is more a syntagma to perform than an episteme to protect? Modern Ayurvedic teaching hospitals tend to subvert the ideological categories (form and content, facade and function, paperwork and process) of modern institutions by drawing attention to their constructedness, to the artificiality of their relationship to Ayurvedic knowledge. If Ayurvedic professionals and their public are not often fooled by institutional appearances, it may be because these appearances are not necessarily taken as separate from an underlying reality.

five Clinical Gazes

In the turn-of-the-century texts examined in chapter 3, the shift of focus in the identification of the crisis facing Ayurveda mirrored the modern shift in the focus of European medical knowledge. Whereas at first the crisis had been attributed to local problems such as adharma and quackery, gradually the crisis was attributed to colonization. Even as the attention of European medicine moved away from host factors onto invasive agents such as germs and viruses as the source of disease, the attention of Ayurvedic practitioners moved away from local ethical malaise to foreign influence as the source of the crisis in Ayurvedic knowledge. This similarity is hardly coincidence since the imagination of the nation as a bounded and discrete entity, mapped into geographic or demographic segments, is epistemically connected to the imagination of the body as a similarly bounded and discrete entity, principally visible through its anatomical structure.[1] Anthropologies of immunology have found that modern discussions of the immune system, both popular and scientific, are saturated with militaristic imagery related to the defense of the nation (Haraway 1991; Martin 1990). Both the modern perception of the body and the modern understanding of the nation are projects of enframing, of enveloping certain processes in the effect of an external framework. The mapping of national space as a delineated section of the earth's surface is a radical departure from earlier cosmographies of sacred sites, networks of trade routes, or land etched with ancestral story lines.[2] Similarly, the somatic space of the modern disciplines as drawn and quartered in anatomical diagrams is a far cry from the cosmo-somatic space of doṣic ebb and flow, which is implicit, if not quite depicted, in the lotus-shaped *yantra* (mystical diagram) discussed in chapter 2 (figure 1).

Has the introduction of modern hospital and educational disciplines discussed in chapter 4 transformed doṣic bodies into docile bodies? Can the anatomical body with its well-defined boundaries, its division into discrete regions, its militaristic defense against viral invasion be mapped onto the body of doṣa, dhātu, agni, and mal? A Marathi textbook published in 1985 offers an Ayurvedic version of the nation-state as a metaphor for the body (figure 7). The sign on the left reads "National Body Consulate Office," while the arrow on the right reads "Entrance: Citizens Only Admitted; Foreigners Forbidden to Enter." Here the militarism of biomedicine seems to be reproduced in modern Ayurveda. The break with biomedicine occurs in the dial on the right, where the needle registers the rasa or flavors of ingested foods and medicines. This dial, along with the very location of the bodily border at the mouth, suggests that the foreigners here are not so much viruses and germs but rather particular foods or medicines. On a similar dial for the metaphorical body of the modern immune system the needle would probably oscillate between positions marked "self" or "not-self" (Haraway 1990). In this chapter I consider the disciplining of bodies and illness in contemporary Ayurvedic hospitals. I am especially concerned with those moments of slippage when the doṣic body overflows the anatomical borderlines and slides out from under modern somatic disciplines. For even at the bodily level, modern Ayurvedic practitioners negotiate a narrative of disease that resists assimilation by a biomedical universalism. Even in the daily activities of diagnosis and treatment, many physicians employ the biomedical techniques that make Ayurveda parallel to biomedicine while circumventing the biomedical epistemologies that would make Ayurveda subordinate to biomedicine.

Doṣic Bodiliness and Docile Bodies

The doṣic body is what I have called in chapter 1 a fluent body, coursing with climates and appetites, messages and passions, winds and tempers. The doṣic body spans the divide between text and world. It is inscribed with signs that are more productively understood as versatile signifiers than visualized as definite objects. To say that it is a fluent body is to say that it is overflowing not only with doṣic currents, but also with polyvalent syntax. The doṣic body bears the imprint of a social matrix, the somato-psychic consequences of living with or against dharma. In this body the heart can be both a center of circulation and a center of con-

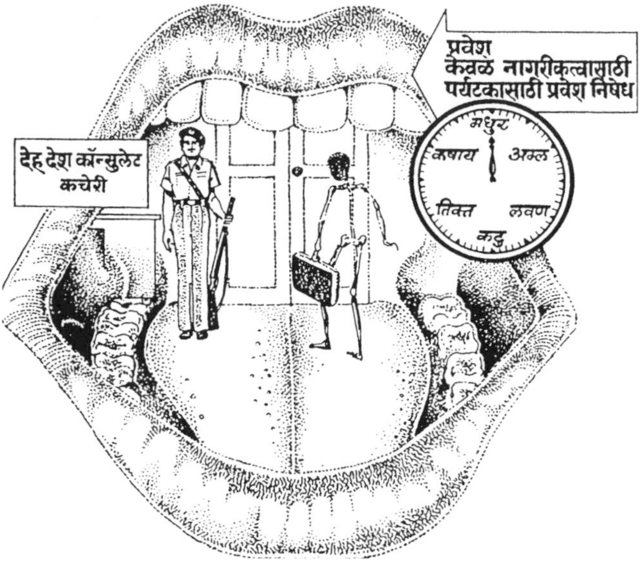

Figure 7. Body as Nation–State. The metaphor of the national body is here depicted in an Ayurvedic textbook (Padyegurjar 1985).

sciousness, while warmth can be simultaneously temperature, temperament, and a somato-environmental agent that eludes modern categories. One M.D. student who was completing a dissertation in English on *kaṭiśūl,* or lower back pain, told me that one of the words he had left in the original Sanskrit was *uṣṇa.* People call it heat, he said, but it is not exactly heat in the sense of temperature. For example, uṣṇa is one of six guṇa that are variously enhanced by six flavors (rasa). Uṣṇa is enhanced by both pungent (*kaṭu*) and sour (*amla*) flavors.[3] Since sourness increases uṣṇa, one professor explained, sour medicines and foods are good for poor digestion. Since sourness also enhances the quality of oiliness (*snigdh*) and, to a lesser extent, lightness (*laghu*), sour medicines and foods are also good for angina: the oily quality decreases the dryness (*rukśa*) that causes the arteries to constrict, and the light quality helps to open up the arterial space.[4] It is for this reason, he said, that pomegranates are good for the heart. The body implicit in such a narrative of heat and sourness, dessication and oiliness, bears more resemblance to a weather pattern than to a biological entity. Doṣic embodiment makes more obvious what might be said of any kind of embodiment: "The body in question is not a

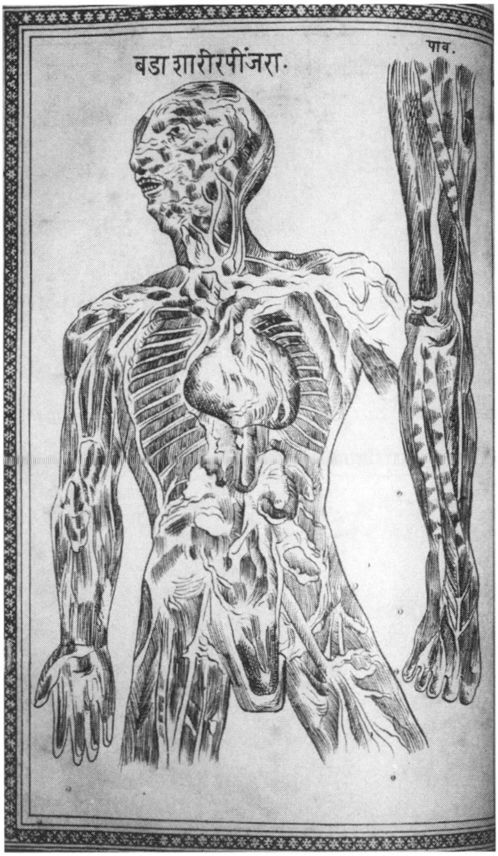

Figure 8. Living Anatomies. "Adult body 'cage' and leg" (Ś. Singh 1912, 1). The word I translate here as "cage" is *pīnjara,* which Monier-Williams (1993 [1899], 625) lists as a "wrong reading" for *pañjara,* meaning "skeleton" or "cage."

hypostatized object . . . but a relation in a system of liaisons. . . . It would be better to speak of a certain 'bodiliness' than of 'the body'" (Barker 1995, 10).

How are we to understand the discourses of doṣic bodiliness in relation to the discourses of docile bodies? In *Śivanātha Sāgar* and other vernacular texts of its era, the bodies depicted are not yet the passive bodies of modern anatomy (figures 8 and 9). They are certainly interiorized, with organs and bones exposed. They are also, however, living

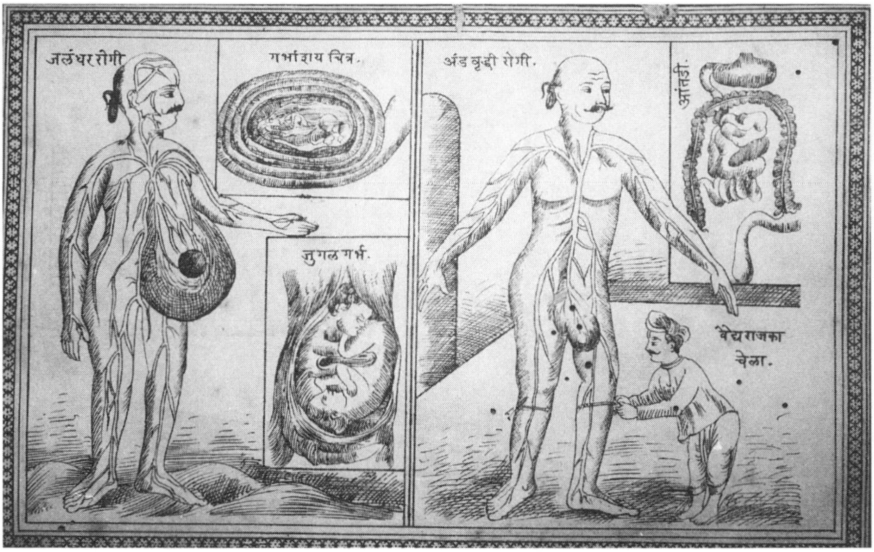

Figure 9. More Living Anatomies. "Patient with water retention" (literally, water inside), "picture of the womb," and "womb with twins" (center). "Patient with enlarged scrotum" being measured by "a student of a vaidyarāj" and "intestines" (right) (Ś. Singh 1912, 6).

bodies, not frozen in anatomical poses, but gesturing and gazing off the page. In modern Ayurvedic anatomy departments, on the other hand, almost the only representations of the body are borrowed from biomedicine—plastic figurines in rigid postures, with inner organs painted in different colors. In one anatomy department, however, I noticed among these items a life-sized model of the ideally proportioned human male, poised in midaction, one arm bent and raised in a fist and one leg stepping forward, eyes open and focused, bones and organs hidden. The dimensions of each part of his body, I soon learned, are in a particular prescribed proportion to the central section of the middle finger. A perfectly proportioned body is an indicator of a long life. It is quite possible that the student depicted in figure 9 is measuring the legs of the patient with the enlarged scrotum in order to predict his life span. Contemporary students still learn the *swanguli pramāṇ* (self-finger measurement), although neither they nor their professors use it clinically. Swanguli pramāṇ is one of the few topics in the Ayurvedic anatomy class that does not correlate to biomedical anatomy. The body of swanguli pramāṇ is not measured out in units of neutral space like an anatomical body, but in units of a self-referential space that mathematically multiplies the length of the body's own middle finger. In contrast to the body parts all around it, this plastic statue represents a body that is ideal rather than normative, dynamic rather than docile, as much engaged in seeing as in being seen and in acting as being acted upon.[5] In fact, despite being an abstract body, a sign of longevity, this body is reminiscent of what Romanyshyn (1989, 108) has called the "pantomimic body" in that it gestures to a world and embodies an emotional situation, if only the situation of glorying in its own health.

As Romanyshyn (1989, 115) has noted, the modern anatomical body is sectioned as if by a grid imposed on a neutral space — as if seen, in other words, through a *camera obscura*. The perfectly proportioned Ayurvedic body is sectioned also, according to a pattern of marmas or vulnerable areas, which are also measured according to swanguli pramāṇ. Suśruta, recognized as the ancient authority on Ayurvedic surgery, identified one hundred seven marmas, which are classified according to both the area of the body in which they appear and the consequences of their injury.[6] The injury of marmas in one category, for example, leads to instantaneous death, while the injury of those in other categories leads to death after seven or fourteen days, to deformity or disability, or simply to pain. Unlike the anatomical body, then, the marmic body is spatialized not so much by a cameralike vision as by possible crises. Romanyshyn speaks of how the anatomical body is actually "lived" only in moments disruptive of the body's ordinary engagement with the world, when, for example, torn muscles, raw bone, and severed veins become visible or painful. Such moments of disruption are, of course, precisely the concern of the physicians and their very motivation for positing marmic or anatomical bodies. However much the anatomical body is projected as a neutral space, independent of anyone's intentions, it is, like the marmic body, an instrumental space in which a surgeon's or anatomist's hands can maneuver. In biomedicine, however, this instrumental space is imagined not in relationship to an injury or a surgeon's work, but as "real," independent of any situation of injury or treatment. In this way, biomedicine creates the naturalized *effect* of an empty homogeneous space in which we locate the organs and systems of the anatomical body, much as nationalism creates the naturalized effect of an empty homogeneous space in which we locate national borders and territories. In marmic embodiment, on the other hand, space is imagined, as in pantomimic embodiment, in relation to possible situations, especially situations of bodily harm.

It is tempting to assimilate doṣic bodiliness to the nondisciplinary bodies of premodern Europe, especially the grotesque Rabelaisian body, spilling out of its boundaries, described by Mikhail Bakhtin. Indeed, Bakhtin (1968, 344) tells us that the grotesque body was inspired partly by accounts of fabulous oriental bodies, with disarranged and half-animal anatomies, that were pictured in popular medieval compilations of stories about India under the name of "Indian Wonders." Is it possible that in such texts Europeans begin to look to other peoples for the counterpoint, the point of release for their own disciplines, in this case a budding anatomical discipline? For the "Indian Wonders" include not only magic herbs, fountains of youth, and devils spitting fire, not only unicorns, phoenixes, and griffins, but also satyrs, centaurs, cyclopes, headless "leumans" with faces on their chests, and so on. "This," as Bakhtin notes, "is an entire gallery of images with bodies of mixed parts. . . . All this constitutes a wild anatomical fantasy" (1968, 345). In the "Indian Wonders," this vision of anatomy run wild is projected away from the bourgeois tidiness of European medicine onto an Indian landscape.[7]

Bakhtin (1968, 319) suggests that the grotesque body encompasses every nonmodern embodiment. He assimilates the grotesque Rabelaisian body to the humoral body of Hippocratic medicine, which is in some respects similar to the doṣic body, insofar as "the confines of the body and the world are effaced" (1968, 355). Yet precisely here and in other passages, as when Bakhtin writes that the "Indian Wonders" primed the medieval imagination for the "*transgression* of the limits dividing the body from the world" (1968, 347; emphasis added), it is possible to glimpse important differences between grotesque and doṣic embodiment. For the grotesque body, at least of Rabelais's time, seems to take its wondrous force from its transgressiveness. It seems to owe its significatory impact to an already intimated separation between body and world and an already initiated parceling of the body into discrete parts. Is this grotesque body not related to the body of the public dissections that marked the transition from spectacular punishments to anatomical discipline? After all, one of these public dissections was performed by Rabelais himself. I suggest, therefore, that the grotesque body plays out the suppressed horrors implied by that public dismemberment that is both entertainment and scientific undertaking. The doṣic body is not, however, transgressive or transgressed in the same way: there is nothing horrible about its ebb and flow. It is not a body reacting to bourgeois boundaries. If the intercourse between the grotesque body and the world is envisioned anatomically through a hyperbolic displacement and replication of organs and orifices, then the intercourse between the doṣic body and the world is imagined dynamically through the continuous flow of qualities such as warmth and coolness; flavors such as sweetness and astringency; or elements such as earth, water, and ether. The grotesque body is fragmented wildly, as befits a body that is almost rebelliously and riotously opposed to a newly dominating anatomical order. The marmic body of swanguli pramāṇ, on the other hand, is fragmented according to an elaborate somatic geometry. This body appears as a harmonious text of interrelated equations.

In Europe it is possible to trace historical development from predisciplinary bodies, which are one with text or world, to docile bodies. In postcolonial India a shift to docile bodies is still being contested. Ayurvedic practitioners, in their need to both parallel and surpass European medicine, necessarily work with bodies that are both doṣic and docile, both fluent and fixed, both text- and material-referent, both coextensive with and apart from the world. In the rest of this chapter I explore the clinical gazes of modern Ayurveda, which perceive one kind of bodiliness or another as the cure requires. I follow these gazes as they focus alternately on doṣa, dhātu, or disease; as they discover doṣa in different etiological moments as entities or as processes; as they allow "symptoms" to double as diseases and "diseases" to double back as symptoms; as they capitalize on the polyvalence of terms to generate health; as they, in short, keep shifting their points of view in pursuit of wellness. First, however, it will be useful to understand how these modern gazes must always maneuver in ways that assume and accommodate the idea of "science."

Doṣa in a Petri Dish

There is scarcely an English Ayurvedic book in print that does not discuss the scientific validity of Ayurvedic knowledge. As Ayurvedic discourse has increasingly taken the form of a dialogue with allopathy, "science" has become a term that assumes extraordinary significance.[8] The name of science is so obviously valorized in certain English works that it is capitalized whenever it appears. "Science" is taken as a sign for a universal knowledge that transcends national and cultural boundaries. Of one book a commentator states, "This book is written with a view to prove the scientific nature of Ayurveda by comparing it with the most developed and scientific western medicine. No attempt is, therefore, made to appeal to sentiment in preference to scientific reasoning as is generally done" (quoted in Ghanekar 1962, afterword:2). A second commentator notes, "The author of this interesting memoir proves to the hilt that Ayurveda is really a scientific system of medicine and is not opposed to the principles and practices of modern medicine" (quoted in Ghanekar 1962, afterword:3).

In Ayurvedic discourse science is the preferred translation for both the word *veda,* which broadly means knowledge, and the word vijñān, which means worldly knowledge or (especially if juxtaposed to unadorned "jñān") specialized knowledge. The author of a Hindi work who wishes to invoke the senses of "science" and "scientific" generally uses the words vijñān and *vaijñānik* respectively. Over the last century "vijñān" has come to be so overshadowed by its translation as science that at least one contemporary Hindi-English dictionary includes no other English definitions except in the field of philosophy, where the word is said to mean "acquired knowledge of the world (as distinct from knowledge of *brahman* acquired by meditation and study)" (McGregor 1995, 920). The latter meaning is listed first to indicate that it arose at a historically earlier period than the second meaning, "science," but the second meaning is starred to indicate that it now predominates. Thus the use of either "science" or "vijñān" in Ayurvedic writing or speech invokes the unquestioned hegemony of a particular mode and method of knowledge.

The criteria for this mode of knowledge are, however, reconstructed and contested in Ayurvedic discourse according to particular local and historically shaped aspirations. Some practitioners advance empiricism as the salient criteria. When I suggested to Dr. Upadhyay that modern science might imply a specific methodology, he replied that science is simply a matter of making observations according to certain preestablished theories. How well this idea of science coincides with the idea of science conveyed in modern science courses is suggested by certain discussions in a class on Ayurveda the Dr. Upadhyay taught for a group of U.S. college students. When he asked early on what "science" meant to them, he received the answer, "reproducibility of results." This he instantly glossed to "universal applicability," which was, he said, a characteristic of Ayurveda. Later on in the class he was describing the properties of different kinds of milk. The milk of water buffalo, he said, is very heavy and hard to digest. Goat's milk is much lighter, more vāta. You can predict the qualities of the milk, he said, by observing the animals' feces and habits. Water buffalo, for example, sleep a great deal, cows are livelier, and goats are the liveliest. When the students realized he was correlating the characteristics of the milk with the behavior of the animals, they started laughing. "This is not a matter of laughing," he corrected them. "This is a matter of observation." While the U.S. students are clearly used to gearing empiricism toward explanations, Dr. Upadhyay is here gearing it rather toward correlations. He reads the signs in a world that they have been trained to test for reasons.

Many contemporary Ayurvedic scholars, like those cited in chapter 3, find eternal truth to be a better criterion for scientific knowledge than falsifiability. Implicitly or explicitly they often criticize European science for its ignorance or exclusion of intuitive knowledge. Hegel had charged, in a manner fully consistent with a modern understanding of the division between matter and spirit, that Hinduism was a pantheism in which "the sensuous is not merely a subservient and compliant expression of the spiritual, but is expanded into the immeasurable and undefined, and the Divine is thereby made bizarre, confused, and ridiculous" (1902, 147). The modern Ayurvedic critics of European science counter such a charge by implicitly arguing rather that the European insistence on removing all spirit from the material world renders the world itself "bizarre and ridiculous." As one Ayurvedic author, H. V. Savnur, wrote, "Philosophy and science are not regarded by Orientals as water-tight compartments, but are permitted to influence each other as part of one organic whole of knowledge" (1984 [1950], 13). European science, Savnur (1984 [1950], 14) suggests, takes only a partial view because "Westerners" are concerned only with "external phenomena," while Hindus, having an "introspective mentality," are concerned with internal phenomena as well. Gananath Sen was quoted as saying, "The spirit of Ayurveda is the spirit of [European] science and something more. It is the spirit of observation and experimental research reinforced by the transcendental intuition (divyajñāna) of the rishis" (quoted in Mukharjee and Narayanarow

1954, 349). The Ayurvedic historians citing this remark went on to explain that this intuition is the fruition of "austerity, solemn meditation and sacrifice" (Mukharjee and Narayanarow 1954, 350). Ancient yogic knowledge complicates not only the progressivism of science, as I discussed in chapter 3, but also the objectivism of science.

Similarly, the author of a 1986 Ph.D. thesis on yoga and Ayurveda (S. P. Mishra 1986, 3–4) notes that "Western science" lacks a "multi-dimensional concept of life" and defines existence merely in physical terms. He argues that the concept of the ātmā is a significant advance over the materialism of European science. Indeed the ātmā is included in the classroom instruction of Ayurvedic anatomy, though it is necessarily excluded from the laboratory demonstrations. One anatomy professor explained that the subject of śarīr racana is divided into the visible or gross (*sthūla*) and invisible or subtle (*sūkśma*) aspects of the body. In a telling conflation of the visible with the dead, she said that ātmā and mana exist in the invisible body, the living body, but are not visible in the corpse. In oral anatomy exams, she would often first ask students to name these two aspects of śarīr and then follow this question with demands for the names of parts of the stomach or the names of the muscles touching a particular pelvic bone. In a lecture to a group of foreign visitors, one hospital director differentiated an Ayurvedic animation of matter from the apparent enervation of matter in European science by using the word śāstra for science in preference to vijñān. He explained that a śāstra is "that which instructs," that which "makes you a disciple." Ayurvedic scientists, he continued, want to learn from and "follow" the universe, while European scientists want rather to exploit it.

Even those who note the limitations of European science, however, may still insist on the compatibility between the basic concepts of biomedicine and Ayurveda. Shiv Sharma (1929, 185–187), the champion of śuddh Ayurveda, who, as noted in chapter 3, faulted European science for its constant self-revisions, also argued that endocrinology is very similar to doṣic theory in that the same factors—diet and drugs, heat and cold, rest and exercise, sleep and waking, and so on—affect both glandular activity and doṣa. In consonance with the views of the authors cited above, Sharma also noted that the difficulty in translating doṣa is due to the "inseparable blending" of the "physical" with the "metaphysical." "The doṣa," he wrote, "are wrongly considered to be 'humors' and should never be translated as 'wind,' 'bile,' and 'phlegm' but rather understood as the bio-motor force, the metabolic activity and the preservative principle of the body, and the vehicles of the qualities of the *Rajas, Sattva* and *Tamas* in the living organism" (1929, 175). Interestingly, a similar explanation of doṣa was offered by Gananath Sen, one of the best-known proponents of miśra Ayurveda during the early part of this century. In 1916 Sen also distinguished doṣa from humors: vāyu, he wrote, refers not to wind but to "functions of life as manifested through cell development in general and through the central and sympathetic Nervous Systems in particular." Pitta refers not to bile but to "the function of metabolism and thermogenesis or heat production comprehending in its scope the process of digestion, metabolism, colouration of blood and formation of the various secretions and excretions which are either the means or the ends of tissue combustion." Finally, kapha does not mean phlegm but rather "the function of cooling and preservation (thermotaxis or heat regulation) and secondarily the production (and products) of the various preserving fluids, e.g., Mucus, Synovia, etcetera" (1916, 13). Shortly thereafter Sen's views were heavily cited in the 1923 Madras Report on indigenous medicine, which also advocated the grafting of the electron theory of matter onto the Saṃkhya theory of "the genesis of atoms" and the grafting of *tridoṣa* (three doṣa) theory onto endocrinology (Government of Madras 1923, part 1:34).

An alternative biomedicalization of doṣa was offered in the same report by M. G. Deshmukh, who wrote that vāta refers to "electrically active bodies that are responsible for the formation of brain, nerve and muscle cells and the exhibition of functions of intelligence, sensation and motion," while pitta refers to "chemically active bodies that are responsible for the formation of cells of the glandular tissues and the secretion of all sorts of ferments that cause digestion and assimilation and the reversible process of breaking down of spent up cells," and kapha refers to "more stable bodies that are responsible for the formation of bone and connective tissue cells entering into the structure of the more stable parts of the body" (quoted in Government of Madras 1923, part 2:74). Several decades later the author of an M.D. thesis suggested an elaborate correlation of doṣa with certain brain chemicals, which he called "neurohumors" (Agrawal 1980). Around the same time, the author of a book on Ayurvedic pediatrics wrote that kapha includes water, protein, fats, and carbohydrates, while pitta includes enzymes, some hormones, and some vitamins, and vāta includes oxygen, carbon dioxide, nervous impulses, and the hormones and vitamins that are not included in pitta (Athavale 1977, 34).

Savnur (1984 [1950], 14, 68) took pains to establish correspondences between biomedical and Ayurvedic understandings of the world at an even more fundamental level. He equated the three qualities (guṇas) rajas, tamas, and sattva with the quasi-Newtonian categories of energy, mass, and essence. He further equated the seven *cakras,* or energy centers in the subtle body, with neurological channels. The author of the book on pediatrics likened Ayurveda and allopathy to two languages that describe the same processes. The Ayurvedic language has five "letters" (elements), the *pancamahābhūta,* while European science has one hundred ten. He concluded, "So long as both can communicate well it does not matter which language one uses" (Athavale 1977, 33). The differences between Ayurveda and European science, then, are simply semantic.

Moreover, Ayurveda is often argued to have anticipated modern science. In his 1916 address, Sen makes the point that the bacterial origin and infectious nature of certain diseases was certainly known to the ancient Ayurvedic scholars. He quotes Suśruta as having written about "various fine organisms which circulate in the blood and are invisible to the naked eye" (quoted in Sen 1916, 16). The ongoing importance of this anticipatory aspect of Ayurveda was brought home to me during a conversation with Dr. Joshi, a friend and hospital practitioner, when he was planning a series of lectures to his M.D. students on *manasik* rog (mental illness). He told me that he planned to lecture on psychiatry first, so that when he lectured on Ayurveda, the students would appreciate its comprehensiveness. I assumed that he meant that Ayurvedic perspectives would seem comprehensive by *contrast* with psychiatric perspectives. A few months later we were discussing the upcoming examination of an M.D. student specializing in mental illness. I mentioned that the student was more worried about the psychiatric part of the exam than the Ayurvedic part. Dr. Joshi responded that this was only natural since psychiatry is a more detailed system. Confused by this remark, I reminded him of his earlier comment about Ayurveda's comprehensiveness in relation to psychiatry. He explained that what he had meant was that by learning Ayurvedic approaches to mental illness after having already learned psychiatry, the students would be able to appreciate how closely Ayurveda approximates psychiatry. While I had assumed that he meant the comparison to convey how Ayurveda surpasses psychiatry, he had meant it rather to emphasize how Ayurveda anticipates psychiatry.

There was nothing apologetic in Dr. Joshi's tone, however. Kakar writes that contemporary Ayurvedic literature is characterized by a defensive note that is an uncomfortable reminder of the "psychological" scars of colonialism (1982:222). Yet such remarks as Dr. Joshi's can be taken less as references to a postcolonial inferiority complex than as allusions to the mythic histories discussed in chapter 3. Once Dr. Joshi and I were having a discussion on the etiology of diabetes, which is usually identified with the Ayurvedic disorder of *madhumeha* (literally, sweet urine). He began to speak about the gaps in Ayurvedic knowledge due to the loss of literature during Mogul and British rules. One of those gaps, he said, is in the pathology of diabetes. The authors of the ancient texts list the causes of madhumeha as defective chromosomes (*bīj* doṣa; literally, a defect in seed), diet, and family. They write that some of the *medh* (fat) and other dhātus liquify and are lost through the urine. Yet they do not explain *why* the dhātus are depleted, even though, he added, they must have known. If they had discussed the dhātu agnis or the pancreas, then we would know exactly how they understood the pathogenesis. As it is, he said, we try to fill the "gaps" with our own theories. What he left implicit is that the theories that fill the gaps are derived in part from modern science. The ancient sages, he added, "had vision; we may only have knowledge." By implication, Ayurveda not only anticipates modern science, but also encompasses it in a wider awareness. In this way contemporary Ayurvedic discourse frequently enfolds physical fact in metaphysics and empiricism in deeper insights. Science, even as it is respectfully capitalized, is also quietly subsumed.

The quest for biomedical correlates of Ayurvedic phenomena therefore continues, despite the failure of earlier correlations to take hold in either clinical practice or classroom discourse. If few authors attempt the elaborate syntheses of Ayurvedic and modern scientific concepts of earlier publications, most still feel compelled to make comparisons between, for instance, doṣa imbalances and pathogens (K. R. S. Murthy 1987, 26) or prakṛti and genetic proclivities (Central Council for Research in Ayurveda and Siddha 1987b, 17). Dr. Pathi, who considered Shiv Sharma's association of doṣa with enzymes to be flawed by Sharma's ignorance of chemistry, argued instead that pitta and kapha should be understood in terms of thermal energy and pH values, while vāta should be understood as the empty medium that allows these energies and values to be shifted from place to place. At the Ayurvedic research conference held in the early 1990s, possible biomedicalizations of Ayurvedic concepts still haunted the discussions. In one presentation the speaker recommended research into the biochemistry of *āma,* usually understood as undigested food residue that contributes to illness. We know the physiology of digestion very minutely today, she said; "Where does āma fit in?" The following speaker pointed out that research into āma would also have to take the agnis into account—that is, the digestive or combustive processes that occur as nutrients are successively converted from one dhātu to another. Research into āma and agni as related to food absorption and enzymes would, he offered, "yield solutions to many problems."

Today many practitioners describe vāta, pitta, and kapha as principles, such as the principles of movement (vāta), heat, metabolism, or conversion (pitta), and material composition or formation (kapha). Dr. Upadhyay cautioned, "Don't think of doṣas as entities. . . . Doṣas are functional systems." A member of the audience at the Ayurvedic research conference asked a speaker on research methodology if there was any way to quantify vāta, pitta, and kapha. In reply, she quoted her Ayurvedic M.D. students, who tell her, "I'm sorry, I cannot bring vāta, pitta, and kapha to you on a petri plate." Even as Shiv Sharma explained the functions of each of the doṣa in roughly biochemical terms, he refused to definitively pin down what doṣa actually *are,* arguing that "whether the Tridosha are energies, forces, principles, humors, or hormones (in their different forms and manifestations), their physiological and pathological significance remains the same" (1929, 191). Similarly the author of one testimonial in the Madras Report wrote that the doṣas exist (like the body) in both gross and subtle states. In the subtle states they are *atīndriya*—that is, beyond the range of the senses. "How then are they known?" this author asks. "They are known . . . by the consequences of the actions for which they are responsible" (quoted in Government of Madras 1923, appendix 1:23).

The author of a 1989 M.D. thesis exploring possible biological correlates for āma noted that patients who were diagnosed with āma and then subjected to biomedical testing procedures were found to have reduced gastrointestinal absorption. He nonetheless concluded, "*Ama* is not one single product but is a host of products of digestion and metabolism responsible for creating a characteristic morbid biological state in the body. Thus *Ama* is both a category of materials and a state of metabolism in the body" (Devalla 1989, 71). When I asked one fourth-generation rural practitioner whether doṣa should be considered *dravya* (substances) or *prakriya* (processes), he just smiled and said that it depends on the context in which they are being discussed. What finally is most interesting is not the question of how doṣa, āma, or agni should be defined, but rather the way this question continues to be raised in professional settings, with an air of both urgency and deferral. There is an almost embarrassed ambivalence among Ayurvedic professionals about the problem of a biomedical referent for doṣa and other Ayurvedic phenomena: this problem should not exist; indeed it is sometimes asserted that it does not exist, and yet it continually reappears. Below I will consider the possibility that the deferral of decision on what doṣa or other Ayurvedic phenomena actually *are* may be clinically useful.

Sonograms and Sphygmographs

The recurrent anxiety about how to translate doṣa into scientific fact is sustained in part by the need to accommodate the somatic imagery of modern diagnostic technologies. In his discussion of the introduction of certain European technologies into India, Prakash draws our attention to the magical underside of these mechanical devices. He recounts that instruments such as the telephone, phonograph, photographic cameras, and X rays were demonstrated with dramatic flair to a Western-educated Indian elite, mixing "science with magic spectacle" and "evoking wondrous response" (1992, 162). Similarly Taussig points out that the colonial use of technology is a celebration of science as "antithetical to 'magic'" *until* the presentation of this technology to colonial subjects, when suddenly "every effort is made to represent the mimeticizing technology as magical" (1992, 207). In this way, science became entangled in the very superstition it was supposed to overcome. Meanwhile, early twentieth-century Ayurvedic scholars stuck to their "superstitions," claiming not to be awed by the mimetic power of new technologies. Some writers implied that these technologies were the means by which European scientists attempted to compensate for their lack of deeper sensory awareness. Nagendra Gupta, for instance, noted in a passage on pulse diagnosis that Europeans used a watch or other instrument to measure the pulse. He cautioned: "The minute knowledge which is the aim of Hindu Medical Science and which is only to be found amongst Ayurvedic physicians can never be acquired by a reference to the watch or the cardiograph. These are mere mechanical appliances which can never help the practitioner to precisely ascertain what particular fault [Gupta's translation of doṣa] has been excited and the precise measure of such excitement" (1919, 28). It is because the Europeans were not able to develop an adequate awareness of pulse, Gupta continued, that they developed instruments to measure pulse, heart, and body heat—that is, the thermometer, the cardiograph, and the sphygmograph. Some seventy years later, however, the first two of these instruments—not to mention stethoscopes, X rays, and sonograms—were routinely used in Ayurvedic hospitals across India. The introduction of modern disciplinary knowledge meant not only the use of tables and timetables, but also the use of new machines and statistical measures. Today's Ayurvedic practitioners have at their command the technologies that mimetically reproduce internal organs, volumes of breath, subtle fluctuations of the heartbeat, or the statistical responses of a patient population to a particular drug. I suggest that the miraculousness of such machines and measurement devices as X rays and sonograms, so widely used and narrowly understood, haunts their materialism even in the societies in which they were invented.[9] The compelling reality effect of the representations produced by such devices may indicate, therefore, not so much a closer grip on reality as a continual power to fascinate.

One day I joined a group of Ayurvedic physicians huddled around a newly acquired sonography machine. We watched ghostly organs shift and turn on the screen as the sonographer searched for an angle of view that would give an identifiable shape to the spleen. Meanwhile, the patient from whom these images were being drawn lay ignored on a cot behind a half-drawn curtain. How do we account for the intense focus on the screen to the exclusion of the woman? Taussig has suggested that the marvelousness of such technologies rests on their "mimetic power" (1993, 208). He notes that while every act of signification carries a memory of sensuous contact between sign and referent, in modern science this memory is obscured by the illusion of an independent copy.[10] The moment of contiguity in the act of signification that constitutes the sonogram is not difficult to detect: the shifting of the instrument against the woman's belly, the sound waves of the machine bouncing back from her organs. Nor are the moments of contiguity hard to detect in many other tools of modern medicine: the handling of the organs by the anatomy student, the light of the X ray penetrating the skin. It is because of this contiguity that Daniel (1983) has argued that most biomedical signification is indexical (in Peircian terms).[11] Yet all these moments of contact are ultimately subordinated to the final pictures that stand in for, substitute for, or supplement body and disease. The intimate contact between the woman and the machine tends to disappear behind the depersonalized image of her finally defined spleen. It is apt, therefore, that Francis Barker calls the modern body a "supplementary body" whose "carnality . . . has been dissolved and dissipated until it can be reconstituted in writing [or in digital images] at a distance from itself" (1995, 57). Taussig's work allows us to understand that the medical reconstitution of the body is a form of sympathetic magic in which the cure is effected partly by means of the body's mimetic copy.

Paradoxically, however, the contiguity of the sonography machine and the woman that lends the image of her spleen its magical power also serves to guarantee its scientific authority. Sonograms have a semiotic status similar to that of photographs, which seem to present uncoded, denotative images. Because it is created mechanically by light reflected off an object and touching the film, a photo creates the impression of a direct picture of nature, unmediated by the photographer. Similarly, a sonogram seems to be direct pictures of the organs because it is produced mechanically by sound ricocheting off the body's interior surfaces.[12] Yet just as photographic images are actually saturated with coded, connotative, and cultural messages (Barthes 1977), so sonograms also carry traces of social meanings. For the intelligibility of such diagnostic images actually depends on a nonmechanical image, the anatomical drawing, which reproduces only what is considered significant in the body: carefully delineated organs or systems. Without the historical priority of anatomical drawings, either a photograph of an open body, with its tangle of nerves, veins, and tendons, or a sonogram, with its shifting shadows, would be highly confusing. The medical intelligibility of these images depends on a history of anatomical drawing. Contemporary Ayurvedic students discover such a body only after they have been trained to see it.

The newly compelling realism and precision of eighteenth-century European anatomical drawings was a consequence not so much of the practice of dissection, which had been going on for centuries, as of a new medical and artistic vision. Foucault tells us that once X. Bichat and his contemporaries began to focus more on bodily locations of disease than on temporal changes, they "felt that they were *rediscovering* pathological anatomy from beyond a shadowy zone" (1973, 126). Similarly, Kuriyama (1992, 23) relates that when the Japanese anatomist Sugita Gempaku began to imitate European anatomical drawings, he felt that he was discovering a clarity that had been "clouded" in earlier representations. Yet earlier representations of the body might have seemed shadowy to Bichat or clouded to Gempaku simply because they attempted to account not only for visual observations of dead bodies, but also for other sensory observations of living bodies. In ancient Chinese and Ayurvedic texts, for instance, bodies were to be known through smell, touch, taste, sensation, and hearing as much as through sight.

Kuriyama also recounts that at the same time Gempaku was drawn to the new realism of European anatomical drawings, Japanese artists were drawn to the new realism of European paintings accomplished by the use of a camera obscura (Kuriyama 1992). The same vision that conjured an anatomical body also conjured a geometric world, sectioning off a neutral, nonsituational space through the technique of linear perspective.[13] It is this linear perspective that made possible the scale drawings, charts, graphs, and diagrams essential to scientific work and to the design of modern technologies. Such exact, mechanically produced images are made intelligible through laboratory conversations, comparison with previously constructed images, or various techniques of visual clarification.[14] For instance, the technique Michael Lynch (1988, 209) has called "upgrading" is used in anatomical models to clearly define the edges of organs, while the technique he calls "uniforming" is used to transform a variegated field of blood and tissue into an undifferentiated monochromatic field that serves as the background against which these organs can be distinguished.

The very mechanical basis of modern diagnostic images gives rise, therefore, to a paradox and potential crisis at the heart of medical scientific authority. On the one hand, these images base their truth effect on contiguous relationships with objects mediated by the mechanical mimesis of the technology. Sound waves bounce off the woman's spleen and are converted into digital data, which in turn are converted to a shadowy presence on a screen. Yet medical scientists and technicians, even those in Ayurvedic hospitals, are driven to obscure the contiguity involved in such representations. Otherwise they risk the possibility of revealing the ways that these images simultaneously (re)construct the object that they touch. The difference between sympathetic magic and medical science is that magical healers freely admit—in fact insist—that they have affected the object in the act of imitation. Medical scientists, however, guard against any possible backwash from the sign toward the referent. It is essential that the woman's sonogram be understood as a picture of her spleen and not a sensuous exchange of substance. Otherwise it might become dangerously obvious that a sonogram takes on a meaning of its own, spilling over the referent, creating the patient out of pale shifting phantoms. Paradoxically, then, it is the very sensuality of such technologies that serves to convey both their scientific authority and their magical power.

In contemporary Ayurvedic hospitals, however, such technologies are marked by a further ambivalence. For even as these instruments produce simultaneously awesome and factual representations of organs and lesions, they persistently fail to illuminate doṣa, āma, prakṛti, and agni. To illuminate these dimensions of illness practitioners must turn away from the technological images back to the living bodies. Practitioners in modern Ayurvedic hospitals, therefore, are often seen vacillating between, arguing over, or alternately privileging the signs of a living body and the signs of an anatomical body. We can trace some of the clinical tension between these two bodies by turning to yet another story of a woman and her sonogram.

I was sitting with Dr. Joshi in an OPD when he met for the first time with a patient who complained of abdominal pain. The reports she had brought from a private biomedical clinic stated that her uterus, liver, pancreas, kidney, and spleen were all normal but that there was "evidence of minimal free fluid in the abdomen." At the bottom of the second page was the request, "Kindly correlate clinically." One of the residents who had seen the sonographic pictures drew a quick sketch of them from memory for Dr. Joshi. Dr. Joshi said that he wanted to see the actual pictures, but meanwhile he led the woman behind a cloth screen for a brief examination. When he emerged, he stated, "Clinically there is no fluid. Sonographically there is fluid." When the resident began to argue with him, he said, "The abdomen is distended, but not from fluid." Nodding toward the resident, he said to me, "His worry is the sonographic report. Our worry is the patient's problem." To the resident he said, "You will unnecessarily produce illness in your mind and the patient's mind also." He prescribed some medicines, saying, "First let us have clinical relief." Then, if necessary, he would worry about the sonographic indicators.[15] Dr. Joshi explained that the medicines he had prescribed (which included *hing* or asafoetida) would accomplish *anuloman* cikitsā, a therapy for disturbances of vāta, the doṣa associated with air and movement. *Lom* means body hair or fur, and anuloman means a combing or movement with the natural direction or grain of an object. Anuloman cikitsā refers to the restoration of what is thought to be the natural downward direction of vāta in the abdomen. Dr. Joshi, then, is treating the woman doṣically, ignoring the specific organ-related problem suggested by the sonogram. Here neither the magical attraction nor the scientific facticity of the mimetic image has managed to eclipse or supersede the practitioner's touch.

One student, who was the son of two vaidya parents, had the following to say during a conversation about modern diagnostic technologies:

> For example, we examine the blood for the hemoglobin percentage. Now in Ayurveda, there is a disease, *pandu* rog. It is very similar—see, I use this word—it is *similar* to anemia. If you want to give one name to pandu in English in modern terms, you have to give anemia. How do you decide whether anemia is there? It's because [the hemoglobin count] is very low, say three grams, four grams; this is what we see in patients. In America it is impossible for you to see three-gram patients. When these patients walk on their own, it is just a *great* thing. The normal person has 14.5 grams. A three-gram person, how is he alive? But still, we see these patients. According to the terms, anemia is very severely there. For pandu [the texts] have given a group of symptoms: sweating, and so many other symptoms. When all those symptoms match, you say it is pandu.
>
> I have seen two patients of anemia, one with three grams, one with

five or six grams. This [second] fellow was sicker. He could not get up. The three-gram [patient] was a bit better. He could get up. He could ask me, "*Namaskār,* doctor, how are you? I am feeling good today." And we could talk. This is what I saw in the wards. If I told you the person had three grams, you would say, oh that is more severe. But according to the symptoms—. So this is how you have to decide whether you are going to depend on the instruments only in order to diagnose pandu or in order to diagnose anemia.

Another example I'll give you is rheumatism. The RA [rheumatoid arthritis] test is positive. The similar disease in Ayurveda is āmavāt. In āmavāt also most of the time RA tests are positive. So many of our practitioners ask the patient to get an RA test if we suspect āmavāt. What happens in āmavāt? Joint loss, swelling, pains, patients cannot use the joint, fever, so many symptoms are given. If these symptoms are present and they are severe, I say āmavāt is there. If the RA test is negative, you have to say the RA factor is not there. Nowadays, modern practitioners are also saying RA test positive means rheumatism present; but RA test negative does *not* mean rheumatism absent. So how will you decide āmavāt is present? If there is no RA test, you should not. Or you should depend on other things—the symptoms, whatever is given in the book, signs and symptoms, the description; that should match. Of course, here also you are not going to get a picture-book picture.

Dr. Joshi told me that modern medical technologies were highly useful in "confirming" diagnoses. What if, however, they contradicted a doṣic diagnosis? In such cases the physician must choose whether to consider the disease or the doṣa. As Dr. Joshi admitted,

The only thing that has now occurred because of this development of modern medical technology is that the practice is going more disease-oriented. By ECG, by electrocardiograph, once it is diagnosed that it is a case of angina, the practitioner who has taken education from the institutions—. One who is traditional would go far away from the technologies; he does not like to use the modern technologies; he says I am traditional, I don't want all this, I will examine according to the Ayurvedic principles. But when we are working in institutions, there are social compulsions. We have to get the ECG done when there is

> heart pain, when there is chest pain, because the patient will take us to task. One who is institutionally educated depends more on modern medical technologies and treats the disease as such. He sometimes forgets the doṣa and prakṛti and other things. He sometimes forgets them.

As one speaker at the Ayurvedic research conference put it, we are always "enamored" of technology, but there is an "immense implication" of anatomy and physiology in this technology. Dr. Joshi's distinction between clinical and sonographic diagnosis was frequently reiterated to his students. Once he told an intern who wanted to order a sonogram, "Go ahead and check. What I wish to stress is *ki* [that] we must be in a position to know clinically: *yah hai, yah nahīṅ* [it is this, it is not this]." Later that day he told me that sometimes the students send a patient for sonography without even knowing which organ they want to examine. Here the sonogram in and of itself, without reference to a particular clinical hypothesis, impresses the students with its mimetic power, which is at once material and magical.

Alongside the introduction of technologies such as stethoscopes and sonograms, which are oriented toward disease, there are also attempts to design technologies that are oriented toward doṣa and prakṛti. The author of a 1986 research report, Sarva Dev Upadhyaya, assessed doṣic values in research subjects using a sphygmograph, a pulse-measuring device strapped on the wrist that has long since fallen out of use in biomedicine. With this instrument he was able to translate the qualitative analyses of pulse types given in Ayurvedic texts and oral lore into quantitative analyses of pulse "waves." Flow-pressure curves plotted on graphs were used to clearly identify the three general types of pulses that characterize the three basic prakṛti. The report accomplishes in a more technical form the transposition of animal movements to curves on a graph, as depicted in figure 10. Upadhyaya writes:

> For example, the movement of Vatika pulse resembling to that of the leech and the snake signifies that the rate of the pulse should be fast, the volume should be smallest and the character should be curvilinear. Similarly, if Paittika pulse jumps like the frog, it indicates that the character of the pulse is of bounding nature and relatively the rate would be slower than Vatika pulse and the volume of the pulse would

be quite high. If Kaphaja pulse moves like a goose, it indicates that the pulse rate would be slowest and amplitude of pulse would occupy the intermediate position between Vatika and Paittika types of pulses (1986, 194).

In Upadhyaya's clinical research, doṣic pulse examination was statistically demonstrated to correlate with pulse measurement and with specific symptom clusters for hypertension and jaundice. The significance of this quantitative study lies not so much in its validation of Ayurvedic pulse diagnosis as in its precise redefinitions of doṣic and disease categories. Upadhyaya (1986, 219) claims that the measurement of pulses with a modern instrument allows for more subtle distinctions both among doṣa and among diseases. For instance, a *vātika* type of hypertension can be easily distinguished from a *paittika* type of hypertension via pulse waves (Upadhyaya 1986, 200).

A decade after Upadhyaya's report, the sphygmograph, despite its apparent promise of greater refinement of the diagnosis of doṣa, had not been introduced into Ayurvedic clinical practice. Yet stories about it circulated among the practitioners I knew. After a visit to Japan, Dr. Upadhyay (my friend and respondent and not the author of the above book on pulse diagnosis) told me that an Ayurvedic research center there had developed a sphygmograph, manufactured by Sony, that measured three pulses called distal, central, and proximal, but corresponding, he thought, to the pulses for vāta, pitta, and kapha. While he was enthusiastic about the research center's promise to send him a machine, he was not overly disappointed when that promise failed to materialize. Dr. Pathi had also seen a Japanese sphygmograph and had not been particularly impressed. These days, he said dismissively, the trend is to "computerize and quantify" everything. On the other hand, a leading doctor at one institution told me that he believed the sphygmograph would yet come into use.

It is not only images generated by diagnostic technology that carry scientific authority, but also the mathematical statistics generated by research methodology. A large portion of contemporary Ayurvedic literature is composed of research reports. Since the establishment of the Central Council for Research in Indian Medicine and Homeopathy in 1971 (since renamed the Central Council for Research in Ayurveda and Siddha), there have been numerous studies into the effectiveness of Ayurveda for

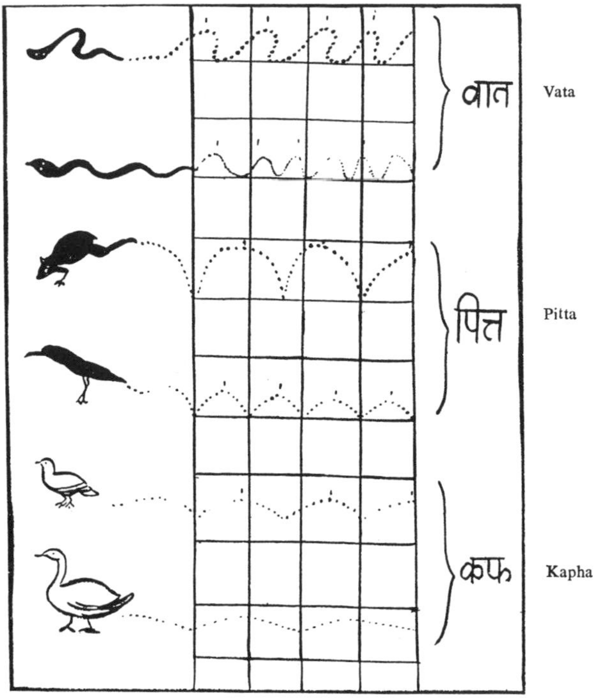

Figure 10. Graphing Doṣic Pulses. The movements of the various pulse descriptions transposed from animal rhythms to laboratory graph (Athavale 1976, 27).

treating specific diseases. In 1987, for example, there appeared a report on the treatment of vision disorders, while in 1988 there appeared a report on the treatment of jaundice and hepatitis (Central Council for Research in Ayurveda and Siddha 1987a; 1988). In each case the researchers conducted clinical trials of specific Ayurvedic formulae, with allopathic drugs used as controls, in the treatment of eye or liver disorders. The research results are quantified in terms of percentage of definite relief or cure, which is measured both by the disappearance of symptoms and by biomedical eye exams and liver function tests. Both studies conclude by claiming the effectiveness of one or more of the Ayurvedic drugs evaluated. Many practitioners, if pressed, agree that there can be no one-to-one correspondence between Ayurvedic and biomedical disease categories. Yet research continues to apply Ayurvedic drugs to biomedically defined disease. When I asked one student what she thought about research focused on drugs and disease, she turned the question back on me: "They are applying allopathic principles and using Ayurvedic medicines. What is that?"

Contemporary Ayurvedic research places a heavy emphasis on the use of pharmaceuticals over other treatment methods such as dietary prescriptions. The research supported by the Central Council for Research on Ayurveda and Siddha focuses almost exclusively on the effectiveness of various drugs as opposed to, for instance, the effectiveness of dietary changes. As one study succinctly puts it, one of the primary purposes of research into Indian medicine is the "discovery" of useful drugs (Udupa et al., 1970, xv). Twenty-five years later at the Ayurvedic research conference I attended, one speaker counted it as a major failing of Ayurvedic research that no drug with the universal appeal of ginseng had yet been launched on the international market. Evaluation of the effectiveness of various drugs is linked to their standardization. In modern times medicinal formulae are more often purchased from middlemen than concocted by the practitioners themselves. This has led to an increasing problem of adulteration and variance in potency, which has led to a call for standardization.

For a while standardization of herbal medicines implied not only the positive identification of plants known by different names in different regions, but also the isolation of the active components of these plants. K. N. Udupa, who headed the committee that wrote the report recommending miśra Ayurveda, advocated that scientists "isolate the correct fractions of [Ayurvedic] drugs which are responsible for providing such beneficial results" (Udupa et al., eds. 1970, xvi). By the early 1990s, however, no practitioner with whom I spoke advocated the isolation of active components. Ayurvedic physicians had backed off from such biomedicalizations, whether because of their infeasibility or because of the danger that Ayurveda would be assimilated by biomedicine or because of a climate of increasing disappointment with biomedical drugs. The prevailing opinion in the early to mid-1990s was that a plant or mineral substance prescribed in the texts should be ingested in its entirety in order that the presumed effects of other ingredients could regulate the specific effect of the active component. As the authors of one study wrote, in Ayurveda the effect of the whole drug is considered to be greater than the effect of the sum of its chemical components (Gair and Gupta 1970, 358–359).

According to Ayurvedic texts, medical substances are considered to have rasa, (e.g., pungent, sweet, sour), guṇa (quality, e.g., heaviness, lightness, dryness), *vīrya* (strength, usually classified as hot or cold), *vipāka* (the rasa rendered after the medicine is metabolized in the body), and *prabhav,* the specific effect, if any, on a particular aspect of the body. All the characteristics of medicines, with the exception of prabhav, can also be applied to foods. The rasa, guṇa, vīrya, and vipāka of foods as well as drugs can be used to diminish or swell the flow of doṣa in the body or to restore the dhātu. This is the reason that one professor, speaking to a group of foreign health practitioners, defined prabhav as "pharmacological activity." "Real drugs in Ayurveda," he went on, "are those with a particular prabhav. Then you can put it in a kind of frame." Other drugs, he said, can be thought of as "specific nutrients for a specific system." Yet rasa and guṇa and so on must still be taken into account even for drugs with a specific prabhav. Thus the administration of Ayurvedic medicines is potentially extraordinarily complex. It is the medicines with a particular prabhav that are most easily assimilable to a modern research methodology, which measures the effects of a particular medicine on a particular disease. Yet such methodology tends to exclude the other characteristics of the medicines.

One speaker at the Ayurvedic research conference commented that clinical method should reflect an Ayurvedic emphasis on "individualization." But the individual that is produced within modern research procedures is one whose individuality is defined by comparability to others according to certain uniform criteria or features. When quantitative research methodologies are applied to Ayurvedic "individuality," certain signs of that individuality such as prakṛti are inevitably singled out and reified. At the Constitution Clinic at Benares Hindu University, research was conducted to connect constitutional types with susceptibility or resistance to various diseases. Vātika types were shown to be prone to tuberculosis and rheumatic fever, while paittika types were shown to be prone to rheumatoid arthritis and kaphaja types to obesity, diabetes, hypertension, heart disease, and osteoarthritis (Dubey and Singh 1970). The researchers argue that constitutional types can be detected through the measurement of biochemical indicators and through psychological examinations (Dubey and Singh 1970, 315).

A 1987 report of the Central Council for Research in Ayurveda and

Siddha (1987a) documents the relationship of doṣa and prakṛti to socioeconomic and demographic factors and the relationship of dietary habits to disease. The report contains tables of statistics on which types of doṣic imbalances and prakṛti are most prevalent among given populations organized by education, gender, age, occupation, and so on. The report (p. 28) claims a statistical link, for instance, between education and certain constitutional types. Ayurveda has been distinguished from biomedicine in part for its consideration of the patient as part of a social field. When this social field is understood not through personal conversation and family involvement in treatment but through statistical survey, it becomes another instance of modern biopower. Here the investigation of prakṛti grades into sociological surveillance. I would like to keep open the possibility, however, that such research exercises are better understood as displays of wondrous methodologies than as directions in clinical practice.[16]

As in biomedical research reports, the authority conveyed by the numerals, equations, tables, and graphs in Ayurvedic research reports does much to obscure the conditions of their manufacture. One afternoon I was sitting with Dr. Joshi and an M.D. candidate from another institution. Dr. Joshi began to fire questions at her about her research on the use of vaginal *vasti* (a kind of medicinal douche) for endometriosis. He advised her to establish a control group who would be given vasti with water or some other placebo. In this way she would be able to assess the specific effects of the remedy. She replied that she had neither the time nor the personnel to establish a control group. When he asked how she would evaluate the effects of the medicine, she answered that she and her students would do biopsies on the tissues. After arguing a little longer for the establishment of a control group, he simply said that controlled research was the ideal, to which she agreed. This conversation adds dimension to the remark made by a speaker at the Ayurvedic research conference that for some reason, nearly all Ayurvedic research undertaken yields positive results. We need, the speaker added, a much stricter peer review of papers; there is a great deal of "fraud." Yet even when they accomplish little else, modern technologies and research methodologies produce a modernity effect that draws on the residual awe of scientific revelations to enforce the authority of medical knowledge. Sen was not necessarily speaking metaphorically, nor simply for Ayurveda, when, in his testimony to the Madras Report, he referred to the "magic expression 'modern scientific' methods" (quoted in Government of Madras 1923, part 2:8).

The Poetics of Clinical Reason

In a 1994 address to the International Association for the Study of Traditional Asian Medicine (IASTAM), Charles Leslie (1994) suggested that an indigenous Asian medicine such as Ayurveda should be validated not by parallelisms to modern science such as those discussed above, but rather by its aesthetic value. Yet biomedicine itself is typically referred to as both a "science" and an "art," the science consisting of facts and evidence such as those produced by diagnostic technologies and the art consisting of judgments about particular cases. Leslie began his talk by pointing out that it was humbling to address a group of doctors as a medical anthropologist. This is a humility I also share; it emerges, I think, not so much in the face of the immense number of physical facts that practitioners have at their disposal, but rather in the face of their vast storehouse of clinical stories. There is a great difference between medical information, such as that produced by sonography machines or statistical measures, and the use of such information to cure a patient. In clinical work, practitioners draw not just on a fund of medical facts, but also on a gestaltic awareness of illness and treatment options that is developed in complicated living contexts.

Deborah Gordon notes that clinical judgment results from a doctor's personal knowledge, gathered through "apprenticeship . . . , oral culture, and the case method" (1988, 260). Arguing against a recent trend to model and standardize clinical judgment, she notes that it is a practical skill, much like speaking a language or playing a musical instrument. In learning such embodied skills, formalized rules are useful to novices but not to experts. Such skills are perfected only through the direct senses of the body when faced with particular situations. They are exercised via intuition, "a situational understanding that occurs effortlessly due to perceiving similarities with prior experiences but without necessarily knowing exactly why." Efforts to model and standardize clinical judgment can therefore result only in the codification of its crudest and most rudimentary elements (Gordon 1988, 278).[17] Medical textbooks provide orderly classifications of disease and schematics of the body and mind but fail to convey the situationally strategic moves of actual treatment (see Rhodes 1993). This problem is not confined to biomedicine. If memorized lists of symptoms cannot teach a future doctor exactly how to diagnose a disease in a particular case, neither can a list of the qualities of doṣa teach an Ayurvedic student how to recognize disturbed vāta, pitta, or kapha in a patient.

Clinical judgment, then, cannot be reduced to a formula but must be understood in its narrative complexity. In contemporary Ayurveda I suggest that this narrative complexity partly involves a continual shift of focus and redefinition of terms. Notice, to begin with, how Dr. Joshi shifts his gaze from disease to dhātu to doṣa as the situation demands:

> There is a big proportion of patients who do not come to us with a particular disease. I think not more than 50 percent of the patients are in a position to be labeled as suffering from a particular disease. . . . There are people who suffer from those diseases which cannot be named as such. . . . Burning in the feet, what would you call it—simply burning in the feet, simply burning in the hands, arms, and shoulders? There's no disease as such. One may say he's developing neuritis, but is it typical neuritis? No, it's not. What would you call it? We say this burning is because pitta is hot, hot in effect, hot in touch, in everything; it is hot. Hot, burning, heat, energy—these are the things which come from pitta, right? So this burning would be named as a symptom of pitta. Now we know it is deranged pitta that is causing problems to this patient. So we start something which brings that pitta back into order so that this burning is gone. So we treat this particular doṣa. Sometimes we treat the particular doṣa.
>
> Now when we treat a disease, sometimes it is directed at treating the doṣa, sometimes it is directed at correcting the dhātu; the particular tissue is to be corrected. We give [medicine] internally; it cures the tissue. Now the tissue is not localized, right? If I say it is muscle tissue, that is prevalent everywhere in the body; it's not localized; each and every organ has got muscles. Sometimes the treatment is directed against doṣa; sometimes it is against dhātu, to correct that particular dhātu. Sometimes it is against that doṣa-dhātu *samuccay* [combination]. Some reaction has taken place: doṣa has come to dhātu; doṣa which was over there has come to this place and has caused a derange-

ment. Now if I have got swelling over here, I will try to find out what the doṣa is and treat against the doṣa. If there is a lot of *mans*, muscle dhātu, I treat for muscle.

Or sometimes I discard doṣa and dhātu. Sometimes I treat only a particular disease. After that interaction [of doṣa and dhātu] it forms a disease. Now sometimes that disease is directly put to treatment. So the first example that I gave you was to treat the doṣa; the doṣa is deranged. Dhātu is deranged? [If] somebody has got muscular wasting, we say there's mansa *dūṣya* [disturbed muscle dhātu]. That is generalized; we don't want to treat it locally; we give internal medicines which increase the muscle tissue in the body, which increase that particular enzyme or pitta, or the particular agni.[18] That particular agni has to be activated so that from the raw materials it is getting in the body, it can manufacture a good amount and good quality of muscle tissue. So that particular tissue is to be treated. So that is [treating] dhātu. If it is *kśay* [wasting, sometimes tuberculosis], then that wasting is to be treated. This was muscle wasting. Now sometimes we give a generalized treatment to cover the whole disease: doṣa, dhātu, everything. So that is directed against the disease.

Over time I began to realize that for Dr. Joshi, deranged doṣa is a facet of every disorder, weakened dhātu is a facet of disorders that have begun to affect particular tissues of the body, and disease is a manifestation of dhātu disorders that have names that are translatable into biomedical terms with a minimum of slippage—e.g., āmavāt / rheumatoid arthritis, affecting the muscle dhātu, or madhumeha / diabetes, affecting all the dhātus but especially the fat dhātu. In order for disease to be physically produced, he clarified in one conversation, dhātu must be affected. Once when he was examining a patient who complained of pain in his legs and hips, he commented that dhātu *dūṣti* (disturbance) had not occurred: there were no discernible problems with the patient's muscles, bones, flesh, or other tissues. All of the man's complaints, however, indicated vāta *prakop* (disturbance): insomnia, pain in various parts of his body, and so on.

The precise relationship of doṣa with dhātu disorder and disease was also clarified in a classroom exchange on mental illness with M.D. students. The students had learned that mental illness involved a disproportion of the three manasik doṣa—sattva, rajas, and tamas (corresponding to the three guṇa of the same names) — which are roughly correlated to equanimity, passion, or inertia. They had also learned that disturbances of manasik doṣa are inevitably accompanied by disturbances of the *śarīrik* (bodily) doṣa — vāta, pitta, and kapha. One day a student asked how, given this fact, any manasik rog (mental illness) could be correlated with neurosis since neurosis has no "demonstrable organic lesion." Dr. Joshi began his reply by saying that where tamasic doṣa is present, kapha doṣa is also present. If an anxious patient exhibits an increased heart rate, vāta and pitta must be involved, and if a patient is depressed, kapha doṣa must be involved. "After all," he said emphatically, "manifestation *has* to be with śarīrik doṣa." There is always a connection, he reiterated, between śarīrik and manasik doṣa. It would have been more appropriate, he went on, to be skeptical about how dhātu dūṣti could be correlated with neurosis. It is true that in neurosis there is no derangement of the dhātus and therefore no lesion. Yet neurosis can easily involve vāta, pitta, and kapha without reaching the dhātu. In stress, for example, pitta alone may be disturbed. If the disturbance of pitta subsequently erodes a particular bodily tissue, only then will it result in a dhātu derangement. Such a case would justifiably be labeled a "psychosomatic" disorder. He repeated: dhātu dūṣti that results from disturbed bodily doṣa associated with disturbed mental doṣa can be considered a "psychosomatic" disorder. In all other physical symptoms of mental illness, "manasik doṣa is expressing itself through śarīrik doṣa." In other words, for Dr. Joshi, any and every complaint, including neurosis, can be understood solely in doṣic terms, while a possible psychosomatic illness such as asthma must be understood in terms of dhātu as well.

After observing Dr. Joshi's practice for a couple of months, I thought I had noticed a particular prioritization of clinical gazes. One day after sitting with him in the OPD, I asked whether it was accurate to say that he treats disease whenever possible as a first resort, dhātu as a second resort, and doṣa as a last resort. He replied, yes, partially. If the disease is unambiguous, then he first tries a "palliation" — that is, a disease-oriented therapy designed to bring relief as quickly as possible. In such cases doṣa may also be affected by the medicine, but it has not been singled out for treatment. An example of the shifting of clinical gaze from doṣa to dhātu is the use in the hospital of *raktmokśan,* or blood-letting, one of the five purification processes known collectively as pancakarma. Raktmokśan is administered for eczema by the use of leeches. For the first forty-eight hours after treatment the itching completely disappears; after a few days, however, it returns. This is because raktmokśan acts directly on the dhātu without treating the doṣa. When doṣa again accumulates in the dhātu, Dr. Joshi explained, the eczema recurs. In this case, then, it is the treatment of dhātu through raktmokśan that is a "palliation."

Different practitioners may differ in their emphasis on doṣa or dhātu, partially according to the leanings of their principal mentors. Dr. Upadhyay told me that the difference in focus on doṣa or dhātu was partly geographical: *Caraka Saṃhitā*, in which doṣa is emphasized, has been more influential in North India; *Aṣṭāṅga Saṁgraha* (considered one of the three most important ancient texts, along with *Caraka Saṃhitā* and *Suśruta Saṃhitā*) has been more influential in South India. Dr. Madhava is a Maharashtrian practitioner who learned clinical Ayurveda primarily from her father, who, she told me, based his practice primarily on *Aṣṭāṅga Saṁgraha*. Following him, she argued that one could not prescribe medicine merely for doṣa, but must treat dhātu as well. For instance, for one patient with throat inflammation she prescribed six different medicines—two to purge the increased doṣa, two to act directly on the disease, and two as "tonics" to restore the dhātu. Dr. Upadhyay, on the other hand, tends to emphasize doṣa in his treatment. One of his patients suffered from migraines, eczema, and fatigue. When she asked him whether the tablets he had prescribed were for her headaches, he replied, "For me there is no difference in your problems. . . . Basically you have excess pitta in your body."

If clinical gazes move quickly from doṣa to dhātu to disease and back again, they also move flexibly among the many possibilities for imagining their object, particularly when focused on doṣa. In narratives of soma and season, doṣa appears to be a substance. It may be said, for example, that the kapha that is accumulated in the winter begins to soften and melt in the spring. Then wherever it accumulates in the body, it causes distress. Dr. Joshi defined doṣa as "functional entities." Of kapha he said, "Wherever there are secretions, body secretions, wherever there is lubrication, wherever there are joints; so joining, lubrication, and the fluid part of the body are maintained by kapha." Yet notice how these "functions" of kapha were substantialized in his discussion of diabetes. In Ayurveda, he began, astringent drugs are a common treatment for madhumeha (diabetes).

Their effect is to reduce the liquification of the dhātu, and they are useful no matter which doṣa is predominant. Diabetes may show a predominance of any of the three doṣa. Patients suffering from kaphaja diabetes are bulky. They should restrict their food intake and spend less time in relaxation. Kaphaja diabetics can also benefit from pancakarma since their diabetes usually involves *śrota* dūṣti (derangement of the bodily channels). Two methods of pancakarma, *vaman* (induced projectile vomiting) and *virecan* (induced purgation or diarrhea), can be used to open up these channels.[19] Before the disturbed doṣa can be removed from the abdomen in these ways, it must first be drawn into the abdomen by one of three means. First, the practitioner can give medicines to increase the doṣa, thus forcing it to overflow the area where it has accumulated and move into the abdomen. Second, the practitioner can attempt to wash the doṣa into the abdomen by saturating the body with oils. Third, if the doṣa is mixed with āma, the practitioner can try to ripen or metabolize the doṣa by giving the patient medicines to increase the agni.[20]

In this narrative doṣa first seems to be inert, a mass to be liquified, and later, when mixed with āma, almost organic, a substance to be ripened or digested. In another conversation Dr. Joshi told me that *dama* or *śwās* (asthma), which is due to vāta and kapha doṣa, can also be treated with pancakarma. First, the excess vāyu is removed by means of purgation, and then vasti is used to stimulate anuloman. Finally, the excess kapha is removed with emesis. Despite the assertion by many practitioners that doṣa is a function and not a substance, it frequently *behaves* as a substance to great clinical purpose in narratives of disease and healing. It is only the imagination of doṣa as a substance that enables treatments in which doṣa can be softened, ripened, redirected, or removed.

At one point when I was struggling, as I periodically did, to understand doṣa, Dr. Tiwari, a professor of śarīr kriya at one of the colleges, took it upon himself to edify me. In the slow sonorous voice that led students to complain of the boredom of his lectures, he began by enumerating the qualities of vāta: dryness, coldness, lightness, roughness, and fineness (*sūkṣmata,* which also means subtlety). The enlargement of the spleen, he explained, is due to the fineness of vāta doṣa. When the *medh* dhātu or fat in the spleen is diminished, the empty space that is left is filled by vāta, which, because of its fineness, is able to penetrate through tiny channels into the organ. The enlargement of any organ, he informed me, is due to vāta. Even in this brief narrative, as in Dr. Joshi's narrative of the role of kapha in diabetes, it is apparent that the various qualities of a doṣa enable it to play particular parts at particular moments of pathogenesis, as well as to be susceptible to particular manipulations at particular moments of treatment.

The versatile way in which the qualities of doṣa can be maneuvered for diagnosis and treatment is further illustrated in Dr. Tiwari's exegesis of angina, which was touched on at the beginning of this chapter. Heart pain, he began methodically, is considered to be kaphaja, pittaja, or vātaja, depending on whether it is experienced during the early stage of digestion associated with kapha, the middle stage associated with pitta, or the final stage associated with vāta. Nonetheless, there is a verse in *Caraka Saṃhitā* that prescribes five medicines for heart pain, regardless of the doṣa involved. You will say, he went on, how is this possible? After all, Caraka "is a big man for vāta, pitta, and kapha." What is the effect of these drugs? He sketched a picture of the heart and pulmonary artery on a scrap of paper. In angina, he said, the artery becomes constricted due to dryness and in some cases due to accumulation of cholesterol. What is the aim of treatment? The artery must be opened. Since rukśa guṇa is obstructive, one must give a snigdh substance that will oppose rukśa and an akāśalike (etheric, here signifying light, subtle) substance that will oppose pṛthvī (in this case, solidity). Such drugs will expand the space within the artery. Since dryness is associated with both vāta and pitta, drugs that act against dryness are effective for both vātika and paittika angina.

In clinical narratives of illness doṣa can fluctuate greatly in substantiality. This is one reason the separation of physiology and anatomy enforced by modern educational structures may interfere with a doṣic diagnosis. At one moment in the narrative of somatic processes doṣa may be considered a substance, while at another moment in that narrative it may be considered a process or principle. Kapha may be physical mucus, for example, or again it may be the principle and process of adhesion that allows a tumor to form. I listened once while a professor tried to drum this paradox of doṣa into his first-year students during a lecture in Hindi on padārth vijñān, the basic principles of Ayurveda:

> So in the body, what increases or what decreases? In the body what substance is "responsible," [English word] what "qualities" are "re-

sponsible," what actions [karma] are "responsible," what do we call them? Doṣa, the qualities [guṇa] of doṣa, the actions of doṣa. It is one of these that increases. It is one of these that decreases. Understand? And in that state what is produced? Disease is produced. So when is disease produced? When there has been an increase of doṣa—whichever doṣa are involved—in the form of substance [dravya], in the form of quality, or in the form of function. Take pitta, for example. Suppose pitta has increased a little, and suppose that the form of pitta that has increased is the "volume." So what do we call this? Substance. Such as "acidity." At other times the amount of substance is exactly what it is supposed to be, and only the quality has increased.

Consider this example: sometimes after one has eaten something or for some other reason, "gas" increases in the body. What do we call that in Ayurveda? What happens because of that? The "volume" of *what* has increased? What do we call "gas"? We call it vāyu right? So vāyu has increased. How did it increase? Its substantiality [*dravyata*] increased. First its "volume" was "one hundred c.c." [cubic centimeters]; now it has become "a hundred and fifty c.c." So the "volume" increased; the substantiality increased.

At other times the quality increases. One person's stomach may inflate. Another person may not have that problem, but his skin may crack and become dry. This often occurs in certain seasons. The body becomes dry; the skin cracks. Dryness occurs. What is that? The substance has not increased. What did then? The quality increased. Understand? The quality increased—that is, the dry quality of vāyu increased. Then at other times the substantiality—that is the "volume"—remains as it is; the quality remains as it is, but the action increases, such as in "Parkinson's," the hand trembles; movement increases; trembling increases. In that instance the substance has not increased; the quality has not increased, so what has increased? There has been an increase in the action [of vāyu].

So how does disease occur? It occurs from increase. How many kinds of increase? Three kinds. Either the substance increases—that is, the doṣa in its substantial form increases—or the quality of the doṣa increases or the action of the doṣa increases. Or two out of the three may increase. Or all three may increase together. It depends on what kind of illness it is.

Such a tidy and systematic division of doṣa into three manifestations of substance, quality, and action is not always discernible in clinical reasoning. There doṣa may seem to straddle such categories in a less organized manner, sliding with more fluidity among materiality, process, and quality. For instance, in speaking to me of the treatment of a patient suffering from gallstones, Dr. Joshi said that it was necessary to manage both kapha and pitta. The gall bladder, he said, is the seat of pitta, but the formation of stones is a kapha problem. The treatment he had prescribed would force the gall bladder to contract. The patient's gall bladder was no longer producing pitta. When he spoke here of managing pitta, he was speaking of a metabolic process, but when he spoke of restoring the gall bladder's ability to produce pitta, he was speaking of a substance. The one-to-one relationship between sign and referent generally enforced in modern science is here diverted into a network of multiple meanings. A polyvalence that might seem, to a scientific mind, to have its true provenance in poetry is here proving itself integral to a train of clinical thought. Here the dominance of relationships of resemblance over relationships of reference that infused poetic Ayurvedic texts is equally important to contemporary clinical reasoning.

In the words of Dr. Vijayan, "Whenever you explain an Ayurvedic principle, you must be fluid in your explanation, in your thinking." Dr. Vijayan once spoke to me in some detail about the neurological illness of one of his patients. After explaining how *sāmakapha* (kapha mixed with āma) was obstructing vāta in the neural pathways, he added that this was his "theoretical understanding" of the illness at that time. Later it might change. Over time I realized that for him diagnosis was the story of an etiology in flux, in which doṣic signs were always available to new narrative constructions. As Dr. Pathi stated in a lecture on Ayurveda before a group of industrial scientists, "The human being is not standardized by God." However, he continued, there must be standardization somewhere. That is why, he said, Ayurveda has divided the somatic continuum into the three doṣa. Doṣa, in other words, are as much heuristic devices as objective facts.

It is therefore understandable that a biomedical doctor who authored a book on Ayurveda quoted to me by a lay friend when I was first wrestling with the idea of doṣa stated that doṣa should be understood as symbols—that is, in this context, metaphorical signs. As symbols, the doctor suggested, doṣa can have different meanings at every instance of reference. Yet how far such an explanation is acceptable to Ayurvedic practitioners themselves is suggested by the following discussion between Dr. Upadhyay and his class of North American college students. As an introduction to the ideas of vāta, pitta, and kapha, he told the students that there are three main "functions" in the universe: "movement, change, and form." He then suggested a correlation between these functions and the sun, moon, and air. Sun, he said, corresponds to change, moon to form, and air to movement. At this, one of the students asked, "You're speaking symbolically?" "No," Dr. Upadhyay responded. "Actually." After several students contested these correspondences, a graduate student in folklore asked whether the sun corresponds to change because it transforms molecules in such great numbers at such great speed. Dr. Upadhyay congratulated her for anticipating one of his points. After more skeptical or confused responses from the students, he stated that heat is always connected to change. A little later he added, "I want you to think beyond physics to philosophy." Here the folklore student interjected, "For me it is poetics. It makes sense if I think of it as metaphor." This time Dr. Upadhyay did not argue but simply went on to say that in Ayurveda, "We talk about sun, moon, and air in the human body." He wrote air, fire, and water on the blackboard and underneath them, vāta, pitta, and kapha.

This was not the only time in exchanges with Ayurvedic doctors when literality seemed to slip into metaphor or metaphor into literality. Dr. Pathi, for example, often made what he called a "comparison" or sometimes a "correlation" between an Ayurvedic phenomenon and a biomedical phenomenon. In a paper on diabetes he stated, "As ojas is sweet in nature it can be correlated to glucose." Similarly in conversation, he told me that the "osmotic pressures" involved in the elimination of waste products (mala) through urine and sweat can be compared to triglycerides in the blood. They are "not exactly like that but can be compared," he emphasized. On later reflection it seemed to me that he was not simply asserting that the osmotic pressures are *like* triglycerides, metaphorically (or iconically, in Peircian terms) sharing certain characteristics with triglycerides. Rather he meant that the osmotic pressures are *almost* triglycerides but *not exactly*. That a comparison with triglycerides can help us to understand osmotic pressures is only part of his point. The other part of his point, which arises from the "not exactly," is that the meaning of osmotic pressures is sliding toward the meaning of triglycerides, coming close to equivalence but falling short. The "not exactly" throws as much doubt on the metaphoricity as it does on the literality.

This seemingly casual slippage between literary figure and reality took on the cast of an ideological stance during one conversation with Dr. Upadhyay. I had asked him what he thought about Leslie's assessment of Ayurveda as an aesthetic rather than a science. He replied that from Leslie's point of view it was perfectly reasonable. Drawing on a familiar cliché of North American life, he argued that Leslie lives in a materialistic society where everything is measured in dollars except for a private realm for emotions off to one side. Therefore, for Leslie and for Americans in general, he went on, to understand Asian medicine as an aesthetic may be necessary. He referred to padārth vijñān, the Ayurvedic subject from which the lecture was quoted above. In secondary school this same term serves as the Hindi gloss for modern physics. Yet this term actually means something closer to the meaning of words. You see, he said, for us everything proceeds from *śabd* (word, sound). Drawing on a cliché myself, I said, "In the West we separate language from matter." "Yes," he agreed, "but *we* do not; the science of language and the science of matter are one in Indian philosophy." Saying this, he brought both hands together over his desk and locked his fingers momentarily. So there you have the aesthetic, he said, holding out his palm to me and then sitting back in his chair with an air of finality.

Indeed Monier-Williams defines *padārtha* as both "the meaning of a word" and "that which corresponds to the meaning of a word, a thing, material object, man, person" (1993 [1899], 583), whereas my Hindi–English dictionary defines it as "1. the meaning of a term. 2. an object. 3. a substance, material; *phys.* matter. 4. a product. 5. aim, end" (McGregor 1993, 598). The professor of padārth quoted above translated padārth for me as "matter" but would not translate padārth vijñān as "physical science." At least some of his students, however, since they had taken modern physics under the same title in secondary school, still thought of his subject as "physical science." This is perhaps partly why they considered it the most difficult and mystifying subject they encountered in their first year of Ayurvedic college. Meanwhile, their professor, after listing the causes of disease in one lecture as *kal* (season), karma (action), and *arth,* described the last in this way:

> So listening is one arth; seeing is one arth. Arth, that is—? Why did I say arth? Who can tell me? Why do we call words and so on arth? I have told you this in class several times. Why do we call sensory objects [*viṣay*] arth? What do we call words? We call them arth also. Arth is the name of what? Whatever thing is taken, is acquired, whatever is sought after [*jijñāsit,* describing an object of curiosity or inquiry], whatever we desire to have, what is it called? It is called arth. Understand? Suppose there is a thing, and suppose that we experience some "curiosity" about it. What happens? Either we touch it or we perceive its appearance or its sound or its "taste" or its "smell." We have five "sensory organs." Therefore we can investigate it in five ways. That investigation can be of how many kinds? Either it is by sound or by touch or by appearance or by flavor or by smell. What do we call the five objects [of this inquiry]? What do we call them? We call them arth.

Arth, then, is an object of sensory awareness; the decision can be endlessly deferred as to whether that object is linguistic or material, meaning or entity. Doṣa and other somatic phenomena surely owe some of their clinically useful ambiguities, moves, and metamorphoses to this philosophical coalescence of word and world.[21]

Symptom and Metonym

The technologies and methodologies introduced into Ayurveda through modern teaching hospitals and pharmaceutical companies encourage a diagnosis that rests on a modern semiotics, a relationship between symptom or medical sign and disease. Indeed practitioners make easy references to "symptom" and "disease" in their talk. Yet I question how far the semiotics of contemporary Ayurvedic diagnosis resembles a modern semiotics of symptoms and disease. In the modern semiotics of diagnosis symptoms signify disease as a nosographic entity that is prior to and distinct from the symptoms themselves. As Barthes states: "Of course the syntagmatic configuration of medical signs, of articulated signs, refers to a signified. This medical signified is a site, a location in the nosographic context." He goes on to point out that this site is "quite simply a name, it is the disease as a name" (1988, 209). This insight is owed, he tells us, to Foucault, and the next insight, we can imagine, though he refers only to "certain philosophers," is owed at least in part to Derrida. For he continues to analyze a certain circularity in the diagnostic process:

> To read disease is to give it a name; and from that moment—it is here moreover that matters become rather subtle—there is a kind of perfect reversibility, which is that of language itself, a dizzying reversibility between the signifier and the signified; the disease is defined as a name, it is defined as a concurrence of signs: but the concurrence of signs is oriented and fulfilled only within the name of the disease, there is an infinite circuit. The diagnostic reading, *i.e.,* the reading of medical signs, seems to conclude by naming: the medical signified exists only when named; here we recognize the critique of the sign made nowadays by certain philosophers: we can manipulate the signifieds of a sign or signs only by naming these signifieds, but, *by this very act of nomination, we reconvert the signified into a signifier* (1988, 210; emphasis added).

Barthes concludes by noting that although the chain of signifiers is therefore theoretically interminable, it can be halted in practice. In biomedicine, diagnostic signification ends with the application of therapy to a particular disease name.

The relationship between symptom and disease is, however, quite different in contemporary Ayurvedic diagnosis. To begin with, consider the Ayurvedic word usually translated as symptom: lakṣaṇ. Lakṣaṇ, as I briefly suggested in chapter 3, can be more simply and aptly translated as "feature" or "characteristic." One speaks not only of the lakṣaṇ of disease, but also of the lakṣaṇ of health, not to mention the lakṣaṇ of physicians, the lakṣaṇ of animals, the lakṣaṇ of chemical elements. One expert lecturing in English to a group of foreign health practitioners listed the "symptoms of health" as the equilibrium of the doṣa, agni, dhātu, and mala. Here the word "symptoms," which we can assume he automatically substitutes for lakṣaṇ when speaking in English, carries the sense of "characteristics." Let us listen in again for a moment to the professor of padārth vijñān as he struggles to convey the meaning of lakṣaṇ to his first-year students, still steeped in the concepts of modern biology, chemistry, and physics that they studied in secondary school:

> What is lakṣaṇ? The "special features" [English words] of something. Understand? Modern science has agreed on certain lakṣaṇ. For example, "chlorine." What are the lakṣaṇ of "chlorine"? Actually, the "periodic table" itself was made up from the lakṣaṇ that should be in one "particular substance," one "element" and not in another. For example, the "number of electrons, atomic number." No other [element] has the same number as "chlorine." Therefore, if you want to "define chlorine," if you want to "define iron," if you want to "define gold," if you want to "define any element," then what do you do? Whatever special dharma [duty] they perform, we call it their lakṣaṇ. Their special dharma is their lakṣaṇ. That is, whatever "peculiar" thing, whatever "specialty," whatever "special features" are in something, those are its lakṣaṇ.

Lakṣaṇ, then, according to this professor, should be understood as the defining characteristics (even the sacred task) of something or someone.

There are several other Sanskrit words that are roughly synonymous with lakṣaṇ and occasionally appear in Ayurvedic texts, including modern textbooks. Caraka lists these terms in chapter 1 of the "Nidānasthānam" (section on etiology and diagnosis) (P. V. Sharma 1981, 1:252). Of these, the ones I have heard or read most often besides lakṣaṇ are *rūpa* and liṅga. Rūpa, which in its broader sense simply means form, appearance, or aspect, is sometimes used because it provides a clearer contrast with *purvarūpa,* early manifestations of oncoming illness indicating an inappropriate accumulation of doṣa somewhere in the body. While the purvarūpa are mild and imply little distress if any to the patient, the rūpa are more pronounced, appearing only when the pathogenic process has resulted in full-blown illness.[22] Liṅga, on the other hand, was defined in the following way by a group of vaidyas in their testimony to the Madras Report: "Liṅga is the extraordinary mark, at the sight of which, we can infer the existence of an object possessing that mark, as we infer the presence of fire in a mountain by merely seeing the smoke" (quoted in Government of Madras 1923, part 2:78).[23] Indeed all of the words translated as symptom seem to refer to a metonymic relationship. This conception of lakṣaṇ as manifest features or metonyms of disease is reminiscent of Foucault's (1973, 91) account of the eighteenth-century European conception of symptoms as visible forms "rooted" in the invisible.

Occasionally the slippage between symptom and lakṣaṇ led to some confused exchanges between me and certain vaidyas, particularly those with little exposure to biomedical usages of symptom and disease. I was observing one small-town practitioner, Vd. Rai, who had learned Ayurveda partly through an apprenticeship and partly through a correspondence course, when he consulted with a woman who complained of weakness, pain in her solar plexus, and shortness of breath. There are "two symptoms," Vd. Rai said, using the English word: first, cholesterol, and second, gastric trouble, which can also put pressure on the heart. He advised her to have her cholesterol level checked and to avoid fried foods, ghee, eggs, and meat. Later, confused by his use of the word symptoms, I asked for the Hindi word and was told "lakṣaṇ." When I asked him to clarify the woman's problem, he told me that heart trouble was the disease and that cholesterol and stomach pain were the lakṣaṇ. I responded that earlier I had understood him to say that heart trouble might be a result of gastric trouble. He said yes, this was possible. The problem is heart pain, but it may result from either cholesterol or gastric trouble.

Later I realized that my confusion stemmed from my expectation that diseases precede and produce symptoms rather than the other way around, just as in a commonsense understanding of semiotics, a referent is presumed to precede its sign. This implicit chronology and therefore confusion is entirely avoided, however, if lakṣaṇ are understood as possible features or characteristics of disease: a *feature* of a heart disorder need not be specified as to whether it is a cause, a result, or simply a correlate. In a later conversation Vd. Rai told me that different "symptoms" (again the English word) are recognized in allopathy than are recognized in Ayurveda. For example, in a patient suffering from a cold, an allopath may observe a vitamin C deficiency, while an Ayurvedic practitioner may observe kaphaja *vikār* (disorder). Each kind of medicine recognizes different lakṣaṇ. Again puzzled, I asked if in that example, the cold was the disease and the kaphaja disorder was the lakṣaṇ. Yes, he said enthusiastically, adding in English, "very good idea." Still puzzled, I asked, "But kaphaja vikār is the *cause* of the cold, right?" Yes, he said. For Vd. Rai, then, lakṣaṇ can as easily refer to causes of disease as to consequences. The priority of the signified is thereby disrupted.

If deciphering the signifying chains of lakṣaṇ does not necessarily render disease as a separate and prior entity, neither does it necessarily end in the disease name and the inception of therapy. We learned above that for Dr. Joshi mere aggravated doṣa that have not yet accumulated in a particular dhātu do not yet constitute a disease. Nonetheless, such a condition can and should be treated *before* it develops into a disease. As one hospital practitioner told me, if no name can be assigned to a particular illness, it can still be treated based on "symptoms" (read lakṣaṇ). A Bengali vaidya testifying in the Madras Report (Roy in Government of Madras 1923) noted that in Ayurveda the fixing of a name to the disease is neither sufficient nor necessary to treatment. Illnesses can assume numerous forms, and illnesses without names must be treated in order to address the derangement of the doṣa.

To complicate matters, something may be a lakṣaṇ in one context and a "disease" in another. This possibility is explicitly acknowledged by Caraka in the last chapter of the "Nidānasthānam" on the diagnosis of *apasmāra* (generally equated with epilepsy): "In the context of wider knowledge, the symptoms [liṅga] gathered here are themselves diseases [rog], but in the present context they are symptoms, and not diseases" (P. V. Sharma 1981, 1:298).[24] A week after the conference on Ayurvedic research I was talking with Dr. Upadhyay. He told me that another speaker at the conference had commented that if Caraka were alive today, he would surely agree that *śoth* (swelling, inflammation) is a symptom and not a disease. Although Dr. Upadhyay had let the comment pass at the time, he strongly disagreed. In allopathy, he told me, śoth is certainly a symptom, but in Ayurveda it can be either a symptom or a disease, depending on the condition. In pandu (anemia) it may be a lakṣaṇ, but in other conditions it may be a disease.

At the conference, Dr. Upadhyay himself made a statement that I heard him repeat in other public settings, to the effect that Ayurvedic understanding of the "disease process" depends on an elaborate network of lakṣaṇ. Does this remark contradict the frequent assertion in twentieth-century Ayurvedic literature (particularly that published in English) and among Ayurvedic practitioners that it is allopathy that treats the symptoms while Ayurveda focuses on the root problem?[25] I think not. A focus on lakṣaṇ does not mean a focus on the less crucial half of the dyadic connection between symptom and disease, but rather a focus on the many significatory linkages between the various stages of the disease process. One professor of kāyacikitsā put it well when, in coaching a student for his upcoming M.D. exam, he said that biomedicine treats either the cause *or* the symptoms, while Ayurveda treats the *saṁprāpti,* the whole course of the disease. Students are taught that there are six stages of saṁprāpti (known also as *kriyākāla*): accumulation of doṣa, spreading of doṣa into other parts of the body, further spreading into the sites of other doṣa, localization in one dhātu or part of the body, the appearance of illness, and finally differentiation, a phase during which the illness gives rise to multiple problems and becomes irreversible. As Dr. Upadhyay stated in one lecture to his foreign students, the practitioner must know which stage of saṁprāpti the illness has reached in order to effectively intervene. If, he said, you treat a vāyu disorder that is not yet localized *as if* it were localized, then it will become localized.

When in a later class Dr. Upadhyay asked his North American students how they understood the six stages of disease, one student said that the first few stages seemed to involve only symptoms, while the later stages involved the full development of the disease. Dr. Upadhyay responded that this was basically correct. This generalization accords with Vd. Rai's recognition of certain symptoms as causes of disease. It also accords with Dr. Joshi's remark that an identifiable disease does not occur until the aggravated doṣa have localized to upset a particular dhātu or organ. Caraka wrote that vikār (one of the words considered synonymous with rog, the usual translation for disease) occurs when all three factors of nidān (here meaning etiology), doṣa, and dūṣya are strongly involved (P. V. Sharma 1981, 1:269).[26] The first disease discussed by Caraka in that same chapter is *jwar,* or fever, which in biomedicine is generally not considered a disease at all but a symptom. In the terms laid down by Caraka, however, jwar qualifies as a rog because in every instance of fever there is a derangement of ras dhātu (usually associated with blood plasma), the first dhātu formed after the digestion of food.

Caraka also states that disease (far from being fully specified in its name) is known through nidān (also known as *hetu*), *purvarūp* (early signs), *rūp* (manifest appearance), *upaśāya* (responsiveness to particular treatments), and saṁprāpti. Fever may, for instance, be due to any of eight causes, seven of which are particular combinations of aggravated doṣa and one of which is an external event such as injury or a neighbor's curse. Each of these causes is associated with a different list of rūp. As Dr. Upadhyay cautioned in another class session, "If it is one symptom, one disease, and one treatment, that is not Ayurveda." In his clinic, he went on, there are ten different patients suffering from "hypertension." Only one or two are on "antihypertensive" drugs as such. Some are receiving antipitta treatment; some are receiving treatment for poor digestion; some are receiving treatment for anxiety. Similarly, cancer, he noted in another session, is a "definite entity" in allopathy. In Ayurveda, on the other hand, each type of cancer falls into a very different category. A metastasized carcinoma, for instance, might be diagnosed as *gulma* (nodule or tumor). "As far as cancer is concerned," he said, "it is only the manifested form of disease." A disease, he concluded, is not just a disease; it is a "manifestation of things that are going on," things, I might add, such as hetu, saṁprāpti, and purvarūp.

The level of attention paid to a disease name, particularly one that can be correlated to a biomedical disease name, differs significantly from one Ayurvedic practice to another, depending on how linked that practice is with modern diagnostic technologies. Recall, for example, how adamant Dr. Karnik in chapter 2 was about the need for a proper identification of disease. This was a position he took again at the research conference when, responding to Dr. Upadhyay's emphasis on lakṣaṇ, he said that the practitioner cannot treat the symptoms in themselves and must diagnose the disease. Even between Dr. Upadhyay, a private practitioner, and Dr. Joshi, a hospital practitioner who daily negotiated between modern and doṣic diagnostic methods, there were significant differences in the importance they gave to particular disease names. I heard Dr. Joshi mention on one occasion that "amoebiasis" is a great problem in India. By contrast, Dr. Upadhyay was quick to dismiss the importance of amoebiasis in an exchange with a patient suffering from diarrhea and cramps. When the patient reported that his stool test was positive for amoebas, Dr. Upadhyay responded, "Our approach is different. We are interested," he said, in the "host factor." It is very rarely, he went on, that he prescribes medicines that are "anti-amoebic." Slapping the lab report with his hand, he said that the loose motions and pain might not result from the amoebas at all. Fifty percent of his patients, he said, probably tested positive for amoebas. In his opinion, he told the man, this was a "chronic āma case." Even after hearing all this, the patient mentioned that the Ayurvedic drug *kuṭaj* had been proven to be anti-amoebic. Dr. Upadhyay replied that he would not prescribe kuṭaj as anti-amoebic per se. In fact, in this case, he could just as well prescribe *bilwa,* which had not been proven to be anti-amoebic. Although the patient protested that every time he had these symptoms, he was diagnosed with amoebas, Dr. Upadhyay remained unimpressed.

The relative unimportance of the name of the disease in certain contemporary Ayurvedic practices plays up the seeming preoccupation with disease nomenclature in biomedicine, where even the sadness resulting from too many gray days, which is little more than a collection of symptoms linked experientially to a possible cause, is rendered into a syndrome. Might this preoccupation have to do with the dependence of diagnosis and treatment on a sign-referent or symptom-disease relationship? Unlike doṣic diagnosis, biomedical diagnosis has difficulty making sense out of multiple stray symptoms unlinked to any one referent. In a kind of medical double-think, disorders such as attention deficit disorder (ADD) or seasonal affective disorder (SAD) or premenstrual syndrome (PMS) or post-traumatic stress disorder (PTSD) are first fashioned out of and then detected through a particular cluster of symptoms, making the disease name itself seem superfluous.[27] It is in such examples, approaching what Barthes (1988) would call autonymy (diseases that are one with their symptoms), that we glimpse most clearly the supplementarity that permits a modern notion of disease. As Derrida has written,

> There is a fatal necessity, inscribed in the very functioning of the sign, that the substitute make one forget the vicariousness of its own function and make itself pass for the plenitude of a speech whose deficiency and infirmity it nevertheless only *supplements.* For the concept of the supplement . . . harbors within itself two significations whose cohabitation is as strange as it is necessary. The supplement adds itself, it is a surplus, a plenitude enriching another plenitude, the *fullest measure* of presence. . . . But the supplement supplements. It adds only to replace. It intervenes or insinuates itself *in-the-place-of;* if it fills it, it is as if one fills a void. If it represents and makes an image, it is by the anterior default of a presence. . . . Somewhere, something can be filled up of itself, can accomplish itself, only by allowing itself to be filled through sign and proxy. The sign is always the supplement of the thing itself (1976, 144–145).

This neatly sums up, it seems to me, the position of disease in biomedicine—that deficient plenitude, that "anterior default of presence," the presumed organic entity that lies *behind* and prior to all manifestation but which, after all, is itself a name, halted at the status of signified only by becoming an object of treatment. By contrast, in Ayurveda, the signifying chain does not end in naming the disease, a definite, if deficient, nosographic entity, but continues along a syntagmatic sequence of signs that are causes, omens, symptoms, manifestations, and pathways in a narrative of doṣic crisis. The inception of a course of treatment does not halt this narrative, sealing the disease into the position of signified, but rather participates in the narrative, keeping the disease open as a sign that can yield further meanings. The fullness of presence of disease as a single prior signified is never pretended. What the ancient and medieval vaidyas most seem to offer contemporary practitioners who wish to avail themselves of it is not exactly a description or representation of disease or the doṣic body, but rather a somatic syntax through which illness can be rewritten as cure.

six Medical Simulations

In chapter 4, I recounted that an Ayurvedic student was upset that an itinerant vaidya dispensing medicines out of his tent might be taken as representative of Ayurveda. Yet even though urban practitioners distance themselves from certain "folk" practitioners with such remarks, they also at times suspect such practitioners of esoteric knowledge. Ayurvedic students speak of secret rural remedies; pharmaceutical agents search for miracle herbs known only to *ādivāsī* ("tribal") peoples. These images arise within national and transnational modernities that necessarily carry ambivalent images of the "folk" and the "primitive." Only within this ambivalence can the noninstitutional practitioner be envisioned as both the vaidya in his tent, which one student laments is the popular image of Ayurveda, and the pulse expert, which, as we learn below, another student regrets that she will never become. Images of "folk" medicine therefore often thrive in metropolitan practices, taking advantage of the way that modern disciplinary knowledge is shadowed by ambivalent desires for that which evades its grasp. The more that professional Ayurveda resembles biomedicine in its particular rationalities, the less prepared it is to satisfy these desires, which are focused on "tradition" or on the promise of cure or—better yet—on a "tradition" that is in itself a promise of cure. There are practitioners, however, working in the interstices between institutional Ayurveda and "folk" practice, who make it their job to satisfy those amorphous desires for a healing tradition, in every sense of that phrase. Dr. Mistry is one such practitioner whose talent is to create the effect of folk medicine and professionalism simultaneously by making use of the symbols and substances of both. If, however, his practice seems a simulation of medicine, it also calls attention to the element of simulation in any medical practice.

Jean Baudrillard has written:

> "Someone who feigns an illness can simply go to bed and pretend he is ill. Someone who simulates an illness produces in himself some of the symptoms" (Littre). Thus feigning or dissimulating leaves the reality principle intact: the difference is always clear, it is only masked; whereas simulation threatens the difference between "true" and "false," between "real" and "imaginary." Since the simulator produces "true" symptoms, is he or she ill or not? The simulator cannot be treated objectively either as ill, or as not ill. Psychology and medicine stop at this point, before a thereafter undiscoverable truth of the illness. . . . What can medicine do with something which floats on either side of illness, on either side of health, or with the reduplication of illness in a discourse that is no longer true or false (Baudrillard 1988, 168)?

Here Baudrillard uses the example of illness to distinguish between mere falseness and simulation. In my discussion of Dr. Mistry the focus is shifted from the example of illness to the example of cure. Baudrillard asks (and, more important, deconstructs) the question of whether a simulating patient who produces "true" symptoms is ill or not. This chapter, in turn, asks the question of whether a simulating doctor who produces "true" wellness is a doctor or a quack. Just as simulated illness tends to erode the distinction between true and false illness, so it may be that simulated cure tends to erode the distinction between true and false medicine.

Actual healing through false medicine has been framed by modern medical science within the concept of the "placebo effect." This concept, however, allows us to bracket simulation off to one side of medical practice, leaving the dichotomy of truth and falseness intact. Baudrillard's analysis of simulation and, even more tellingly, Taussig's (1993) analysis of the mimesis involved in any act of signification suggest, on the contrary, that simulation is integral to medical practice and is already troubling the binary of truth and falsehood, which is a foundation of scientific knowledge. I draw here on these analyses to trace the mimetic intricacies of medical simulation in Dr. Mistry's Ayurvedic practice in an Indian metropolis. The "magical" ability of the sign, identified by Taussig (1993, 233), to "spill over" and reconfigure the referent accounts for the miraculous ability of the doctor's pulse diagnosis to reconfigure the patient's illness. Simultaneously, the commodity value of pulse reading as a sign of traditional wisdom and the political value of pulse reading as a precolonial practice not assimilable to European-styled medical training account in part for the doctor's enormous popularity and commercial success. In his own way, then, Dr. Mistry participates, like other practitioners, in addressing, or perhaps exploiting, the political imbalances inherited from the colonial era. My interest in his story is, once again, not to determine or police the boundaries of "true" Ayurveda, but rather to examine more closely how the effects of "true" Ayurveda are created. I am interested in tracing how the effects of authenticity are generated rather than in establishing the boundaries beyond which something must be considered inauthentic. Ultimately, the market-driven and politically motivated mimesis at the heart of Dr. Mistry's signifying practice disturbs not only a notion of medical authenticity that is crucial to biomedicine, but also a notion of cultural authenticity that is crucial to anthropology.[1]

Undisciplined Pulses

I first heard about Dr. Mistry from one of his patients. The patient told me that Dr. Mistry was a specialist in nāḍī parikśan, or pulse examination. Through pulse he was able to diagnose not only which of the three doṣa were disturbed, but also the exact symptoms the patient was experiencing. The patient said that Dr. Mistry had accurately diagnosed his problems and had given him medicines that had an immediate beneficial effect. I was intrigued. I was, after all, committed to tracing the differences between the standardized Ayurveda taught and practiced in modern institutional settings and any Ayurveda that might be eluding that standardized version. Since the elaborate type of pulse diagnosis Dr. Mistry was reputed to practice is not taught in Ayurvedic institutions, he seemed to fall into the second group. Even so, I did not assume that Dr. Mistry could be considered a "traditional" vaidya. Although some doctors I knew referred to "traditional" vaidyas, I was skeptical of this category for both theoretical and practical reasons. Theoretically I, like many of us, had come to understand that "tradition" is a category invented in recent times as a counterpoint to modernity, while practically I knew that Ayurvedic hospitals and colleges modeled on biomedical institutions had existed for the better part of a century. It was very rare to meet a cosmopolitan practitioner who had had no encounters with such institutions.[2] Nonetheless Dr. Mistry's exclusive reliance on pulse diagnosis was clear evidence of his distance from institutional Ayurveda.

The pulse diagnosis of particular illnesses was introduced into Ayurveda relatively late, with the appearance in the thirteenth century of a text on nāḍī parikśan entitled the *Śarangadhara Saṃhitā,* believed to have been developed primarily from Tantric and Unani sources (Upadhyaya 1986; Rai et al. 1981). Even pulse examination to detect excess doṣa was introduced into Ayurveda as part of an eightfold diagnosis only in 600 A.D., long after *Caraka Saṃhitā* had been first composed.[3] One prominent Ayurvedic practitioner and scholar with whom I spoke scorned practitioners who diagnosed only through pulse. "These are not Ayurvedic doctors. I'll tell you: Ayurveda is a more thorough, elaborate examination."

Nonetheless, a practitioner's ability to diagnose a patient's illness simply by feeling his or her pulse is often taken as the quintessential sign of "traditional" Ayurveda. The powerful mystique of this diagnosis is pervasive among rural and metropolitan Indians and foreigners alike. One North American told me that he had been accurately diagnosed as having recovered from hepatitis six months earlier by a vaidya who examined only his pulse. In the hill station where Vd. Rai and Vd. Shastri practiced, a Sikh "sexologist" (as one of his multilingual signboards read) diagnosed solely through pulse, dispensing medicines prepared according to his family's secret formulae for every kind of sexual and reproductive disorder.[4] Vd. Rai, who had learned much of his Ayurvedic theory and pharmacopoeia from a correspondence course and from drug companies but his pulse diagnosis from apprenticeship, confidently rattled off the problems he detected in a patient's pulse often before hearing his or her complaints. He patiently tried to describe to me the pulse movements that signified such illnesses as viral fever, stomach problems, cough, burning hands, or headache. Outside of town, in villages half a day's journey away, I was told that Vd. Rai could diagnose any illness through pulse. This mystique haunts even the imagination of certain urban professionals. One Ayurvedic professor in his fifties told me that he had known only one teacher who was able to diagnose illness through pulse and that teacher had never taught the technique to any of his students. This type of diagnosis, he went on, is not described in the classics. How do you think it developed then? I asked. Maybe from god, from siddhis, he replied.[5] A professor at another institution confirmed this view, saying of pulse-reading vaidyas, "Here in India some meditation, some siddhis, some yogic exercises they know, so they can diagnose, they can see anything. That is supernatural power."

On the other hand, Dr. Trivedi, an urban practitioner who routinely reads diseases in pulse, consistently denied that he possesses a mystical power. One day a patient in her forties arrived in his clinic, saying that she had heard that he did nāḍī parikśan. He replied that only veterinarians diagnose by examination only. Our patients, he told her, talk to us, so tell me what is wrong with you. In conversation Dr. Trivedi told me that he no longer diagnoses only from the pulse precisely because patients believe that pulse reading is a siddhi. He is wary of becoming a maharaj, someone of legendary stature. Besides, he said, patients want someone to listen patiently to their complaints; 50 percent of the cure occurs in the listening. (His own nāḍī guru, however, had not allowed patients to tell him anything until he had read their pulse.) Dr. Trivedi was quick to dismiss other parts of nāḍī lore as well. It is said that a patient's pulse should be read on an empty stomach. This is a practice that some vaidyas, including a pulse reader from Rishikesh (introduced below) follow religiously. According to Dr. Trivedi, this practice was simply "dogma." "You can examine pulse at any time," he said. He explained that fasting was once customary because a vaidya worked as a farmer in the afternoon and a pharmacist in the evening. Therefore the work of seeing patients had to be completed in the morning. If the patient was told to come with an empty stomach, then he would come early. Food does cause some variation in pulse, he said, but its effect can be detected and accounted for.

The mystique surrounding pulse diagnosis is enhanced by the fact that it is not, and presumably cannot be, taught in Ayurvedic colleges. Nonetheless, certain institutional practitioners argue that it should be. When I asked Dr. Joshi once whether he thought that Ayurvedic knowledge needed to be more standardized, he replied,

> It's not standardization; it is getting more of the traditions into the institutions; for example, we have heard a lot about pulse examination; we hear about vaidyas who still diagnose anything with the pulse.

They used to keep everything secret; that's one [thing]; they were afraid somebody else would learn it and their livelihood would be in danger. We hear of many good vaidyas who die without [teaching] anything to any of their disciples. But pulse examination — nāḍī vidya they used to call it — is no more in the institutions; that is a big zero in the institutions. If you ask me, "Please examine my pulse," I'll take your pulse rate and I'll take your rhythm. I'll not be able to tell you what you have eaten in the morning.

Jean: But doṣa?

Dr. Joshi: Yes, that is the only information that we get from pulse, but that much information is quite insufficient as compared to the information those people claimed to have gathered by pulse examination. You see, they used to tell you what you had for breakfast; each and every detail of your breakfast they used to tell you. How was it possible? We don't know. We do not really know that. I don't think there are many people living who can diagnose with nāḍī. Now it is very difficult to find the genuine vaidyas also, you see. Some maintain a livelihood simply by making a hoax of it. They claim they are vaidyas. But to find out who are the real vaidyas, the traditional vaidyas who have that knowledge of nāḍī, is really difficult. That effort must be made by the institutions. And we must procure those vaidyas, at least hear some lectures from them. That we are not able to do in institutions. Probably either the institutions have ego problems or the tradition is shy of interacting with institutions. Either they don't want to come to the institutions or institutions have got [too much of] an ego to go to them.

The thorny problem of how to distinguish the "real, traditional" practitioners from the imitators will be considered more fully below. Here what is forced onto our attention is how institutional Ayurveda is haunted by the possibility of a profound expertise that it necessarily excludes.

One day I was sitting with Dr. Trivedi and one of his daughters, an allopathic practitioner, in his clinic off a crowded side street in a major city. I asked about the possibility of teaching nāḍī parikśan in the colleges.

Dr. Trivedi: It should be taught.

Daughter: Because you have to pass it on to the future generation. Otherwise it's going to be a great loss.

Jean: But how will they teach it with the present educational structure?

Dr. Trivedi: Exactly, exactly, exactly. If it is a gurukula type, where the students sit for two years, three years. Now my son-in-law has been sitting here for seven years. That is why he has mastered that subject. Even if a student sits here for two years, he can pick it up. But this present system of education will not teach it.

Daughter: I have seen my father telling the exact blood sugar from nāḍī parikśan. Maybe a few milligrams off here and there. But usually it comes up alongside.

Jean: I remember once or twice you've said, oh it must be 130 or something like that.

Dr. Trivedi: Yes [laughter].

Daughter: There are patients who hide the report. I've seen this in front of my eyes. They hide the report and first ask, what is the blood sugar? And then they show him the report.

Dr. Trivedi: There is one lady, she has her blood sugar examined every six months. And she asked me to tell the report with the pulse. Now she has decided not to go for that pathology [lab report]. And not spend that sixty rupees. She says, "I can get it in no time." [Laughter.]

Jean: Why is it that nāḍī parikśan got left out of the colleges?

Dr. Trivedi: It is a painstaking job. Easy education is accepted. Painstaking means that you have to think constantly. When I used to study it, I used to always have this habit of looking at my pulse. So I concentrated constantly. Then sometimes on my wife, I used to just observe it. But it's a painstaking job, no doubt.

Daughter: And the other thing is, you know, if somebody is an expert in this nāḍī parikśan, they may not want to pass it on to their children. They want to keep it to themselves.

Jean: [Gesturing to Dr. Trivedi] But he is not that way.

Daughter: No, he is not that way. But there are people.

Jean: What is the reason for that attitude?

Dr. Trivedi: I don't know. I don't know. Actually when I ask them why they are not giving it to somebody, they say that no one is well prepared to accept it. It is as good as giving an M.A. education to a twelve-standard boy. So [the students] must be ready to accept it. They must have zeal to accept it, and then [the vaidyas] will teach it. Otherwise it will go to waste. But let it go to waste. At least one out of a hundred will accept it.

Daughter: I've seen people who do nāḍī parikśan but who keep it to themselves. Maybe two or three whom I know. It's become a subject of awe you know, like [in awed tone] "*Are* [Oh], it's nāḍī parikśan."
Dr. Trivedi: It is as good as becoming a maharaj. So I just stopped that thing. They used to say, "Some siddhi is there with Dr. Trivedi." They don't believe that it is a science. "Dr. Trivedi tells everything without asking any single question." . . . The way of education is different. Ayurvedic people think that to sit with a guru and study is not a proper way of studying. And they want everything quick. And it is impossible. Any knowledge which is quick is impossible.

Several of the contemporary meanings of pulse diagnosis flash forth in this conversation. There is the desire of the patient population for a divinatory diagnosis that is independent of modern techniques or history taking. There is the refusal of certain pulse aficionados to enter the flow of the modern historical record, allowing a subtle experience to be codified into a rational system, submitting their knowledge to modern institutional discipline at the expense of rigorous discipleship. There is the defensiveness of Ayurvedic students, who want an education as similar to biomedical education as possible. Finally, there are the subtle but telling shifts of attitude on the part of Dr. Trivedi and his allopathic daughter. In one moment she voices her awe, and he his delight, at his accurate diagnoses of blood sugar, while in the next moment she makes a detached assessment of the awe of the public and he speaks of his distaste for being a maharaj.

When I asked Dr. Trivedi, in another conversation, whether nāḍī could be explained physiologically, he replied:

No. That is a personal study. It cannot be explained in words or books. It can be experienced. Even if I tell my student that this is vāta, this is pitta or kapha, and this is its potency, this is the strength of its movements, the person who is studying has to have his own personal judgment of it. And how is this [judgment] made? My guru discusses the symptoms with the patient. My guru tells me that this nāḍī is showing pitta, and these are the symptoms. Then I feel that nāḍī; I know the symptoms, so I understand this particular type of feeling of nāḍī. My guru has not told me; he has only shown me the place: that under this finger, pitta is there. How much strength is there, he has not explained to me. Whether it is tat-tat-tat-tat-tat-tat-tat-tat. Or whether it is tāḍa,

> tāḍa, tāḍa, he has not explained. But he has asked me to see the nāḍī. When I see the nāḍī, my personal feeling is that it is daḍ, daḍ, daḍ, daḍ, daḍ, like that. My guru has not explained anything. But I am feeling it. My guru has told me all the symptoms of that person. Now when those symptoms are there, I correlate my feeling of this nāḍī with them. Then he tells me that this is pittaja *meha* [pitta-related urinary disorder]. The patient tells all these symptoms, pittaja meha. I understand daḍ, daḍ, daḍ, daḍ, this feeling. Then I correlate it with *prameha* [urinary disorder], pittaja meha. But this is a personal experience. Physiologically we can't explain anything. As we cannot explain it, it is a science of feeling. It is as good as music. You are saying, "I am getting happiness by hearing that music." What [occurs] physiologically, we can't say.

He went on to say that the skills of the practitioner develop through meditation and yogic concentration:

> Yoga means Patanjali yoga, not hatha yoga, not *āsanas.* Yoga also has disciplines like the discipline of *dinacarya* [daily discipline], *ṛtucarya* [seasonal discipline]. If you maintain those disciplines, then [you develop] power in your fingers and feeling. Now sometimes we can understand [the illness] without touching the patient or anything. How? Ayurveda, or yoga, describes it as a close rapport with the patient. And I just explain it as how the mother in the hospital can understand the cry of her own child without seeing the child. There are thirty just-born babies, but the mother can understand the cry of her own child. How? We can't explain. But that feeling is there. So similarly if that feeling is created between the doctor and the patient, [we know] the symptoms easily.

In pulse diagnosis, the discipline of hospital procedure is superseded by the discipline of mental asceticism. In addition, the practice of nāḍī parikśan is embedded not only within an incalculable sensory experience, but also within a quasimaternal empathy. Pulse reading belongs not to a contractual medicine, where doctor-patient relationships are shaped by legally defined rights and responsibilities, but to a paternalistic healing, where doctor-patient relationships are shaped by emotional dependence and parental nurturance.

The ideal of paternalistic care is found in the oldest Ayurvedic texts and is occasionally still echoed by the most modern institutional practitioners. As one Ayurvedic surgeon told me, when a patient comes to the hospital for treatment, he "surrenders" himself. If he does not surrender himself, the doctor cannot feel "confident." The patient cannot hide anything from the doctor. All this, he went on to say, is especially true in surgery. Surgery is dangerous; under anesthesia the patient is almost dead. It is the surgeon's duty to take care of him. He can do this only if he develops an intimate relationship with him. According to some physicians, the relationship between vaidya and patient, like the relationship between guru and disciple, is ideally more affective than contractual. Pulse reading draws some of its value from its power to establish closeness and foster confidence. As one institutional practitioner told me, "Nāḍī parikśan also gives some faith to the patient. When you touch a patient, he thinks, 'This doctor is going to do something for me; definitely he will do something for me.'"

Mahadeva Sastri corroborates many of Dr. Trivedi's ideas about pulse in a recent article on nāḍī in an Ayurvedic journal. First, Sastri argues that in pulse reading, experience alone counts, while rational explanation is futile: "The yogi is able to understand the fineness in the movement of blood and the control on it. The physician has to learn this art by practice, without which mere explanation of theory serves no purpose" (1989, 673). By implication, the physician, then, must develop the sensory awareness of a yogi. Sastri goes on to elaborate the relationship between pulse and music:

> The movement of the pulse is often compared to a string of a musical instrument in action. During the vibrations of the string, the harmonic movement can be seen causing nodes along the string at different points. The musician presses his fingers at the nodes to produce different pitch or notes. A veena or a violin is an example for this. Pulse beat is synchronous with the heartbeat. Just like the string in the instrument producing waves by each harp [*sic*], for every beat of the heart there is a corresponding pulse beat. . . . It is only the expert musicologist who can detect the slightest error among the notes of sound while all his attention is pointed in all the aspects of music, which may not be found with others. This analogy holds good in pulse examination (1989, 674).

Dr. Trivedi said that he himself had been well prepared for pulse reading because he played the tabla; after learning one set of complex rhythms, it was easier to learn the other. (Coincidentally or not, Vd. Rai, the young rural pulse-reading vaidya, also played tabla.)

When I asked one Ayurvedic student from a family of practitioners the difference between his training and that of his parents, the last difference he mentioned was nāḍī parikśan:

Student: In Ayurveda is studied the nāḍī parikśan: the pulse is felt by the vaidya, and the vaidya can diagnose anything. . . . This is a great diagnostic feature which we, the students of Ayurveda now, have totally lost. Totally lost. We cannot diagnose anything from it; I can personally because of my father. But if you see him, if you meet him personally, he can tell you anything. He just holds your pulse and starts telling, just like a miracle! He can tell you so many things; we cannot.
Jean: Normally when you would give a patient an exam in this hospital, you wouldn't do pulse diagnosis?
Student: Yes, yes, we do pulse diagnosis. We see all the basic things. You know the basic elements in Ayurveda—vāta, pitta, and kapha. We go for that much—whether the vāta is more, or whether the pitta pulse shows, whether the form of the pulse is good. That much, the very basic things, we can do. But at this moment, I cannot diagnose a disease or a very critical condition just by seeing, by feeling the pulse.
Jean: But your father can.
Student: Yes, he can. And he does in front of everyone.

In conversations such as this and the one with Dr. Trivedi and his daughter above, we see how easily knowledge that has not been transposed into the tabular and disciplined rationalities of college curricula or hospital routines passes over into miracle. One frustrated student complained that not only are Ayurvedic graduates regarded as inferior to allopathic graduates, but they are not even considered proper Ayurvedic doctors. When people think of Ayurveda, she said, they think about pulse readers who can diagnose any illness through pulse. But we are not taught to do this, she exclaimed. Yet the very fact that this kind of pulse reading is not taught in the institutions marks it as a healing practice that has not been subjected to modern discipline. It is a semiotics that is not constrained into a one-to-one, measurable, and duplicable correspondence between sign and referent.[6] How much is its popular appeal due to its very quality of being nonstandardized? Nāḍī vijñān signals its practitioner not as a person trained in a standard science according to an institutional discipline, but as a person of particular caliber following a mental or supramental discipline.

Quackery and Excess

Dr. Mistry does not share Dr. Trivedi's scruples about exploiting popular longings for miraculous diagnoses or cures. Some months after first hearing of Dr. Mistry from a patient, I met a young Ayurvedic practitioner who had trained with Dr. Mistry for a few years after completing her Bachelor of Ayurvedic Medical Science. She encouraged me to observe his practice but cautioned me that he would not be able to explain his method of reading pulse. This was one of the frustrations that was prompting her to leave his employ. When she handed me one of his cards, I noticed a long string of letters after his name. The familiar BAMS, held by his assistant, or the M.D. or Ph.D., held by most senior doctors of Ayurveda in his generation, were missing. Instead there were other letters with unknown referents. There was also the word Ayurvedacarya, a credential granted to some practitioners of previous generations who, in the early days of institutionalization, had either received licenses based on long years of practice or had taken the standard Vidyapīth exam established in 1907, usually studying under the guidance of a senior vaidya.[7] According to other doctors with whom I spoke, this exam had become almost totally corrupt by the 1950s. Dr. Mistry, I later discovered, had taken the exam in 1974 or 1975. When I asked the young doctor to explain the string of letters, she said, "That is another problem. He doesn't have a degree in Ayurveda; this I know." She went on to say, however, that she had learned a great deal about pulse diagnosis in his clinic simply because she had had the opportunity to examine a hundred or more patients in a day. Later I mentioned the mysterious garland of degrees to Dr. Upadhyay, who is well respected in institutional Ayurvedic circles. "I know," he said. "Actually he's a fraud."

When I finally met Dr. Mistry and received permission to observe his medical practice, I was very aware of all this contradictory hearsay—the testimonial of the satisfied patient, the qualified recommendation of the partly dissatisfied employee, and the out-and-out denunciation of another Ayurvedic doctor. In other words, I was, in spite of myself, already caught up in the question of whether Dr. Mistry was a "true" Ayurvedic doctor or a quack. I say in spite of myself because my training in medical anthropology had instilled in me a certain discomfort with the concept of quackery. As I understood it, quackery was a concept used to discredit medical practices other than biomedicine. Some biomedical doctors consider all Ayurveda to be a kind of quackery, based on a bogus view of the body and dispensing treatment the biological effects of which are scientifically unproven. My training in medical anthropology, however, had influenced me to put biological efficacy aside in favor of symbolic efficacy. Medical anthropologists are generally less interested in whether or not a particular treatment actually cures disease than with the question of how that treatment constructs or reproduces the physical or social body. Following Lévi-Strauss's (1963a) seminal analysis of a Cuna healing song in "The Effectiveness of Symbols," we place an emphasis on cultural efficacy, achieved through symbolic manipulations, which overshadows or explains physical efficacy. It is perhaps partly for this reason that the question of quackery has rarely been addressed in medical anthropology. Quackery seems to have as much claim to cultural efficacy as any scientifically validated medical practice.

Yet this view of quackery, which assimilates it to descriptive accounts of cultural belief, overlooks the contested nature of medical truths at the local level. Pigg (1996) has pointed out that while outsiders may tend to assume a seamless social consensus regarding the efficacy of a particular local medicine, local people themselves often sustain a lively discourse on the genuineness or falseness of particular practitioners or instances of cure. Such discourses raise the possibility of another level of quackery. Ayurveda or any other nonbiomedical practice may be considered generically true or false by a whole host of authorities, including biomedical doctors and development workers. But particular Ayurvedic doctors or other types of practitioners may also be considered true or false within their own social field. According to what criteria should an anthropologist interpret these claims of truth or falseness? What, moreover, is the connection between such claims and the commodification of cures or the cultural politics of medical systems? These were the questions that haunted me when I visited Dr. Mistry's clinic for the first time.

The clinic is on a shady suburban street of a North Indian city. Even before the clinic opens at 11:00 A.M., a crowd of patients gathers on the steps and spills out into the street. Within a few hours there are forty or fifty people milling in the waiting room, collecting their case forms at the reception desk, or picking up bottles of pills from the dispensary counter. In small consultation rooms off the waiting room Dr. Mistry's assistant doctors, numbering two or three at any given time, talk to patients and take their pulse. Above the crowd is a large digital display that flashes luminous red numbers corresponding to the tickets held by waiting patients. Similar to displays seen in Indian banks or fast food restaurants, it announces the number of the patient who will be seen next. On the walls are enlarged copies of notification letters for awards that Dr. Mistry has received. Most of these read like letters from the vanity publishers of biological reference works. Also on the walls are a number of framed color photographs. All of them feature Dr. Mistry with some prominent political or religious figure. In one he is taking the pulse of a past winner of the Nobel Peace Prize. There are also copies of articles about Dr. Mistry from a number of different tabloids in English, Hindi, or regional languages.

While I was waiting to meet Dr. Mistry for the first time, one of his assistants brought me a pile of several tabloid articles. The reportage was based on interviews with Dr. Mistry and with enthusiastic patients. A few of the articles described Dr. Mistry's relationship with his guru, identified as a Tibetan who, until his death, had practiced Ayurveda in a village outside the city. The story of Dr. Mistry's apprenticeship was later elaborated in conversations with Dr. Mistry and his partner, Dr. Lal, whom he considers the expert in the theoretical and pharmaceutical sides of the practice. When Dr. Mistry first opened his practice, he was frustrated by the hit-and-miss diagnostic process. Then one of his ex-patients told him about a swami who diagnosed simply by touching the patient's pulse. Every day this swami was visited by three hundred patients. According to Dr. Mistry, the vaidya once lived at the borders of India and Tibet, where he had picked up medical tips from wandering sadhus (renunciants). Dr. Mistry became determined to learn the swami's method. As reported in one of the tabloid articles, it took three months to convince the swami of his sincerity. The guru continually put him off, saying, tomorrow, tomorrow. Finally, Dr. Mistry said, no, today. The story goes: "The swami searched his eyes for a full second. And then he said, 'Learning, teaching is for later. First take this broom and clean the floor. So [Mistry] picked up the broom and became absorbed in cleaning the house. Some days passed in this way. Then one day Baba became fully persuaded that the ego inside his disciple had softened and dissolved. Mistry studied pulse exam at the feet of his guru for one thousand days and became an expert." Dr. Mistry's partner told me that Dr. Mistry studied nāḍī parikśan with the swami for three years, "whenever he could get time and all that." After the swami felt a patient's pulse, Dr. Mistry would feel it himself and try to reconstruct his guru's reading. Today his own students use the same method to learn pulse reading from him.

The purpose of the advance publicity handed to me and posted around the lobby for the patients was clearly to sell Dr. Mistry as a particular kind of healer trained by a guru in secret powers. While promotion in some form is a necessary part of any medical practice, Dr. Mistry's tactics seemed heavy-handed to me even at this first visit. As I will discuss further below, his commercialism lacked the subtlety and seeming objectivity of most professional medical services. This is partly due to the fact that in the subtext of his publicity, the commodity for sale was not so much the medicines and therapies as the doctor himself. Both he himself and certain signs of traditional authority, such as the forest-dwelling guru, the charismatic religious leaders, and the esoteric ability to read the pulse, were fetishized. Thus the imperatives of capitalism make it possible for the use value of his practice (healing illness) to be obscured by the dense semiotics of the exchange value.

When I was at last ushered into Dr. Mistry's office that first day, I witnessed the method of patient consultation that I was to observe over and over during the coming weeks. Dr. Mistry's consultations with patients rarely take more than five minutes. He greets them with a smile and reaches for their pulse across the table. He presses three fingers close to the outside bone of the wrist, much the way any Ayurvedic doctor can be observed to do. After a few seconds of silence he offers the diagnosis. The patient generally agrees to the diagnosis and then adds a few more complaints. Following the pulse reading of a new patient, Dr. Mistry records the results on the case form with a series of specialized notations. There are close to fifteen different notations, of which probably half are commonly used. Each one refers to a particular characteristic of the pulse, which in turn refers to a particular condition of the body. In addition to the pulse characteristics pertaining to the three doṣa, there are characteristics pertaining to moisture, dryness, and pace, as well as conditions such as low immunity, poor circulation, liver problems, or arthritis. Later I learned that particular combinations of the more general characteristics may encode a particular disease. In a box on the case form Dr. Mistry writes down the main complaints agreed to or volunteered by the patient. The pulse reading is recorded only on the first visit. On the opposite page of the case form a running tab is kept on improvements and changes in medicine.

For new patients or patients with new complaints Dr. Mistry quickly selects one of fourteen prescription slips stacked in slots against the wall. Each one is organized around a related group of illness problems. For example, one is entitled "Heart Mind Blood Pressure"; another, "Kidney Liver"; another, simply "Vāyu"; another, "Pitta"; another, "Prameha/ Madhumeha," the Sanskrit terms associated with urinary disorders and diabetes respectively. On each slip is a list of anywhere from eight to thirty-five medicines. Some of the most common medicines are found on several slips. The names and formulae have been developed by Dr. Mistry and Dr. Lal. Dr. Lal told me that the medicines are based on classical recipes in early Ayurvedic texts but vary from these recipes in specific ways. During the patient consultation Dr. Mistry rapidly checks off six or seven medicines on the chosen list, inserts it in the case folder, and hands it to the patient, who will collect the medicines from the dispensary counter in the lobby. For return patients he usually makes any necessary adjustments on a previous prescription slip already stapled into the case folder.

Dr. Mistry nearly always makes some promise regarding the cure. In one case he told a diabetic woman that she would gradually be able to stop taking insulin. "I promise you diabetes will disappear," he assured her. "And the pain in her legs?" her son asked. "The pain in her legs will go away within fifteen days," Dr. Mistry replied. He does not always promise absolute cure. Once he cautioned the parents of a mentally disabled boy that he could produce only 75 percent improvement, not 100 percent. The boy will grow taller, he promised; he will be able to work by himself. The parents commented that there was no treatment in allopathy. Dr. Mistry agreed but added, "We can treat." There is, in fact, no illness that Dr. Mistry refuses to treat. He even claims some success at curing AIDS. His patients are discouraged from talking at length to him about their illness. Dr. Mistry told me at one point, "I don't listen to people. What is important is what the pulse is telling me." He believes that the patients are prejudiced by allopathic notions. When a reporter for a Hindi newspaper asked him why he never questioned the patient about his complaints, he replied that the symptoms fluctuate according to the individual and his psychological state. "Through pulse exam," he was quoted as saying, "I can disentangle the symptoms and find the root." At the end of the consultation Dr. Mistry rings a bell under his desk, signaling his assistant to send in the next patient and makes a mark on a ledger on his desk where he records the number of patients seen each day. His record, I was told, exceeds four hundred.

The first several times I visited Dr. Mistry, he repeatedly sent me into a side room to hear stories of cures from patients of his choice. These stories all had at least two twists of plot in common. At the beginning of the stories Dr. Mistry amazed the patients by reeling off their symptoms after simply feeling their pulse. At the end of the stories he cured their illnesses, either completely or 80 to 95 percent. Over time I learned that Dr. Mistry encourages his patients to measure their cure in terms of percentages. "How much *fayda* [benefit, improvement]?" he would ask, "70 percent, 80 percent, 90 percent?" He wrote the patient's reply on the case form and circled it. While other doctors I observed also requested patients to rate their cures in percentages, Dr. Mistry requested this more consistently. Usually he suggested very large percentages as answers. The lowest percentage of improvement I ever observed him record was 15 percent in the case of a brain tumor.

The day I met Dr. Mistry, he showed me a photo album documenting a recent trip to Europe. Some of his European patients had brought animals for treatment, including a large python. In the album was a photograph of him holding the animal and smiling broadly. He explained that at first he had searched for the snake's pulse near the head but had finally found it near the tail. Some days later he told me that his friends in Europe had written that the python was much improved. At that time I thought to ask him the animal's problem. He said that the python was suffering from excess pitta, the doṣa associated with heat. I joked, "Can a snake suffer from excess pitta? It's cold-blooded." He laughed and said that it must have eaten a mouse, which in turn must have eaten some pitta-aggravating food.

I left Dr. Mistry's clinic that first day, and on many subsequent days, in a state of wonder. Compared to the other Ayurvedic practices I had observed, his practice had, for me, a surreal quality. His clinic was simultaneously evocative of a number of contradictory images. The digital display was reminiscent of fast food restaurants in Delhi. The speedy patient consultation was reminiscent of hectic OPDs in Ayurvedic hospitals. Perhaps the strangest and most unnerving resemblance, given the clinic's urban setting and professional appearance, was to a colorful tent in a Himalayan hill station where I met an itinerant vaidya, Kaviraj Kumar. Framing this tent was a banner advertising the illnesses for which he offered a cure, many of which were related to sexual virility (see figures 11 and 12).

In North India Kaviraj was a widely used title for vaidyas up until the twentieth century. It is still in use by a few vaidyas, usually those who have no university education. There were several ways in which Dr. Mistry reminded me of Kaviraj Kumar. For one thing, both of them had decorated their clinical spaces with various kinds of testimonials. Some of these testimonials were framed degrees and certificates issued by dubious institutions, mimicking the signs of authority to be found in the offices of professional doctors, whether allopathic or Ayurvedic. But there were other forms of testimonials as well. Like Dr. Mistry, Kaviraj Kumar had photo albums full of pictures of himself with famous people. Both were shown with politicians, but Dr. Mistry was also shown with world religious leaders, while Kaviraj Kumar was shown with Hindi film stars. This difference in choice of authority was appropriate to the difference in their personal styles and clientele. Kaviraj Kumar identified himself with charismatic heroes and catered to villagers with minimal education. Dr. Mistry identified himself with saints and catered to urbanites with spiritual leanings. The basic method of appeal, however, the evocation of a higher cultural authority, was much the same. Like Dr. Mistry, Kaviraj Kumar made what seemed to be extravagant promises of cures for difficult diseases. He even offered, in his promotional flyer, a contract whereby the patient would pay nothing until the cure was achieved. In the next sentence, however, he stated that patients with faith would certainly pay

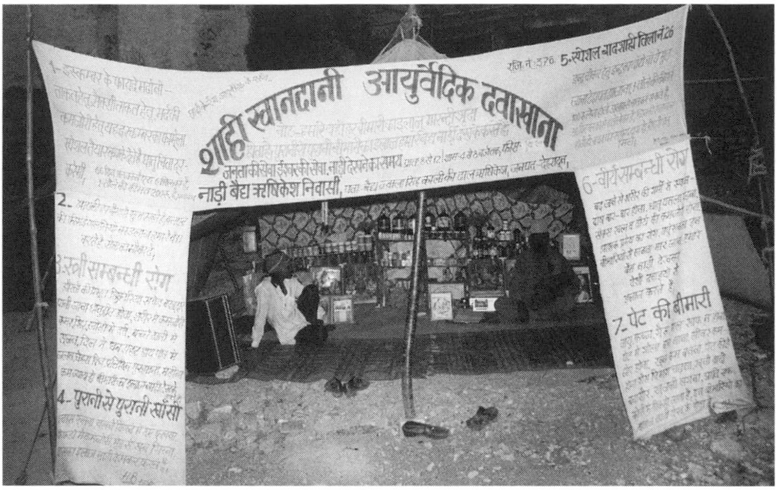

Figure 11. Itinerant Vaidya's Tent. The banner reads "Royal Family Ayurvedic Dispensary" and boasts that the vaidya in this tent offers guaranteed cures of all illnesses, even very old illnesses, after examining the pulse. Underneath, a line reads, "In the service of the people, in the service of God," and then lists the times of reading pulse and the fee. On the sides are listed a sampling of the problems that can be cured.

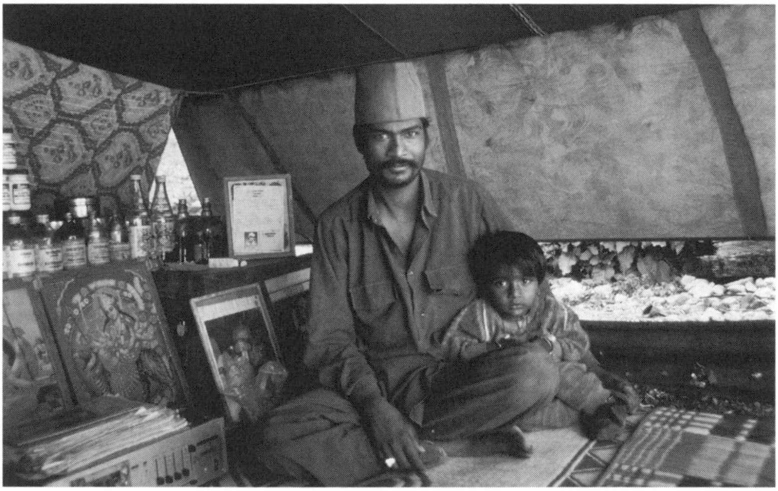

Figure 12. Itinerant Vaidya. The vaidya is surrounded by jars of jaḍī-būṭī, pictures of gods and goddesses, and a stereo system that blasts out *bhajans* (devotional songs).

cash. Both Dr. Mistry and Kaviraj Kumar claimed to diagnose solely according to pulse, and both insisted on reading the pulse when the patient's stomach was empty. Both of them maintained that they had learned nāḍī parikśan during apprenticeship to an adept.

Kaviraj Kumar was the first Ayurvedic practitioner I had met who practiced amid rumors of his quackery. One of my Indian friends told me that he would never go to a doctor "like that." Another said that a friend's condition had worsened after taking Kaviraj Kumar's medicines. Others simply laughed when I told them I was observing his practice. Like Dr. Mistry, Kaviraj Kumar had his own formulae for particular ailments. In his case, however, they had been passed down from Himalayan ṛṣi who lived six hundred years ago. They were written on laminated pages in a booklet entitled (in Hindi) "The Catalog of Indian *Śilajīt* Tonics of the Himalayas," a book that, according to Kaviraj Kumar, can be copied only once in five years. Śilajīt is a medicinal mineral found in the rocks of high mountain ranges such as the Himalayas. In Ayurveda it is used for a number of different complaints, ranging from diabetes to sexual debility. In one of my conversations with Kaviraj Kumar he showed me a chunk of śilajīt, to which he referred (though we were speaking in Hindi) with the English word "refined." It was a polished black rock, astonishingly light, with smooth, glassy facets, breaking easily like flint. He suggested that I should take some to strengthen my brain since I am a scholar. After some hesitation I agreed. He weighed out a chunk and ground it for me into a coppery black powder. He told me to take it twice a day with milk and cautioned me not to eat lemon in the meantime. As a matter of fact, I had no intention of ingesting the śilajīt. What I wanted to do was test it. A few days later I took the powder to another Ayurvedic doctor, who had been raised in a reputable Ayurvedic household and was well acquainted with the Ayurvedic pharmacopoeia. He smelled the powder, tasted it, mixed it with a little water in his palm, and told me that it was not śilajīt. He said that real śilajīt smelled different, tasted different, and did not dissolve so easily. He also said that real śilajīt was as black as tar, even when ground. He said that the śilajīt I had bought was probably boiled sugar with a few other ingredients. I concluded, with some reluctance, that Kaviraj Kumar was a quack.

I still found myself, however, faced by a troubling question: What did it mean to say that Kaviraj Kumar was a quack? Suppose he himself believed the śilajīt was authentic and had been cheated by his suppliers. Or suppose he had sold me fake śilajīt only because I was a rich foreigner who was not seriously ill. In those cases would I still consider him a quack? Moreover, if the śilajīt was false, did that mean that the recipes in the book were also false? Did it mean that he had no knowledge whatsoever about Ayurveda? While I was sitting in his tent, he told one patient to come back after 5:00 P.M. because the pulse had to be checked on an empty stomach. Surely that was a piece of information that was "true." That is to say, it was information recorded in revered Ayurvedic texts on pulse diagnosis and information that could be confirmed in conversation with other vaidyas. If his śilajīt was false, was his background equally suspect? Was his relationship with his guru as fictive or distorted as the relationships he claimed to have had with ex-chief ministers and movie stars? Was his practice mythologized? Or was his falseness localized and confined to the śilajīt itself? Where did his quackery reside?

I decided that Kaviraj Kumar was a quack because the medicine he sold me was not the real article but an imitation. Whether I (or rather someone who had not been taught to mistrust the use of photo albums in medicine) could nonetheless have experienced a curative effect from that medicine, a sudden clarity of mind, perhaps due to Kaviraj Kumar's considerable charisma, or to the persuasive authority of six-hundred-year-old formulae developed by a ṛṣi in a cave, or to the sheer glassy beauty of the śilajīt in my hand, was irrelevant. There had been a serious slippage between the sign, the name śilajīt, and its referent, a chunk of boiled sugar.

Taussig's extensive investigation of mimicry, no less than Baudrillard's analysis of the commodity as sign (which both owe much to Karl Marx's analysis of commodity fetishism) allow us to understand that the śilajīt disappointed me because it turned out to be no more than a simulacrum. According to Baudrillard (1988, 22), an object's exchange value is never exhausted in its function. Any object has what he calls "an excess of presence," an extra value as a sign of cultural capital. In Taussig's (1993, 233) terminology, the commodity "spills over its referent" in what he refers to as a "mimetic excess." Until it proved to be sugar, the medicine I purchased had all the fetishistic glow of śilajīt,—its name, its glassy elegance, catching the light of calculated ancient wisdom in Kaviraj Kumar's eyes. It had, in fact, the full exchange value of śilajīt. Had I not paid one hundred rupees? Because it was the wrong chemical compound, however, the use value had been, in one instant, deflated. If I had not tested the śilajīt, it would have remained an object that was culturally, if not also medically, potent.

Where Baudrillard and Taussig differ is that Baudrillard suggests that the commodity's excess of presence is exhausted in the expression of social prestige or status. Taussig, on the other hand, suggests that the commodity's excess of presence is nothing less than a kind of magic in which the commodity, its fetishistic advertisable glow, asserts power over the object of which it is supposedly a commodification. To put it crudely, śilajīt as an Ayurvedic commodity asserts power over śilajīt as a rock. In fact (though perhaps "fact" is not exactly the right word), at some level imitation śilajīt asserts power over real śilajīt. A well-educated layperson once commented to me that he did not believe that śilajīt was actually an ingredient of all the Ayurvedic medicines for which it was listed as an ingredient. He believed that even reputable Ayurvedic drug companies must be substituting other ingredients. This may or may not be true of śilajīt. However, this mimetic excess of the medical label is probably true of other Ayurvedic medicines, such as *brahmi,* which is widely used for neurological disorders, among other things. One Ayurvedic doctor told me that there was not enough brahmi in the world to account for the amounts of brahmi listed on hair oil labels. Of course every commodity is not an imitation in the same way that Kaviraj Kumar's śilajīt was an imitation. But the imitative qualities of commodities in general make it that much more difficult to identify the particular imitativeness of the śilajīt. The question becomes even more complex when indicators of falseness more subtle than chemical substances are considered—indicators, that is, such as photo albums.

Mimetic Vertigo

A few weeks before my purchase of the śilajīt, a friend and I had watched a group of traveling snake charmers, playing their sonorous instruments to entice serpents out of baskets, inviting the crowd to offer rupees to the king cobra, the representative of Śiva, and, at the same time, charging ten rupees to a foreign woman for a snapshot. My friend commented that it was always the poorest village people who were scammed by the snake charmers. It occurred to me, however, that these people were not simply being scammed but were paying the snake charmers to put on a show and officiate at an act of worship. Perhaps Kaviraj Kumar also was selling a performance and a mystical relationship, if not to gods, then to one's own body. Medical anthropologists routinely discover the value of ritual medicine in such psychological or social effects. The problem was that Kaviraj Kumar did not seem to be practicing ritual medicine, but rather Ayurveda, which is argued to be a science. The problem was that he had bottles of medicine sporting the labels of a reputable Ayurvedic pharmacy arrayed alongside other bottles containing fake śilajīt and other jaḍī-būtī. The problem was that juxtaposed to his colored pictures of gods and goddesses were framed certificates that mimicked the gilt-edged degrees in the offices of professional doctors. Professional medical science is not expected by most of us to involve overt showmanship, which, insofar as it is instrumental, is expected to be the province of magic. The fact is, of course, as medical anthropologists have demonstrated, medical science does involve showmanship, from the color-enhanced photographs of microscopic pathology to the opening of the draped body in the operating theater. Professional medicine's show does not, however, usually include photo albums full of famous patients. Medical science, as will be elaborated below, usually disguises its simulacra as natural or functional objects — as bodily organs, for example, or surgical tools. It is not expected to display them with casual ingenuousness, like obvious advertising ploys. It might be said that science's most dazzling show is its illusion of objectivity.[8]

This brings me to a second troubling question: what had motivated me to test the śilajīt? By the time I met Kaviraj Kumar, I had already spoken to numerous vaidyas and sat in numerous dispensaries, and yet I had never before been moved to test any practitioner's knowledge or medicines for their truth. There may have been many motives for testing the śilajīt, but prominent among them were surely Kaviraj Kumar's framed certificates from obscure and dubious medical associations and his testimonial photo albums. It is unlikely that I would have thought to test his medical authenticity had his cultural authenticity been clearly intact. Kaviraj Kumar was, however, neither pure Ayurvedic doctor nor pure pulse reader; neither pure professional nor pure folk practitioner; neither pure scientist nor pure magician. I have pursued this diversion into Kaviraj Kumar's tent because the same thing that motivated me to test the śilajīt also led me to continually ponder the truth or falseness of Dr. Mistry. Here also were the suspect certificates and boasting photographs. Here were the prototypical guru story and the mystique of pulse diagnosis, coexisting with Ayurvedic degrees and Ayurvedic drugs. Might not Dr. Mistry, like Kaviraj Kumar, prove to be an imitation?

Just as more educated Ayurvedic practitioners sought legitimacy by reproducing European medical institutions, so inevitably "folk" practitioners seek legitimacy by imitating professional Ayurveda. Kaviraj Kumar, with his framed certificates and rows of jars bearing pharmaceutical company labels, is a case in point. Closer scrutiny might well reveal that he and others have also begun to imitate themselves, or rather the image of themselves projected back at them by a cosmopolitan populace undergoing a wave of interest in folk medicine. When, for instance, I first asked Kaviraj Kumar where he learned Ayurveda, he gestured toward one of his suspect certificates. When I asked later if he had also learned from a guru, he said yes. A few days later when I asked who had taught him nāḍī parikśan, he replied, "An old man." It occurred to me that he might have begun to realize that I thought that a genuine pulse reader would have learned his art from an old man rather than from, say, a correspondence course. It may be a modern inevitability that we all, learning over time what constitutes our authenticity, begin to imitate it.[9] The old man guru becomes a legitimating sign just as much as the book of recipes, the framed certificate, or the photographs.

In Dr. Mistry's practice the levels of mimicry become even more entangled. If Kaviraj Kumar is, through his suspect certificates, mimicking the accoutrements of professional Ayurveda, then Dr. Mistry, through his equally suspect certificates, seems to mimic the folk practitioner's mimicry of the accoutrements of professional Ayurveda. He also mimics the professional practitioner directly—for example, in his extremely modern factory, where gloved and uniformed workers operate shiny steel machines to turn out uniform rows of capsules. He further mimics the folk practitioner directly not only through his photo albums, but through his privileging of pulse diagnosis and discipleship to a guru.

Any Ayurvedic student can read the predominant doṣa in the body through the pulse, but none of them can diagnose three hundred different diseases, or detect a history of homosexuality or the onset of arthritis, or trace the entire etiological narrative of the illness entirely from pulse, as Dr. Mistry claims to do. Above I mentioned an Ayurvedic student who worried aloud to me that the public would not accept her and her fellow students as Ayurvedic doctors because they could not diagnose diseases solely from pulse. When I asked her if she knew of any Ayurvedic doctors who could, she promptly named Dr. Mistry. While Dr. Upadhyay was convinced that Dr. Mistry was a fraud, curious Ayurvedic professors sometimes asked me whether he could really read pulse. While Dr. Trivedi was concerned only to detect the underlying pathology through the pulse, Dr. Mistry considered it important to predict the symptoms from the pulse. He used pulse not simply as a diagnostic tool, but as a sales pitch and a psychological boost to healing.

In addition to pulse reading, Dr. Mistry sometimes mixes bits and pieces of other folk and professional practices into his own particular healing concoction. Several times, for example, I observed him practicing what he called marma cikitsā, which he compared to acupressure. In the standard Ayurvedic syllabus the theory of marmas occupies a small place in the study of anatomy, as noted in chapter 5. Students are taught that marmas are points that are particularly susceptible to injury and should be known and avoided by surgeons. However, there is also some mention in the early texts of a treatment involving marma. In South India in particular there are practitioners known as marma specialists who treat certain ailments by stimulating particular marma points. Dr. Mistry's comparison of marma cikitsā to acupressure is not far-fetched: marma cikitsā and acupuncture are extensively compared in a theoretical work by one of the foremost authorities on marmas in Ayurveda (Thatte 1988). Today, however, marma cikitsā is rarely, if at all, practiced outside of South India, where it is practiced for the most part by independently trained specialists.

Marma therapy remains, like elaborate pulse diagnosis, among those marginally Ayurvedic practices that are not taught in modern institutions. Treatment of marmas generally involves tapping and thereby precisely stimulating particular marmas. One lecturer at the Arya Vaidya Sala in Kerala, speaking before a group of European health practitioners, divided Keraliyan marma cikitsā into three strands: one based on Ayurveda, another based on Siddha healing, and a third related to Kalahari martial art. When Kalahari fighters are taught "traditional warfare," they are also taught about marmas as specifically vulnerable areas in the body. Each of these strands of marma cikitsā organizes and enumerates the marmas somewhat differently. Practitioners of these three strands have borrowed so heavily from one another that, as the speaker went on to say, "There is no clear demarcation nowadays." This scholar also cautioned the foreigners that in marma cikitsā, "Attainment of perfection comes only by experience and training." He warned: "Don't try to practice what I have told you." The management of marmas is a "very complex process." The improper management of marmas — and even sometimes the proper management of marmas — can lead to illnesses of excess vāta. Although the foreigners asked for a demonstration of marma cikitsā, they were not given one. Later, in North India, another Ayurvedic pundit told the same group about a certain demonstration for which the Arya Vaidya Sala is famous. In this demonstration some roosters are put on a table. When trauma is induced by stimulating certain marma points, the roosters fall over limp. When "countertrauma" is induced by stimulating corresponding antidotal points, called *adankal,* the roosters revive and run around again. "They didn't show you?" he asked. "Then they are misers."

In South India, marma cikitsā is often practiced by healers who also practice bone setting and massage. Dr. Vijayan's stories of these practitioners conveyed a mingled romanticism and social distance. Although he practiced an innovative form of marma stimulation himself, he told me that "marma is really in the hands of local people; if you give them one million dollars, they won't tell you. Those people who have real information [about marmas] are rare. They don't even teach these things to their children." Marma practitioners learn from gurus, who test them in several ways. One test, Dr. Vijayan said, involves threatening the pupil. If the pupil responds to the threat by running away, he will be taught marma cikitsā, while if he responds to the threat by fighting back, he will be sent away. Marma gurus want only disciples with a noncombative temperament since knowledge of marmas can easily be used to harm people. These people, he said, work at a "feeling" level, not an "intellectual" level. They use a particular seed, smaller than a fingertip, which they grip between their thumb and the side of their second knuckle. With this tiny seed, he said, they can stimulate marma points very accurately: "They can concentrate like a laser beam." Sometimes, Dr. Vijayan said, these marma experts even walk on their patients. Most of these people, he said, are "heavy drinkers" who are "not living a sattvic life." "Well," he amended, "maybe it is sattvic to them."

Some of these adepts were invited to work in the marmas department of the local Ayurvedic hospital, essentially a department of orthopedics. There they are called "marma technicians." Once, when Dr. Vijayan was working as a student in the orthopedic OPD at the Ayurvedic hospital, there was a traffic jam on the street outside. The villagers in one car were taking a friend to the allopathic hospital. He had been unconscious for more than two weeks following an accident. Since they were stuck in traffic, they decided to bring the patient into the Ayurvedic hospital. Soon after he was brought into the marma unit, the "marma technician" arrived, drunk as usual. He took the patient's pulse. "These people," Dr. Vijayan said, "take pulse in a different way." He demonstrated by carelessly grabbing my wrist, resting his fingers loosely across it for a moment, and then dropping it abruptly. The friends undressed the patient, and the technician threw a sheet over him so no one could view his technique. After he pressed a few points, the patient opened his eyes. The patient's friends gave the technician a wad of money, and he left. This story is important not so much for what it tells us about marma therapy as for what it tells us about modern Indian perceptions of marma therapy. Here is a practice in which the precision of a laser beam is achieved with a rustic tool, a subtle savant arrives disguised as a drunkard, and a precise pulse examination masquerades as an indifferent brush of the patient's wrist. Here is a healing practice, in other words, that, for modern observers, seems to draw its authority from the mystery with which it cloaks a sophisticated esoteric knowledge in apparently "primitive" practices. Such a practice is therefore perfectly suited to Dr. Mistry's simultaneous evocation of "folk" medicine and science.

One of the patients who received marma cikitsā from Dr. Mistry was a nonresident Indian who periodically came to India on business. He had been seeing Dr. Mistry for several years. After examining his pulse, Dr. Mistry told him that his "center" was misaligned. He asked him to take off his shirt and lie down on his back on the floor. With a ruled tape he quickly measured the distance from the patient's right nipple to his navel and then the distance from his left nipple to his navel. He said that one distance was an inch longer than the other. (I could not corroborate this since his thumbs and fingers were covering the rulings on the tape, and the tape was covering the nipples and navel.) Then he had the patient turn over on his stomach, and in a few jerky motions he wrenched his back with two hands. When he again measured the distances from the two nipples to the navel, he found them to be equal. Then he showed his audience, which included two or three of his assistants as well as me, a swollen place on one side of the patient's lower back. He invited us to feel the swelling by touching first that spot and then the corresponding spot on the other side. Dr. Mistry pinched the skin around the swollen area and then rubbed in a medicinal powder emptied out of one of his capsules. He called on us to note how the powder had been absorbed by the skin. He applied a second capsuleful of powder and then a third. Finally, he declared that the skin was no longer absorbing the powder. Then he repeated the procedure on another swelling on the man's shoulder. He explained that pinching the skin created a space into which the powder could penetrate. Before the patient left, he reminded Dr. Mistry of another health problem he was experiencing. Dr. Mistry promised they would address it at his next visit. He assured the patient that this off-centeredness had been the most serious problem. "Now," he said, "I am not worried."

Dr. Mistry's marma cikitsā, which he later told me he had learned from his Tibetan guru, seems to be a peculiar selection of North and South Indian medical treatments offered by a wide variety of noninstitutional practitioners. The diagnosis of off-centeredness, together with the measurement of the distances from nipples to navel, is strongly reminiscent of a diagnosis of navel displacement common in some areas in North India. I have observed village healers make this diagnosis when a patient experiences a severe pain in his or her lower torso, often after straining to lift or carry a heavy load. These healers realigned the slipped navels by reciting mantras and tying particular roots onto the patient's body. I have also heard of North Indian sadhus who realign displaced navels by measuring the distances between the nipples and navel of the prone patient and then drawing a properly centered adjacent body on the ground beside them. I have never heard, however, of any practitioner attempting to heal this problem with massage. In any case, Dr. Mistry's jerking of the muscles of the back resembles chiropractic treatment more than it resembles most Ayurvedic massage, which is designed not so much to manipulate muscles as to saturate the tissues with medicinal oils. The marma treatments practiced by Keraliyan specialists, on the other hand, involve the application of pressure to very small points rather than the twisting of muscles or joints. Furthermore, in Keraliyan Ayurveda the misalignment of the navel is an unrecognized ailment, while the rubbing of dry powder into the skin is considered appropriate only for patients who have been diagnosed with excess kapha, the doṣa associated with coolness and moisture. Dr. Mistry, as I discuss below, never diagnoses anyone with excess kapha. It is difficult, then, to make sense of his marma cikitsā except as his own innovation, drawing freely on this and that "folk" practice with which he has come into contact.

Ordinarily medical anthropologists interpret this kind of eclecticism as medical syncretism. The concept of syncretism implies, however, that two or more distinct and internally consistent traditions meet and intermingle in a largely mechanistic process. Taussig (1987, 218) has outlined a different way of understanding those medical practices that draw their imagery from diverse cultural practices. He suggests that what seems like syncretism is actually a particular moment in an ongoing mimetic and countermimetic reverberation bearing the traces of political memory.[10] Nineteenth-century orientalists, as noted above, preferred to conceive of Ayurveda as a secular and empirical medicine that confirmed the notion of classical and secular origins of modern civilization. Ayurvedic knowledge involving "fabulous" animals or possession by, for example, celestial musicians was bracketed out as "magical" and projected into the realm of folk medicine. Thus the study of Ayurveda became a site for the consolidation of modern science against superstition. As discussed in chapter 5, Prakash (1992) has noted that this dichotomy was subtly displaced in certain Indian settings, where displays of scientific knowledge tended to evoke not only objectivity, but also a sense of wonder. Yet contemporary cosmopolitan Ayurvedic practitioners continue to reproduce this dichotomy, dividing Ayurveda as secular and empirical from the magic of "folk medicine." Dr. Mistry plays on this binarism in outrageous ways, the signs of professional and folk medicine circulating dizzily through his clinical landscape.

One day a teenage girl suffering from liver cancer came to the clinic with her parents. The parents were worried because the girl had recently been in a lot of pain. Dr. Mistry predicted that the pain would lessen. Her parents said that she did not like the diet that Dr. Mistry had prescribed. Then Dr. Mistry sent the parents out of the room. He began to ask the girl about her enjoyments, her pleasures, her happy memories. Eventually she told him about a time that a close friend embraced her. As they spoke, Dr. Mistry pressed a place on her wrist with his finger. Then he admonished her to eat a simple diet of rice, dal, and vegetables. He sent her out of the room, called the parents, and promised them that she would now eat properly. He called the girl back into the room, pressed the point on her wrist, and asked her to recite the foods she should eat, which she did. He told the parents not to worry. After the girl left, Dr. Mistry turned to me and asked if I had heard of "anchoring." When I said no, he informed me that there were four parts to Ayurveda: medicines, pancakarma, marma cikitsā, and "anchoring." He said that 80 percent of illness is psychological. This patient's parents, he told me, are totally "negative." He said, "They have been anchoring the girl that she is not going to live." By pressing on her wrist while she remembered the experience of her friend's embrace, he had "anchored" her in a positive memory. Whenever she feels discouraged or disinclined to eat her rice and dal, she can press the same point and relive the happiness of embracing her friend. Then she will want to live.

Afterward I was amazed that Dr. Mistry thought I would accept his assertion that "anchoring" was one of the four parts of Ayurveda (which, in any case, is classically divided into eight parts, none of which happen to be either pancakarma or marma cikitsā).[11] Much later I asked his partner, Dr. Lal, where he had learned this technique. She laughed and said that he was fond of reading self-help literature published in the United States. She said that he had learned the technique from an American patient who practices neurolinguistic programming (NLP). She added that Caraka discusses some of the psychologically oriented methods used by Dr. Mistry. For example, Caraka wrote that a physician should always sit up straight and smile. NLP is one of a host of new-age therapies of the West that work to reenchant medical professionalism. Like many other such therapies, it works on the body via the mind. Dr. Mistry's repetition of such practices suggests yet another level of mimetic vertigo: the imitation of new-age practitioners who themselves seem to imitate assorted idioms of "folk" healing. Not the least astonishing aspect of this last mimicry is that Dr. Mistry presents "anchoring" as one of the *original* parts of Ayurveda.

At some point during my observation of Dr. Mistry, I had a long conversation with Dr. Upadhyay, who had warned me that Dr. Mistry was a fraud. I hesitantly voiced the idea that Dr. Mistry might be only partly a fraud. I reminded Dr. Upadhyay that many Ayurvedic graduates with perfectly legitimate degrees might actually be ill-qualified to practice Ayurveda. Dr. Upadhyay replied that we were talking about someone who, unlike Ayurvedic graduates, might not know the locations of the liver and the spleen. I mentioned that hundreds of doctors with minimal Ayurvedic knowledge had received degrees during the early years of modern Ayurvedic education. Dr. Upadhyay countered that doctors who had obtained questionable degrees for the sake of the survival of Ayurveda could not be compared to someone who had obtained questionable degrees for the sake of "commercialization," or making money. Dr. Upadhyay also contrasted Dr. Mistry with rural practitioners who have some knowledge of local plants but no formal Ayurvedic education. Such practitioners, he said, are legitimate because they are healing people in areas where other doctors are not available. In Dr. Upadhyay's view, then, Dr. Mistry's mimicry of both professional Ayurvedic doctors and bona fide rural practitioners is quackery because, as he argues, it is driven by mercenary motives.

Dr. Mistry, on the other hand, declared to me that he has made enough money and that he is now simply on a mission to save Ayurveda. In that mission he feels that his detachment from a medical knowledge based on the location of livers and spleens is one of his strongest qualifications. He believes it is he who is saving Ayurveda by not allowing it to be contaminated by modern pathology. He says that his guru taught him to "forget allopathy." One day a patient arrived whose arm was trembling severely. He was convinced that he had Parkinson's disease and malaria. Dr. Mistry had his assistants massage his arms and feet with a powder containing ginger and with warm bundles of herbs. Dr. Mistry told me that the patient's feet were cold while his head was hot. Therefore he had to be "rebalanced." Otherwise he would become paralyzed. After warming the feet, the assistants cooled the head with an application of ghee. Later Dr. Mistry explained that what the patient thought was all a "game." The problem was not Parkinson's or malaria but an increase in the patient's *apāna* vāyu (the type of vāyu considered to regulate the release of urine, feces, semen, menses, and fetuses). Once his feet had been warmed and his head cooled, he felt much better.

Dr. Mistry then launched into a crusader's spiel. He said that a physician should "think in Ayurveda, dream in Ayurveda. Whatever we do, we write Ayurvedic diagnosis, Ayurvedic treatment. Otherwise, we'll all start thinking this way [i.e., allopathically], and the whole Ayurveda will be lost." He said he had started a campaign to return to the "basic principles" of Ayurveda. During an emergency, he said, most doctors begin to think in allopathic terms. He, however, does not think that way. He considers where the vāyu is moving, what the pitta is doing, and so on. When someone asked him at a conference whether he could cure alloplasia, he replied, "Why are you calling it alloplasia?" He finished up his impassioned speech to me by declaring that if he treated a patient according to allopathy, he would be "cheating" him. The criticism of Ayurvedic institutional practice, where allopathic diagnoses are frequently integrated with Ayurvedic diagnoses, is implicit. According to Dr. Mistry, it is the mimicry of allopathy found in institutional Ayurveda that is a kind of quackery. One of Dr. Mistry's former assistants, who also knows Dr. Upadhyay from lectures, told me that Dr. Mistry's knowledge of Ayurveda was actually very superficial compared to that of Dr. Upadhyay. This may well be true, and yet it is, interestingly, not Dr. Mistry's ignorance of Ayurveda per se that Dr. Upadhyay has criticized, but rather his ignorance of anatomy.

In a later conversation Dr. Upadhyay compared Dr. Mistry's practice to that of a "shaman" or a "Zulu healer." When I commented that there might be some benefit in such healing practices, he agreed but said that what he objected to was the mixing of such practices with "systems" such as Ayurveda. He said Dr. Mistry reminded him of some healers from the United States who had given a presentation at a conference on holistic medicine. These healers had horrified him by telling the audience in prissy tones, which he imitated for my benefit, "Now put your arms over your head and imagine that you are flying like a bird." He was appalled that such people could consider themselves practitioners of "holistic medicine." Dr. Upadhyay said that if Dr. Mistry called himself a "faith healer," he would not find him so objectionable, but "he is using the name of Ayurveda." Dr. Upadhyay feels that Dr. Mistry's faith-based practice is a misrepresentation of the scientific and systematic essence of Ayurveda. He believes that Dr. Mistry's Ayurvedic signboard and professional facade belie his folk-medical content. He does not deny the possibility that Dr. Mistry's practice could have medical efficacy. He concedes that he may have somehow learned something about pulse diagnosis; he concedes that some of the large number of medicines Dr. Mistry dispenses to any given patient in what Dr. Upadhyay terms a "shotgun approach" are bound to be beneficial; he even concedes that the faith Dr. Mistry inspires in patients probably contributes to their cure. What disturbs him, finally, is not Dr. Mistry's medical inauthenticity, but rather his cultural inauthenticity. What disturbs him is what disturbed me about the fake śilajīt, the slippage between sign and referent, because in this case the sign, Ayurveda, is one that is invested for him with a very particular meaning. Dr. Upadhyay believes that "true" Ayurveda is a practice purged of any magic associated with what he calls "faith healing." Dr. Mistry, on the other hand, feels that "true" Ayurveda is a practice purged of any trace of allopathy.

Dr. Mistry was fond of saying that he practiced "110 percent Ayurveda." Ultimately it is this extra 10 percent, this excess of meaning "spilling over the referent" (Taussig 1993) that challenges scientific and social scientific rituals of signification. The two aspects of Dr. Mistry's practice that make him most susceptible to the charge of quackery are his recruitment of images from magical medicine and his commercialistic style. Like magic, the techniques of advertising make obvious the sensuous aspects of signification that are more hidden in modern science (as discussed in chapter 5). The advertising image explodes with a tactile force on the mind. The sign is not simply representation: it is barrage, impression, physical sensation. Significantly biomedical doctors in private practice, with the exception of cosmetic doctors (who are selling not so much health as appearance), have typically not advertised themselves in a way that bombards the subconscious with imagery. In clinical visits we are bombarded, to be sure, by the icons of stethoscopes and anatomical diagrams and plastic intravenous tubes. These objects, however, are supposed to be entirely functional, and without fetishistic glow. That is, they are supposed to tidily serve and correspond to the act of breathing, the pumping of the heart, the circulation of life-giving sugars in the blood. Baudrillard could be referring to modern medicine, as well as political economy, when he notes, "It is the cunning of form to veil itself continually in the evidence of content. . . . That is its peculiar magic" (1981, 145). Pharmaceutical companies do advertise, of course, either directly to the public via television or magazines, or through salesmen who sit in doctors' offices, flicking through glossy, full-color schematics of the effects of drugs on the body, a blur of curving arrows, cross-sectioned kidneys, block-print letter claims.[12] Biomedical doctors themselves, however, generally do not advertise, except by a discreet listing of services. Such discretion has become a sign of professionalism for urban Ayurvedic doctors as well. Practitioners who advertise more extravagantly are suspected of being quacks.[13] The Udupa Report of 1959, in its attempt to bring Ayurveda into professional parallel with biomedicine, admonished that it was improper for medical practitioners to advertise themselves and that too many vaidyas disregarded this precept (Government of India 1959, 160). I suggest that the restriction of advertising in retail medicine is designed partly to protect the signs of science from fetishization, thus consolidating their special, objective relationship with natural objects. When these signs are recruited in advertising images, they risk seeming like simulacra, manipulated solely for the purpose of making money.

Dr. Mistry, however, has no compunction about advertising. He hands sheafs of xeroxed articles about himself to his patients. These articles compile not discreet listings of services, but hyperbolic listings of personal attributes. When Dr. Mistry demonstrates marma cikitsā to me and to his apprentices, he reminds me uncannily of a salesman demonstrating a product, deftly and efficiently working his magic, calling his audience to witness with a speed and positivity that sweeps all doubts under the carpet of the next dazzling feat. Indeed Dr. Upadhyay told me that Dr. Mistry worked in advertising before he turned to medicine, although Dr. Mistry never confirmed it. On several occasions he commented to me that he was not a businessman. Yet one of his patients once told me that when he had asked Dr. Mistry why Ayurveda, despite its antiquity, was so little known and appreciated, Dr. Mistry had replied that Ayurveda was not adequately advertised. When I asked Dr. Lal about this, she tactfully replied, "Advertising wouldn't be the proper meaning." She explained that Ayurvedic doctors need to have faith in Ayurveda. She assured me that all Dr. Mistry's publicity arises by word of mouth. Dr. Upadhyay, on the other hand, informed me that the head of a particular Ayurvedic professional association had told him that Dr. Mistry paid him 10,000 rupees in exchange for every invitation he received to participate in a scientific seminar. Dr. Mistry once showed me a video he had produced of a seminar on pulse diagnosis, promising that it would explain many things. At least 50 percent of the video was devoted, however, not to information about pulse but to testimonials by apprentices and patients, many of them Europeans or North Americans, of Dr. Mistry's fabulous cures.

From Function to Fetish

The apparent ambivalence about advertising is probably to be expected in a medical practice that wanders between the master categories of science and magic, the effectiveness of substance and the effectiveness of symbols. One day when I arrived at Dr. Mistry's clinic, he told me that he had had a "horrible experience" the previous day. For the first time in his life, he said, he was afraid. "I never get afraid normally," he said. "I stay very— ." He hesitated then and I suggested the word "calm," and he said yes. On this occasion, however, a woman had arrived with very advanced kidney stones. Her stomach was distended, and she had not urinated for two days. She started screaming from the pain while sitting in Dr. Mistry's office. Dr. Mistry told me, laughing, that her family had expected him to perform some "magic." Fortunately, he suddenly remembered a treatment his guru used to do for kidney stones involving an oil massage and a medicine to redirect vāyu in a downward direction. A few minutes after Dr. Mistry had administered this treatment, the woman went into the bathroom and passed out two or three small stones in her urine. She was smiling and dancing, Dr. Mistry said, and he was giving thanks to God. Here, although Dr. Mistry implicitly denies that he performs magic, he manages also to hint that he actually does perform magic.

On another of my visits a dialysis patient arrived from a distant city. His allopathic doctors had recommended a transplant for his one remaining kidney. He had come to Dr. Mistry because he did not want surgery, yet he did not want to remain on dialysis. Dr. Mistry promised that through his medicines the kidney would eventually regain its function. He cautioned, however, that the patient must continue dialysis for the time being. A few days later the patient returned, complaining of nausea. When Dr. Mistry asked if he had received dialysis, the patient said no.

Dr. Mistry became stern, saying, "I told you very clearly. You must take dialysis. Repairing the kidney will take time." Then he said he would give the patient a medicine to add to his bath that would immediately induce urination. He told him, however, that this was a one-time, temporary solution and that he should arrange for dialysis the very next day. Two days later the man returned to the clinic a third time. He claimed that he had still not received dialysis. He said he was urinating and eating and felt no need of dialysis. Dr. Mistry said, "Wonderful." He turned to me and said, "Magic." He still insisted to the patient that he should get dialysis when he returned to his home. Meanwhile, he sold him six months' worth of medicine. After the patient left, Dr. Mistry told me that his guru used to tell patients to use the therapy he had prescribed instead of dialysis. Now, for the first time, Dr. Mistry had tried it and it worked. "It's magic," he repeated again. He said that when he had discussed the case with Dr. Lal, she had told him, "You are killing that man. You should force him [to undergo dialysis]." "How can I force him?" he asked. He said he had also consulted with a kidney specialist who had predicted that without dialysis the man's feet and stomach would swell. When Dr. Mistry informed the specialist that these symptoms had not occurred, the specialist was amazed. He asked, "What did you do?" and added, "It's magic."

One day over lunch Dr. Mistry told one of his students and me a whole series of stories that had the effect of simultaneously asserting and denying his magical abilities. One infertility patient told him that her guru had told her that if Dr. Mistry simply touched her stomach, she would become pregnant. Dr. Mistry told us that since she believed this, he had to touch her stomach, even though he thought to himself, "This is horrible, illogical, nonscientific." Then, he said, she became pregnant. Only after his student asked did he tell us that the woman had also taken medicines for infertility. He told us that his guru had warned him that at a certain stage of his career, patients would believe he possessed some siddhi or paranormal power. If he began to believe this himself, he would lose his "gift," and he would have to start practicing "wrong tricks." He went on to say that eventually one actually did develop siddhis.[14] He himself used to materialize jewels in his hand like Sai Baba (a well-known spiritual guru) but he stopped because, he asked us rhetorically, what is the point? Dr. Mistry's messages about magic, then, are mixed. Patients believe he performs magic, and so he pretends he does; if he begins to believe in his magic, he will lose it; if he loses his magic, he will have to start faking it; magic is horrible and unscientific, but it works; he gave up performing magic years ago. The oscillation here between magic and science, between real magic and pretend magic, is itself slightly hypnotic.[15]

Dr. Mistry also reinforces the sense of magical performance in his practice with bursts of playfulness or laughter at extreme moments. When Dr. Mistry's assistant informed us that the kidney patient still had not taken dialysis, Dr. Mistry turned to me, laughing, and said he did not know what the problem was and that he would have to find out. Another time a suicidally depressed patient in his office was crying and threatening to throw himself under a truck if he was asked to leave the clinic. Dr. Mistry sent him into another room with a second depressed patient who had been taking his medications for ten days. He said to me, "I will make them mix, talk. Something might come out, I don't know," and he laughed. At that moment, and at those moments when he turned to me palms up, helplessly, and said, "Magic," I had the disorienting feeling that we were joined as twin spectators at his amazing, not-to-be-believed clinic, where anything might happen. His surprise and amusement at these times lent a certain unexpectedness, superfluity, excessiveness to his cures.

It is not only Dr. Mistry's medical treatment that takes on a certain fetishistic aura in his discourse, but also he himself. After sitting in his clinic for several days, I realized that he never diagnosed any patients with excess kapha, even when they suffered from asthma and other upper respiratory problems that other doctors considered to be classic kapha disorders. When I asked why he never detected excess kapha, he replied, "There are no kapha people on this planet." He went on to say that 80 percent of the people in the world had excess pitta. Only one in two hundred thousand people had a predominance of kapha. Those people, he added, were so healthy that they did not require medicine. The only problem kapha people experienced was a slight tendency toward bulkiness, he said, gesturing to himself. He explained that the reason there were so few kapha people was because of the pollution and chemicals in the environment. Chemicals are hot, whereas kapha is cold. Then he told me about certain techniques he had devised for conceiving kapha children. He characterized these children as calm and cheerful. He said that because he himself was kapha, he was able to remain very fresh and energetic. A kapha person, he asserted, could work for hours without becoming irritated. "It is like a Zen master," he said. Thus Dr. Mistry is not simply a purveyor of health but an embodiment of health. He warned us over lunch of the pitfalls of believing that one was god. He implied that he had personally seen too many godmen fall to be tempted to be one himself. What he lacked in godliness, however, he projected in a splendid iconicity, glowing with kapha, the source not only of a disease-free life, but also of the transnational serenities of "Zen."

Dr. Mistry's ambivalence about magic and equivocation about advertising intersect in his clinical method at the importance of faith. Dr. Lal had implied to me that the impression of advertising arose from Dr. Mistry's faith in himself, and in the conversations cited above he sometimes seemed to imply that the impression of magic arose from his patients' faith in him. This faith is largely inspired by pulse reading. When I entered his office for the first time, he was with a married couple and a small child. After taking the child's pulse, he told the father that the boy was suffering from asthma. After the family left, he informed me that now the father had full confidence in him because he had correctly assessed the child's problem. Weeks later his partner was listing the most important aspects of pulse examination. The first item on the list was to instill the patient's trust. The patient, she told me, must believe that he will be healed. "Pulse in a way is a tool to bring that faith, mainly," she said. Part of Dr. Mistry's great popularity, she said, was due to the fact that "instantly he can produce that faith." She added, "To generate confidence in the patient that he is going to be cured, that itself generates the healing process."[16] Later Dr. Lal said that the people who came to their clinic had usually been suffering for so long that they had lost any hope of being cured. The moment they are given faith, "things start working." She confirmed what Dr. Mistry had told me earlier — that 80 percent of illness is psychological. All of the aspects of Dr. Mistry's practice that smack of quackery can be understood as working to construct an atmosphere of faith: the photographs, the effusive newspaper articles, the suggestions of magical powers, even the vanity-publisher awards. It is pulse reading, the sign of the quintessential and missing "traditional" vaidya, that is the centerpiece of this collection of faith-inspiring objects.

Dr. Mistry told me his guru used to call the ordinary Ayurvedic diagnosis the "maybe" diagnosis. Now, Dr. Mistry claims, his diagnosis is totally without guesswork. Many patients, including a few who had not been hand-picked to talk to me, told me Dr. Mistry's diagnosis was amazingly accurate. A few ex-patients told me that his diagnosis had seemed vague. Dr. Mistry himself once said that the pulse is like a computer: if one knows how to operate it, one can operate it; it is not "magic." While Dr. Trivedi and others, as noted above, compared pulse reading to understanding or playing music, Dr. Mistry frequently compared pulse reading to the operation of a television set. In order to receive the information broadcast through a particular channel, it is necessary to know which button to push. Similarly, in order to receive the information moving through the body, it is necessary to know where and how to press the patient's wrist. Although it hardly exhausts Dr. Mistry's phenomenology of pulse, the analogy is intriguing, not least because the televised media are one of those instances of signification that evoke the hidden sensuosity of the sign. They are also a form of signification based in the photographic image, which, through editing, manipulation, juxtaposition, and so on, accumulates meanings that exceed its subject. Dr. Mistry's pulse readings are not simply or even primarily diagnoses but rather, as his partner told me, the first acts of healing. The pulse reading sparks the faith that fires the healing process. When Dr. Mistry, from the pulse, successfully predicts the patient's current symptoms, he gains the credibility to predict the course of the cure. The sign or the copy that is the pulse reading seeps back to affect the original, the illness, exactly as in sympathetic magic or the powerful images of advertising. Once a patient told me that although she had been warned against Dr. Mistry, she continued to see him because he, unlike other doctors, had correctly assessed her problems. I commented that he seemed to be an expert at inspiring faith in his patients. "Yes," she exclaimed. "So what if he has a big ego? I give thanks for his big ego." It is his "big ego" that has enabled him to cure her migraines. Even Dr. Mistry's self-aggrandizement, then, his own excessiveness as a sign, is vital to the healing process. What Lévi-Strauss wrote of the Brazilian "sorcerer" applies equally to Dr. Mistry: "Quesalid did not become a great shaman because he cured his patients; he cured his patients because he had become a great shaman" (1963b:180).

In the video he showed me of one of his pulse seminars, Dr. Mistry explained that "pulse reading has nothing to do with logic"; it is not "figuring out." It is not the kind of knowledge whereby a person sees smoke and concludes there is fire.[17] He asserted that the "basic principle is awareness, and it comes from meditation." Meditation, he further explained, means to focus on one thing without being distracted by others. Then he switched off the video for a moment to explain that if he is distracted by other things when he is examining the patients, then "I'm just trying to impress them, and trying to impress is a dangerous thing. Everything becomes like a gimmick and not genuine." Later he repeated this idea and added that there is a "subtle line between gimmick and truth." It seemed that he was alerting me to the fact that he walks this subtle line in his practice. If for one instant he loses his meditative focus, his ability to read pulse might dissolve into gimmickry.

Over the weeks I had become increasingly puzzled by the fact that Dr. Mistry recorded the patient's pulse only on the first visit and not on any subsequent visits. Finally I asked him how he was able to assess the patient's improvement without referring to an entire sequence of pulse readings. He said, "Ah yes, good question, good question." He seemed not to have considered this problem before. After a pause he replied that he was concerned only with what was happening in the patient's body at the moment. Later I asked the same question of Dr. Lal and received much the same answer. She said, "Pulse is what is going on at that moment," adding that pulse reading is like "Zen." Through pulse, Dr. Mistry told me, he was able to reconstruct the whole chain of events, the entire etiology of the illness, from first cause to immediate complaint.

Given this explanation, the question then becomes why Dr. Mistry bothers to record the pulse on the first visit. The most obvious reason would be to allow Dr. Mistry's several students to compare their diagnoses with his and with the patient's litany of complaints. Once I was observing Dr. Mistry's partner with a patient. In the box on the case form reserved for pulse notations she wrote p+++ for excess pitta and v+++ for excess vāyu. After hearing the diagnosis, the patient said she was not suffering from acidity but rather from gas. Dr. Mistry's partner then moved the symbol for excess pitta, which is considered to be a source of acidity, below the symbol for excess vāyu, which is considered to be a source of gas. I realized then that the pulse code on the case form is expected to precisely parallel the complaints of the patient. Because Dr. Mistry fills out the case form after discussing the complaints with the patient, he is able to assure that the pulse symbols as recorded for his students perfectly predict the symptoms. Ultimately it seems that the pulse symbols refer less to the referent, to the illness or even the aggravated doṣa, than to those other signs, the discomforts of the patient. The importance of pulse is not so much to signify the disorder as to divine the complaints. In Dr. Mistry's practice, then, the pulse neatly exemplifies the self-referentiality of the sign discussed by Baudrillard. Pulse is a simulacrum that owes its meaning not to its use value, its relationship with the illness, but to its exchange value, its relationship with those other signifiers, the symptoms.

When Dr. Upadhyay and I were discussing whether Dr. Mistry could really be considered a quack, he said at one point, irritated by my equivocations, "A fraud is a fraud is a fraud." In the successive moments between the repetitions of the word "fraud," however, a whole landslide of slippage can occur. During my association with Dr. Mistry one definition of quackery after another had to be discarded. Quackery could hardly mean simply a mimicry of medicines or methods or qualifications since such mimesis is essential to the training and identification of any medical practitioner. Quackery could also hardly mean a mimicry with intent to deceive since deception may be used to inspire the trust of the patient. An Indian friend told me once that the family and the family allopath had deliberately refrained from telling her mother-in-law that she was suffering from cancer because the word itself would have killed her at once. The deceptive manipulation of certain potent signs may occur in any kind of medicine. Finally, quackery could not even be mimicry with intent to deceive for mercenary motives since any doctor can be expected to have a few such motives. Quackery seems to be composed of qualities that slip back and forth between falseness and authenticity, continuously infusing one with the other.

The problem of Dr. Mistry's "quackery," like that of Don Juan's deceit, as acutely analyzed by Shoshana Felman (1983), can be greatly elucidated by a consideration of the different powers attributed to language. Dr. Upadhyay, like Don Juan's critics and lovers, epitomizes the constative power of language, committed to the division of the true from the false, while Dr. Mistry, like Don Juan himself, epitomizes the performative power. Indeed, as we have seen, the promise, the quintessential performative statement, is essential to Dr. Mistry's cures. The performativity of language undermines the distinction between truth and falseness as surely as does simulation in Baudrillard's scheme. For, as Felman notes, truth and falsehood do not apply to a language that is designed not to inform but to perform, to accomplish by pronouncement. Dr. Mistry's promises of cure, like Don Juan's promises of love, cannot be true or false, but only successful or unsuccessful.

Yet even the apparently more informative speech acts of Dr. Upadhyay, like the seemingly objective discourse of science, betray a hidden performativity. Felman notes that any utterance is always "in excess" of its statement. This excess is responsible for the performative "force" of even the most patently constative speech acts. In Dr. Upadhyay's emphatically informative statement, "A fraud is a fraud is a fraud," notice how the successive repetitions of the constative produce the very excess that constitutes the performative, his forceful effort to convince me that Dr. Mistry is a quack. Just as Dr. Mistry's promises of cure are designed to modify the prognosis of his patients, so Dr. Upadhyay's comment was designed to modify my opinion of Dr. Mistry. His performative intention leaves its urgent trace on his constative meaning.

Even as the partial resemblances of nationalist institutions produced in the colonies inevitably parodied the monumentality of history (as discussed in chapter 1), so the partial resemblances of professional and "folk" medicine, of modernity and "tradition" in Dr. Mistry's clinic, parody the monumentality of both science and culture. In the play of simulacra in his practice, the originals of either scientific medicine or ritual medicine become impossible to retrieve. Nordstrom (1988) has pointed out that much Ayurvedic practice defies classification as either "folk" or professional medicine. What I have tried to unravel here are some of the mimetic plays that may be involved in this defiance. Baudrillard (1988, 172) has commented that Disneyland exists to conceal the fact that the United States is Disneyland. Similarly we could say that magical medicine exists to conceal the fact that professional medicine is also magical. As a possible technician of magic who has entered the world of professional medicine, Dr. Mistry seriously upsets this act of concealment.

Because Dr. Mistry mimics not only the professional doctor honored by science, but also the folk doctor essentialized by anthropology, the force of his mimicry extends beyond medicine to social science. Dr. Upadhyay had forewarned me about allowing my picture to be taken with Dr. Mistry. I myself, having noticed several photos of Dr. Mistry with Europeans and North Americans in one of the tabloid articles handed to me on my first visit to his clinic, was quite aware of my own potential as a marketing tool. Yet if I recruit doctors in my knowledge-making practices, how can I object if they reciprocate? If I write this chapter on Dr. Mistry to try to argue certain insights about the politics of authenticity, then why should he not take my photograph to try to sell his drugs, each of us milking the other for all our possible exoticism? I did not object, therefore, when Dr. Mistry's assistant took a picture of me sitting next to Dr. Mistry listening to a patient. Taussig (1993, 248) tells of the jolt he experienced when he saw the plastic IV tubes and bluish X ray lamps hung against the walls of a mystical healing center in Columbia. These signs of science, drained so thoroughly of functional meanings, were glowing all the more excessively with fetishistic meanings. If there is anything comparable in Dr. Mistry's clinic—any sign that, for me, spills over its referent so completely as to erase it—perhaps it is the photograph I have not yet seen of me sitting with Dr. Mistry, the photograph of the interested white foreigner, one more legitimating sign glimmering from the photo album, arousing in patients the faith that allows them to be healed.

seven Parodies of Selfhood

In this last chapter I take the story of Ayurvedic responses to postcolonial imbalance back into the hospitals, where contemporary practitioners subversively reconfigure a psychological universalism, particularly through the development of Ayurvedic psychotherapy. I explore why the practice of Ayurvedic psychotherapy seems to trouble and even parody North American conceptions of the purpose and narrative course of psychotherapeutic practice. I argue that such sessions as I recount here disrupt one of modernity's central assumptions, an essential interiorized self, at what would ordinarily be a key site in its deployment, the confessional form of psychotherapeutic consultation.

While the elaboration of Ayurvedic psychotherapy is only a couple of decades old, the reworking of the modern interior self is tellingly foreshadowed by earlier engagements between yogic and psychoanalytic theory. In the small yoga departments found in most Ayurvedic hospitals, yoga usually means hatha yoga—that is, physical postures (āsanas) and breathing exercises (*prāṇayāma*) to ease tension, enhance relaxation, or strengthen particular parts of the body. For some practitioners, however, yoga means a more comprehensive mental discipline. Dr. Trivedi, for instance, considered hatha yoga by itself little more than "gymnastics." He argued that it should be taught and prescribed only within a larger yogic practice involving strengthening of the mind through meditation (*dhyān*), mantra repetition, and other techniques discussed in Patanjali's *Yoga Sūtras*. It is useful, therefore, to turn briefly to a non-Ayurvedic literature on yogic anticipations of modern psychology, particularly yogic theorizations of the unconscious.

In 1976 C. T. Kenghe observed, "It is usually believed that S. Freud brought about a revolution in psychological thought by introducing the concept of the unconscious mind. This is certainly true as far as Western psychology is concerned. However, the unconscious mind is not at all a new concept to Indian psychological thinkers. From times immemorial, they have been aware of such a force and references to it can be found even in the earliest Vedic literature" (1976, 37). Other writers have linked the unconscious to the *saṃskāras,* the impressions left on the mind from the experiences and deeds of previous incarnations (H. L. Sharma 1979, xii; Kumar 1966, 111.) In one detailed elaboration of this linkage, Swami Ajaya writes:

> Samskaras can cluster together and become active, either in response to an external situation or as a result of their own ripening. When they become active, they motivate actions and create external circumstances, so that what is unfinished and important can be completed and thereby transcended. . . . They are like tiny seeds that can sprout and create a painful melodrama. . . . One's complexes are thought to be dissolved in successful psychotherapy. Similarly, in the process of self-realization through yoga, the samskaras are metaphorically described as being "roasted." They become like burnt seeds that can no longer sprout; they can no longer lead to impelled and unregulated action through unconscious motivation (1983, 67–68).

What is interesting here is that actions are identified as the manifestations or signs of latent impressions in the mind, which are in turn the consequences or signs of previous actions. Like the Lacanian unconscious, these clusters of seeds that compose the "unconscious" of Patanjali's yoga tend to unsettle a distinction between acts and signs. One can imagine a virtually endless cycle (in Sanskrit nomenclature, a *samsāra,* or wheel of existence) where actions signify and signifiers act. Here action becomes a kind of speech, a sequence of signs communicating meaning to the depth psychologist. Since the saṃskāras are merely the products of previous experiences and deeds, they are not in themselves "natural" or inherent contents of the mind (as, for example, the instincts of a later Freud). Rather, the saṃskāras are as relative and mutable as the social masks of the ego. Kenghe therefore concludes, "Yoga does not consider any instincts to be natural and hence, whereas according to Freud the instincts cannot be completely removed and can only be kept under rational control at the best, according to Yoga they can be completely removed and thereby the whole of the unconscious can also be conquered" (1976, 46). While this more easily conquered unconscious posited by yogic theorists is not, to my knowledge, directly theorized by Ayurvedic practitioners, it is nonetheless implicit within certain moments of contemporary practice. Before turning to these moments, however, I consider the aspects of the mind that *have* been theorized by Ayurvedic practitioners.

Mental Substance

Ayurvedic ideas about mentality frequently draw on Sāṃkhya philosophy, which organizes the phenomenal universe into thirty-six tattvas. At the level of the twelfth tattva is *purūṣa* (also known as ātmā or *jīva*), the personal soul or awareness, consciousness without content or quality, knowing but unknowable, not subject to illness. All of the tattvas beyond the twelfth compose prakṛti, the knowable aspect of creation, which is imbued with the three qualities of sattva, rajas, and tamas. Included in prakṛti are the three mental faculties: *buddhi* (discriminating intellect), ahaṃkāra (self-identification, often translated as ego), and *mānas* (the aspect of mind that comprehends sensory objects). Also within prakṛti are the five senses and their objects (sound, flavor, and so on); the five powers of action (speaking, touching, and so on), associated with the five organs of action (voice, hands, and so on); and the five elements (fire, air, water, earth, ether).[1] In other words, the three psychic faculties identified within Sāṃkhya are part of prakṛti, the objective world, rather than part of consciousness, subjective awareness. It is not so much that Sāṃkhya is nondualistic as that it posits a differently configured dualism than Cartesianism. Rather than locating a split between mind and body, it locates a split between awareness and matter, or knower and known, the latter *including* the mind and all its faculties. As Agehananda Bharati has written, "From the canonical manifestations of mind (*buddhi,* 'intellect') via mānas, 'the thinking organ,' conative energizer, to the body of flesh, all these are conceived of as matter, albeit of different degrees of subtlety and density—the body is the crudest, thickest of these material entities, *buddhi* the subtlest" (1985, 193). Thus a predominantly mental illness, like a predominantly physical illness, can be understood in terms of relationships between volumes and properties of matter.

It may be partly for this reason that Gananath Obeyesekere (1977) has argued that Ayurvedic treatment of mental illness is "somato-psychic" in that it interprets psychological ailments in terms of physical—that is, doṣic—processes. At the same time, he notes that in Sri Lanka this interpretation accords well with the tendency of Sinhalese patients to "somatize" psychological conflicts. In a somewhat similar argument Mark Nichter (1981b) finds that in Sri Lanka interpersonal problems are often expressed in bodily symptoms. While the Ayurvedic practitioners he discusses are aware of their patients' social difficulties, they project them onto a humoral stage (1981b, 9). Neither of these arguments questions the idea of somatization itself. That is, each rests on an assumption that the somatic illnesses under consideration are secondary, while the "real" or primary illnesses are either intrapsychic (for Obeyesekere) or psychosocial (for Nichter). Laurence Kirmayer (1988), on the other hand, has argued that the idea of somatization simply confirms the Cartesianism of other aspects of biomedicine in that it presumes the domination of mind over body.

Evidence of apparent "somatization" can certainly be found in Indian Ayurvedic practices. In the OPD of one Ayurvedic hospital, patients who were being treated for predominantly mental illness reported such ailments as stomach pain, constipation, loss of appetite, a sensation of choking, weakness, flatulence, chest pain, shortness of breath, heart palpitations, and low blood pressure. Only rarely would a patient mention sadness, indifference, or nervousness among his or her complaints. In this hospital, however, unlike in the practices discussed by Obeyesekere and Nichter, such instances of "somatization" are routinely diagnosed with psychiatric categories such as depression, anxiety-depression, neurosis, and schizophrenia. Practitioners at this hospital told me, for instance, that belching is often a sign of depression since patients feel that by releasing gas they can relieve the heavy feeling of sadness in their chests.[2]

On the face of it, then, the somatic complaints of many of the patients at this hospital appear to be secondary effects of psychiatrically defined problems. Consider the diagnosis of one young man in the OPD who reported that his problem began when he donated blood to his sister a year before. He complained of giddiness, stomach pain, eye pain, flatulence, headache in his temples, low blood pressure, occasional trembling, leg pain, and nervousness, especially when alone. When I asked why he had donated blood to his sister, he told me that she was having a difficult delivery. The doctor who was attending him told me that like many patients, he believed that blood loss resulted in low blood pressure. When I asked the patient if his sister was well now, he said that she had died. Yet to consider this patient's illness as a simple case of depressive somatization seems to overlook its persuasive symbolic logic. If in donating blood to his sister, the young man offered her a part of his heart, his life's substance, then has he not lost that portion of his personal substance in her death? The idea that his grief is expressed in physical symptoms not only subordinates his body to his mind, as Kirmayer suggests, but also medicalizes his sadness as depression, disregards his own etiological knowledge, and creates a split between his "imaginary" illness and his "real" disease. A more helpful interpretation is suggested by Nancy Scheper-Hughes (1992), who notes that the poor and marginalized tend to communicate their distress through a somatic medium. To call this communication a "somatization" of emotional problems is to project a middle-class language of psychic pain onto a working-class or underclass language of physical pain.

Meanwhile, the language of urban Ayurvedic practitioners often moves very freely between somatic and psychological "idioms of distress" (Nichter 1981a). In this language psychiatric categories and psychosomatic insights are singular moments rather than final conclusions in an unfolding understanding of illness. A split between mind and body is rarely sustained since even when psychic or social disturbance is given a psychiatric name, it is still, as Obeyesekere notes, diagnosed as overflowing doṣa. One could conceivably argue that a mind-body split is also not sustained in contemporary psychoneurology, which emphasizes the biological genesis and treatment of illnesses such as depression. The location of mental illness in brain chemistry and neurological function, however, still confines physical problems to the mind, linking them to chemicals, such as seratonin and dopamine, that are exclusively associated with mental function. In Ayurvedic practices, on the other hand, predominantly mental illnesses are traced to the same physical elements as predominantly somatic illnesses. Even so, Obeyesekere's assessment of Ayurvedic treatment as somatopsychic does not quite convey the relationship of psyche and soma in Ayurvedic practice as I observed it. For if mind is substantial, doṣa is also mental and susceptible to social disturbance.

According to ancient texts, doṣic derangement originates with the improper engagement of the senses with sensory objects (*prājñāparādha*).

This improper engagement can include everything from eating unsuitable food to abusing one's elders to feeling excessive fear or joy in response to an event. Caraka wrote that impure food; insults to gods, teachers, or brahmin; mental shock due to fear or elation; and difficult postures are all possible causes of insanity. Any of these may disturb the doṣa, which then directly affect the heart (*hṛday*), the seat of the intellect, thus deranging the mind.[3] *Caraka Saṃhitā* contains a litany of the signs of vatika paittika and kaphaja insanity, which range freely through physical condition, action, and feeling. One suffering from paittika insanity, for instance, is characterized by intolerance, agitation, nakedness, terrorizing actions, excessive movement, heat, fury, desire for shade and cold food or drink, and a yellowish cast to the skin (P. V. Sharma 1981, 2:161). One suffering from kaphaja insanity is characterized by slowness of speech and movement, excessive thinness, desire for women, loneliness, excessive sleep, nausea, salivation, and white fingernails (ibid.).[4] Although many of these signs of insanity have ceased to hold much meaning for urban practitioners—despite their almost verbatim appearance in a 1990 Hindi book shown to me by Kaviraj Kumar entitled *Modern Ayurvedic Guide* (Śuklan 1990)—mental illnesses are still classified according to doṣa. Depression without agitation, for instance, is typically considered a kapha disorder, while sociopathology is typically considered a pitta disorder. In an M.D. thesis published in 1994 (R. Kumar 1994, 72) the pathogenesis of "depression" was traced along a path that essentially followed that charted by Caraka for mental illness. Aggravated doṣa gather in the heart (hṛday) and *manovaha* śrotas (literally, mind-carrying channels) and eventually produce depression. Note how mind is enough of a substance here to move like fluid through bodily channels.

The circulation of doṣa between mental faculties and bodily organs or tissues is one instance of the intermingling of mental substance and other substances, the incessant migration of qualities. The circulation of the *triguṇa* (sattva, rajas, and tamas) between world and mind is another. In illnesses that primarily affect the mind, both the bodily doṣa (vāta, pitta, and kapha) and what are called the mental doṣa (characterized according to the triguṇa as sattva, rajas, and tamas) may be disturbed. As qualities of mind, sattva, rajas, and tamas are associated with clarity and equanimity, desire and initiative, and inertia and inhibition respectively. One professor explained that sattva is responsible for knowledge, rajas for action, and tamas for confusion or fear. Drawing a picture of a radio on the blackboard, he said that at all times we are receiving and responding to various signals from the universe, just as a radio receives input and responds with sound. Sattva, rajas, and tamas refer to the three possible responses we can have to the world. All three are necessary, but ideally sattva should exist in the greatest proportion since it fosters tranquillity and detachment. It is useful to recall that these qualities apply not only to mind, but to every other kind of matter as well. Food may be more or less sattvic, rajasic, or tamasic, as may particular activities, living environments, and so on.

The word "psychosomatic" is usually used to translate the word *manodaihika,* an adjective meaning "related to mind and body." According to some sources, including Dr. Joshi's lectures to his M.D. students, manodaihika (or *manośarīra*) disorders are mental in origin and somatic in manifestation (Tripathy 1981, 136; S. S. Mishra 1980, 50). In this category scholars have included hypertension, āmavāt, certain diarrheas and fevers, the illness usually glossed as asthma, and so on. Here, the concept of psychosoma does not enforce a split between "imaginary" illness and "real" disease but simply identifies the involvement of mental factors at a certain stage of pathogenesis. While technically the category of psychosoma within biomedicine is also used to refer to such illnesses, clinically it is also frequently used to refer to hypochondria, mysterious aches and pains, and a host of ailments prefaced with the prefix "pseudo"—for example, pseudoangina and pseudoepilepsy (Kirmayer 1988, 66). On the other hand, for many Ayurvedic physicians I met, hypochondria, or the tendency to invent or exaggerate illness, is itself taken as evidence for aggravated doṣa (usually vāta). The way that ailments fluctuate between mental and somatic manifestations at different points in a pathogenic narrative is therefore hardly grasped by the word psychosomatic.

In keeping with the understanding of mind as mental substance, vaidyas frequently treat particular mental complaints with medicinal substances. For example, *sirodhāra,* a form of pancakarma in which a warm medicinal oil or milk-based liquid is dripped in a slow stream onto the forehead, is used in Ayurvedic clinics and hospitals throughout India for diagnoses such as insomnia, depression, headache, neurosis, and schizophrenia (see figure 13). Dr. Vijayan, who routinely uses sirodhāra with his patients, told me that it alleviates vāta disorders of the head and

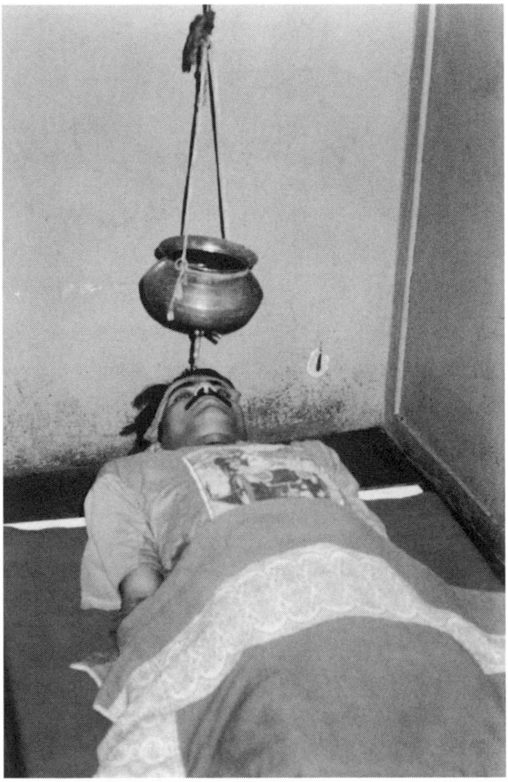

Figure 13. Sirodhāra. A patient in an urban Ayurvedic hospital is treated for insomnia.

stimulates the cranial nerves. Here the "organic" (as some Ayurvedic physicians refer to the biomedical, organ-related, visible) and the doṣic (the guṇa-saturated, invisible) seem to be joined in one domain. Noticing that sirodhāra induces a kind of meditation, Dr. Vijayan also concluded that it disengages the conscious mind, allowing the unconscious to surface. Other forms of pancakarma, such as emesis, vasti, and nasal drops, are also used to cleanse the doṣa in mental illness, particularly psychosis (unmād), in which both mental and physical doṣa are considered to be severely disturbed.

In addition to the application of medicines through pancakarma, there are two classes of ingested medicines that are especially used for mental complaints. One is called *vājīkaraṇa* (which, as mentioned in chapter 4, is one of the eight branches of Ayurveda listed in the early texts). These medicines have been understood for centuries as aphrodisiacs and correctives to sexual dysfunction. In the last decade they have begun to be used for the treatment of depression at a certain Ayurvedic hospital (of which more will be said below). As R. H. Singh, the doctor responsible for this development, explained, "We are using these drugs for mood elevation." It had occurred to him that since much of sexual dysfunction is related to the mind, the drugs for sexual problems might also work for mental illness, specifically depression. In his M.D. thesis, one of Singh's students (Tripathy 1981, 98) reported that two Ayurvedic aphrodisiacs (*aśvagandha* and *kapikacchu*) were found to be effective in anxiety and depression.

The other class of medicines in use at this institution and elsewhere for mental problems is known as *medhya* rasāyan, a name that suggests renewal of the intellect. Medhya rasāyan medicines are considered to improve both intelligence and memory. Practitioners frequently point out that modern medicine has no equivalent of medhya rasāyan. In the hospital just mentioned, these medicines are commonly used to treat anxiety. Several of Singh's students note in their M.D. theses that medhya rasāyan drugs are predominantly cool in effect and sweet and pungent in taste. Very few of these substances are bitter, sour, or astringent, but many of them are oily. Since coolness, sweetness, and oiliness increase kapha, the students speculated that these drugs might be largely kaphaja in effect, improving the bodily physique and soothing the mind (Shetty 1991, 85–86; S. S. Mishra 1980, 65–66; A. K. Mehta 1976, 92–93). While these researchers all observed that a tranquil mind is a clear mind, they drew different conclusions from this correlation, perhaps reflecting the changing views of their mentor. A. K. Mehta first noted that modern medicine had no drugs to improve intelligence and only drugs to relieve anxiety and depression and then wrote: "However, a study of the phenomenon of stress, anxiety and tension indicates that the basic intelligence, memory and other attributes in a man are greatly masked by mental tension; accordingly if a person is tranquilised and made free from tension and anxiety his mental performance improves. . . . Thus an ideal tranquiliser or an anti-anxiety drug may be treated as a *Medhya* agent" (1976, 93). Ashwini Shetty, on the other hand, wrote: "It will be relevant to mention here, that a tranquilised mind in the present context is fundamentally different than the tranquillity as afforded by modern tranquilisers which basically suppress the brain hyperactivity. A *Medhya Rasayana* improves the micronutrition of brain cells and gradually removes the state of hypoxia in the brain, which is the main cause of the hyperactivity" (1991, 86). Another student, who was just completing his degree in 1995, also under Singh's supervision, disagreed that the improvement of intellect was a secondary effect of the reduction of anxiety. In his opinion, it was equally possible that the reduction of anxiety was a secondary effect of the improvement of the intellect. When I asked him if any psychiatric drugs could be considered medhya rasāyan, he replied that no drug that is composed only of an active ingredient can be considered a medhya rasāyan. Rasāyan always implies a therapy that directly improves the nourishment of the tissues (dhātu). When I asked Singh himself if he thought the effect of the medhya rasāyan drugs was due to the enhancement of kapha, he replied that he would prefer to say that their effect might be due to the calming of vāta. He added that he and his students had not yet been able to determine whether the improvement of the intellect through medya rasāyan is due to the reduction of anxiety or the other way around.

What is intriguing here is that the Ayurvedic substances being used to treat mental illness are not oriented toward restoring a "normal" mental state but rather to developing an enhanced mental state. While the vājīkaraṇ medicines produce happiness, the medhya medicines produce a stronger intellect. Unlike antidepressants or tranquilizers, these medicines are potentially beneficial for the healthy as well as the ill. Despite the psychiatric nomenclature, the idea of the normal, which is so central to psychiatric constructions of mental health, is entirely absent in these constructions of Ayurvedic mental health. Perhaps the medicinal treatment for mental illness can be said to resemble the psychotherapeutic treatment for mental illness at this institution. For if the Ayurvedic psychiatry practiced there is missing the seemingly crucial pivot of normality, then similarly the Ayurvedic psychotherapy practiced there is missing the seemingly crucial pivot of a true and prior interior self.

Sattvāvajaya

In a passage of the "Sūtrasthānam" of the *Caraka Saṃhitā,* there is reference to three types of therapy, *daivya* therapy, *yukti* therapy, and sattvāvajaya. In one relatively literal translation this verse reads: "There are three types of therapy—spiritual, rational and psychological. The spiritual therapy consists of recitation of mantras, wearing roots and gems, auspicious acts, offerings, gifts, oblations, following religious precepts, atonement, fasting, invoking blessings, falling on (the feet of) the gods, pilgrimage, etc. The rational therapy consists of rational administration of diet and drugs. Psychological therapy [sattvāvajaya] is restraint of mind from the unwholesome objects" (P. V. Sharma 1981, 1:79).[5] Outside of this one verse, there is no other mention of sattvāvajaya in any of the seminal Ayurvedic texts. Yet Singh, a prominent physician noted for his work in the field of mental health, has developed sattvāvajaya as an Ayurvedic specialization that he translates as psychotherapy. At the institution where he practices and teaches, Ayurvedic psychotherapy is conducted not only by him, but also by a psychologist I will call Dr. Nandi, who was jointly trained in psychiatry and kāyacikitsā, and by Ayurvedic M.D. students specializing in mental health.[6]

Prior to 1981, theses on mental health written by Singh's students concentrated for the most part on the mind-strengthening drugs discussed above (e.g., Malviya 1976; A. K. Mehta 1976). S. S. Mishra (1980) evaluated the effectiveness of "traditional mental health promoting practices," which he identified as health regimens (swasthavṛtt), correct behavior (*sadvṛtt*), and yoga. The research subjects underwent a program of "mental health education," which included meditation on the god of their choice for a few minutes each morning, regular bathing, a visit to a temple for meditation, prāṇayama in the evening, truthfulness and piety, and some degree of *brahmācarya* (sexual self-discipline). Mishra concluded that such practices "do promote the mental peace and induce a feeling of well-being." He added that unfortunately he had great difficulty persuading people to undertake the program: "Even the educated persons did not know that the practices like visiting a temple and meditation or worship may bring mental peace and well-being." Most people believed that such practices were meant only for spiritual benefit. According to Mishra, the neglect of such practices "even in traditional families in rural areas . . . is leading in turn to deterioration of mental health superadded with the rising incidence of anxiety and stress in today's society due to rapid population turnover, urbanisation, and industrial development which are the main causes of the deterioration of mental health in urban areas" (S. S.

Mishra 1980, 133). Mishra does not mention sattvāvajaya. Yet perhaps it was partly the reluctance of his patients to understand yoga as a mental health therapy that led Dr. Singh and some of his later students to discover psychotherapy as one of the three types of therapy.

The translation of sattvāvajaya as psychotherapy first appears in Rajkishore Tripathy's 1981 thesis, devoted to the use of certain Ayurvedic drugs for anxiety and depression. After defining sattvāvajaya as psychotherapy, Tripathy comments that the mental restraint — or, as he translates it, "mind control" — referred to in the above passage of *Caraka Saṃhitā* is achieved through "spiritual knowledge, philosophy, fortitude, remembrance and concentration" (1981, 25).[7] He goes on to say that according to Ayurveda, "volitional transgression (prājñāparādha) [is] the main etiopathological factor" in mental illness and can be corrected through psychotherapy.[8] Following certain verses in *Caraka Saṃhitā,* he suggests that psychotherapy involves encouraging the patient to behave appropriately and to understand the truth and pursue "self-realization." "By this," he writes, "he stands clear of egoism and he gives up taking refuge in anything and becomes able to understand the reality." Tripathy also defines *samādhi,* usually understood as a deep state of meditation, as "mental equanimity." In his thesis, then, the path to mental health has not yet diverged from the path to liberation. It is not until five years later that sattvāvajaya was first used in M.D. research at this university. During the interim the concept seems to have been fleshed out by Singh and his students until, along with drugs, it became a primary treatment for mental disorders at the university's Ayurvedic hospital.

In Singh's 1986 book on Ayurvedic mental science, the discussion of sattvāvajaya is less than a page long, suggesting that at the time of writing he was just beginning to elaborate his ideas on the subject. In that section, referring to the above-mentioned sutra from *Caraka Saṃhitā,* he writes, "Sattvāvajaya is that method of treatment through which one tries to bring the intellect [*dhī*], mental fortitude [*dhṛti*] and memory [*smṛti*] of the patient into a proper condition" (R. Singh 1986, 139). He draws on sutra elsewhere in *Caraka Saṃhitā* to identify two methods of sattvāvajaya: assurance to the patient of the return of lost objects or persons and inducement of emotions opposite to those associated with the patient's distress.[9] In *Caraka Saṃhitā* it is written, "If the mind is affected due to loss of some liked thing, it should be pacified by consoling and assuring [the patient] to provide a similar thing" (P. V. Sharma 1981, 2:170). The first of Singh's students to do research on sattvāvajaya, A. R. V. Murthy, writes in his 1986 thesis, "If the cause of a mental disorder is the separation from a close friend or a relative or loss of a very dear object, then [the patient] has to be treated either by providing him with the object or by assurance of the same" (1986, 53).

In a paper written jointly by Singh and Karel Nespor, a Czech psychiatrist (Nespor and Singh 1986, 29), another method of sattvāvajaya, psychoshock therapy, whereby patients are suddenly frightened to jolt them into another mental state, is added to this list.[10] According to one South Indian practitioner, psychoshock is used with psychotic patients at an Ayurvedic hospital for the mentally ill with which he used to be affiliated. A version of it was also used by Dr. Pathi when one of his patients was distressed that he could not satisfy his parents' high expectations for his academic achievement. "Having once heard someone refer to 'split personality,' he developed it," Dr. Pathi told me. He used to go out and return with no memory of where he had been. One day Dr. Pathi pretended he was about to kick him, and the young man was suddenly reintegrated. In Murthy's thesis, which is about the use of group sattvāvajaya for irritable bowel syndrome, another five techniques of sattvāvajaya are listed: regulation of thought, reframing of ideas, channeling of assumptions, refining of objectives and ideals, and proper guidance in decisions (A. R. V. Murthy 1986, 53). In a list posted in Singh's office in 1995, there was only one addition to this list: the inducement of patience in the mentally ill person. Privately Singh informed me that reassurance and replacement of emotions are the two most important techniques of sattvāvajaya.

Addressing the fact that sattvāvajaya has been mentioned only once in the ancient texts, Murthy writes, "All these facts reflect one thing—psychotherapy including sattvāvajaya was done by some specialists at the time of Caraka" (A. R. V. Murthy 1986, 55). He refers to another passage, in which Caraka advises persons with mental disorders to visit specialists—apparently verses 46 and 47 of chapter 11 of "Sūtrasthānam," where solutions for mental disorders are identified as the proper pursuit of righteousness; possessions and pleasure; service to experts; and knowing oneself, including one's place, time, strength, and abilities (P. V. Sharma 1981, 1:77–78). Murthy goes on to explain that most of the texts extant from that time are from the kāyacikitsā branch of Ayurveda, which concentrates on corporeal treatment. "However," he writes, "whatever is available is very concrete and fundamental on the basis of which the whole concept of psychotherapy as prevailed in those days can be pictured very easily" (A. R. V. Murthy 1986, 55).

The reconstruction of Ayurvedic sattvāvajaya mirrors the reconstruction of Ayurveda itself. In the case of sattvāvajaya, not only is an entire field of specialization elaborated from one verse, but this field is also found to correspond to and anticipate a modern therapeutic technique. Like the various practitioners discussed in chapter 5 who translated Ayurvedic processes into biomedical terms, Singh collaborated with Nespor (Nespor and Singh 1985, 29) to translate the techniques of sattvāvajaya into modern psychological terms, comparing the replacement of emotion to shuttling in Gestalt therapy and the reframing of ideas to Ericksonian hypnosis.

Since sattvāvajaya literally means "winning the mind," the single reference to sattvāvajaya from which Ayurvedic psychotherapy has been (re)constituted could easily be interpreted to mean not a relationship between doctor and patient, but rather a mental discipline. In fact, of the three types of therapy listed in the verse, only one, yukti, translated above as "rational" therapy, seems to require the interventions of a healing technician. The others appear to refer to therapies that can be administered by oneself, one's family or community, or a practitioner who specializes in mediations with unseen realms. In the passage in *Caraka Saṃhitā* that describes the treatment for unmād it is suggested that a friend of the ill person console or shock the patient, while in the passage on apasmāra, it is suggested that a friend should talk to the patient about righteousness, wealth, and so on (P. V. Sharma 1981, 2:170, 177). In his thesis, Murthy acknowledges that sattvāvajaya could signify "subjective mind control" but argues that Caraka is speaking of "objective" mind control involving the doctor's "interference" (A. R. V. Murthy 1986, 112). Singh confirmed this in conversation, saying that in sattvāvajaya "a physician wins the mind of the patient."

An element of such "sattvāvajaya" is, of course, common to many Ayurvedic practices since, for most practitioners, mental and physical health cannot be separated. In a lecture on mental illness to his M.D. students Dr. Joshi said that there was no psychological specialty in Ayurveda because mind is a factor in every disease. After noting that there is no "separate psychology" in Ayurveda, another professor added that this was not a deficiency since "everything in Ayurveda is connected with psychology." Later on he reiterated that "informal" psychotherapy was part of everyday Ayurvedic practice. Every Ayurvedic practitioner I observed was treating mental and physical problems conjointly, just as we observed Dr. Upadhyay do in chapter 2. Frequently the treatment of the mental component of disease involved an intervention in a patient's social relations. Once Dr. Upadhyay advised a mother to send her son away from home for two years. "His dependence on you is part of the problem," he said. One of Dr. Pathi's patients suffered from headache and acidity. His problem, Dr. Pathi told me, was that he believed that his boss had given him extra work because he disliked him. Dr. Pathi told the boss to go to the man's house and explain that he was giving him extra work because he considered him a good worker. Soon after, the patient's condition improved. Dr. Pathi told another "psychic" patient, who was "harassing" his family, to plant trees by the side of the road. All the harassment stopped, he said. One professor recounted that he cured the schizophrenia of one of his patients simply by instructing his wife to treat him differently.

When I asked one of Singh's students about the psychotherapy he used in his research, he said that it involved detailed discussion of the patient's problems. For example, he said, if a patient was worried about a land dispute, he would ask him if he really deserved the land in question. If the patient said yes, then he would invite the other party in the dispute to the next therapy session and offer a compromise solution. Here the psychotherapist seems to stand in for a *pancāyat,* village elder, or dispute mediator. Whereas a North American intervention would focus on the self-esteem and willful action of the patient, these Ayurvedic practitioners focus on alterations in the social environment. Even a son's greater independence is to be achieved not by his own epiphany and will, but by his mother's actions. The emphasis is not on reconciling the patient to his loss and strengthening his resilience, as in North American psychology, but on intervening directly and effectively in his situation. In my first conversation with Dr. Nandi, she volunteered that her psychotherapy was different from European or North American psychotherapy in that her patients required a great deal of advice. Alan Roland, a psychoanalyst who has practiced extensively in India, notes that his Indian clients frequently relate to him in much the same way that they might relate to a guru (1988, 60, 63).

Dr. Singh himself told me that there is no fundamental difference between sattvāvajaya and modern psychotherapy. In his opinion both involve the removal of the mind from harmful sense objects. In his thesis, Murthy claims that in his research for the first time "a comprehensive regimen of sattvāvajaya, an Ayurvedic method of psychotherapy, was employed with satisfactory outcome" (A. R. V. Murthy 1986, 109). In a section entitled "Modern Concept of Psychotherapy" he distinguishes supportive psychotherapy, which includes advice, reassurance, encouragement, and social intervention, from psychodynamic psychotherapy, which includes psychoanalysis, behavior modification, and a "client-controlled" therapy not focused on the patient's early history (1986, 67–69). He says that he employed "dynamically oriented short term group psychotherapy," which was "mainly supportive . . . with resource for insight" (1986, 92).[11] Does the emphasis on social (or sometimes spiritual) interventions over intrapsychic interventions in this hospital reflect an assumption of a more sociocentric, cosmocentric, or even decentered personal identity? In the discourses radiating from Dr. Singh's (re)invention of sattvāvajaya, I could find no reference to the mining of the mind to reveal a true interior self.

Imported Interiority

Genealogies of modern selfhood suggest that psychotherapy is an institution in which authentic interior selves are constructed at the same time as and by means of the epiphany of their repression and the move toward their recovery. Psychotherapy is only one of many modern institutions infused with what Foucault has called pastoral power, a form of power that "cannot be exercised without knowing the inside of people's minds, without exploring their souls, without making them reveal their innermost secrets" (1982, 214). This mode of power is an "individualizing tactic" that produces "the truth of the individual," which, for psychotherapy, is the interior self, complete with hidden conflicts and feelings. Psychotherapy is therefore one of several confessional idioms that reinforce a modern expressivism wherein revealed emotions become signs of an inner and nonrhetorical "real" self. According to Charles Taylor (1989, 379), who has traced this modern expressivism from Romanticism to Freudianism and on to contemporary human potential movements, the turn toward expressivism involves a shift to an understanding of art as expression rather than mimesis. I suggest more broadly that the turn toward expressivism also involves a shift to an understanding of personal identity as expression rather than mimesis. Thus the source of personal identity is to be found within, as one's true nature, rather than in the social realm, as learned or strategically developed personae. In this modern expressivism, then, the ways in which personal identity and emotions are constructed through social interchange are necessarily obscured (Taylor 1985, 278; Lutz 1988, 224). Whereas individuality in Europe was once marked by ceremony, gift-giving, lineage, and alliance—i.e., locating the subject in relation to ancestors—now it is marked by techniques of surveillance—i.e., locating the subject in relation to a norm (Foucault 1982).

What I wish to emphasize here is that the modern narrative of the interior subject is noticeably akin to the modern narrative of national culture discussed in earlier chapters: both narratives naturalize an identity that they simultaneously construct; both narratives assign primordial depth to something that is an effect of certain modern political exercises. As I mentioned in chapter 1 these are parallel stories, the first concealing the historical construction of interiorized individuals and the second concealing the historical construction of cultures. Ayurvedic psychotherapy evokes both these narratives of recovery—first, as a revival of ancient medical science, the exercise of a practice with an assumed primordial dimension, and second, as a discovery of authentic subjectivity, the revelation of a self with an assumed interior depth.

The extent to which the private self is transposable into Indian settings has been often questioned. It has become almost axiomatic in anthropology to note that while European and North American selves are said to be autonomous and contained within fixed boundaries, South Asian selves are sociocentric, permeable, and even, at times, transpersonal (White and Marsella, eds. 1982, 21; Shweder and Bourne 1982, 106–107). Many scholars of South Asia speak eloquently and ethnographically of a continuous flow of substances from person to person or between person and physical world (Ramanujan 1989; Marriott and Inden 1973; Daniel

1984). From an Ayurvedic perspective, one crucial aspect of personality is prakṛti, which refers to the patient's dominant doṣa. While the determination of prakṛti is based partly on what we think of as psychological characteristics, it does not necessarily require the personal revelations associated with a modern confessionalism. Practitioners have told me that they assess the temperament of the patient more through observation than through interrogation. North American patients oriented toward a more confessional mode of psychological diagnosis are sometimes puzzled or disappointed by the lack of it in Ayurvedic consultations. In chapter 2 I suggested that for North American consumers of holism, prakṛti takes on connotations of a true inner self to be expressed. As used by Indian practitioners, however, prakṛti seems to be more a characterization of physical substance than psychic essence. It is useful here to recall the linguistic connection between Ayurvedic prakṛti and the prakṛti that means "nature" or "matter," that which is not purūṣa in the Saṃkhya cosmos.

Dr. Joshi once spoke to me frankly about his own prakṛti:

> I know my body structure and my mental makeup is of vāta and pitta prakṛti. Now pitta is hot; I am very hot-tempered, right? I get excited at the smallest of the nonsense that is done everywhere. I have seen people—there may be hell of things going on anywhere—they don't get angry—that is the sign of having a kapha prakṛti. Any damn thing that happens in front of them, they are not moved at all. They will go silently "Okay, it is going on." But it bothers me; even the smallest thing bothers me a lot. That means I am pitta. One who is vāta is always modulating. Vāta would rather deviate [the] mind from one place to the other. . . . So if you're not able to concentrate, that is because of vāta, and if you get angry, that is because of pitta.

In this comment Dr. Joshi treats his prakṛti less as an aspect of his personality than as the somatic matter responsible for his personality. He also assesses his prakṛti more in terms of his reactions to events than in terms of an inner essence.

While it is doubtful that Indian selves can be essentialized as sociocentric, it is clear that modern institutions that typically enforce the experience of a private, bounded self have tended to have different effects in Indian settings. For instance, although such signs of the bourgeois private self as novels, diaries, letters, and autobiographies were introduced in India during the mid-nineteenth century, "they seldom yield pictures of an endlessly interiorized subject" (Chakrabarty 1992b, 9). In colonial and postcolonial India, the same institutions that have allowed Europeans and North Americans to imagine modern interiorized and expressivist selves seem to serve rather to proliferate new kinds of socially centered and mimetic selves. A handful of ethnographic vignettes from the Ayurvedic hospital mentioned above demonstrates this process. They suggest that while interior selves are certainly evoked in contemporary Ayurvedic psychotherapy, they are never authorized as authentic, prior, or central. The casual subversion of the status of interior selves is not due to any lack of gesturing toward interiority, but rather to a relativization, even trivializing, of interiority. The narrative I read in these stories is one in which the invention of a true inner self at the moment of the awareness of its repression seems to be not mystified but delightedly announced. Thus the artificiality of this "authentic" self is made visible, and the interiority of this self becomes one more ephemera playing over the surface.

Rhetorical Selves

Two young men arrived for group therapy. Seated around the table were Dr. Nandi, the psychologist, another doctor, the anthropologist, and, off and on, the office assistant. The first patient, in his early twenties, complained of chronic weakness, stomach pain, muscular tightness, and constipation. Dr. Nandi questioned him about his future plans in relation to his family's means and expectations, probing for a conflict between the two, which he denied. She then asked about his dreams. When he said that he dreamed mostly about religious themes, holy rivers, and temples but sometimes about taking exams, Dr. Nandi and the doctor exchanged glances, smiling, nodding, and saying in English, "anxiety, anxiety." Again Dr. Nandi asked if he felt pressure from his family about his future, and again he said no and returned to the topic of his digestion. Dr. Nandi informed him that the source of the problem was vāyu, which was not circulating properly. She and the other doctor then spent fifteen or twenty minutes discussing his diet, recommending, at various points, dried fruits, warm milk with sugar and cardamom, lemon water to wash out his digestive tract, and so on.

Then the patient volunteered that he also had a history of piles. Here the office assistant, who was avidly following the session, chimed in, telling the patient which hospital clinic he should consult for piles. No one seemed surprised at or disapproving of the assistant's participation. After examining case records about the piles, Dr. Nandi briefly discussed diet again and then referred to the worry "inside" the patient. She suggested once more that he was experiencing tension because of a lack of parental support to continue his studies. He told her that actually when he was twelve, he had been forced to have sexual relations with a man. He wondered if this might be the root cause of his piles. The conversation ranged then from the possible relationship between male homosexual behavior and piles to remedies for piles. When Dr. Nandi said the patient was afraid, he disagreed with her. The other doctor informed him then of his unconscious mind, and Dr. Nandi explained that there is a "conscious," an "unconscious," and an "in between," using the English words. Then she told him to apply calendula ointment to his piles. "You don't have a big problem," she said. "Your weakness results from improper diet." She told him to drink warm milk with turmeric, repeating, "You don't have any special problem."

Dr. Nandi then talked briefly with a second young man, a return patient who was still suffering from lack of appetite, back pain, weakness, and nightly discharges.[12] She asked whether there had been any improvement from the Ayurvedic medicines she had prescribed earlier. He said that one of them had been effective and the other had not. She leafed through his chart and asked what he considered to be his greatest problem. He told her it was lower back pain. They discussed his family and educational situation. She pointed out that since he was from a large family with a small income, he must be worried about what he would do when he finished his degree. "You will have to get a job," she said. She told him to keep taking the medicines and reassured him that the nocturnal emissions were not causing his weakness. She advised him to follow the same diet she had prescribed for the first young man. Then she spread a cloth on the floor to demonstrate two hatha yoga āsanas that would be good for digestion. She showed the two young men a picture of the āsanas and then guided the first young man through the movements.

Following this psychotherapy session in some detail enables us to notice certain twists and turns in the diagnostic narrative. To begin with, the first patient reported what those raised in the aura of biomedicine would consider physical complaints. When traced to mental causes, such complaints are framed as somatization, as discussed above. Yet while Dr. Nandi suspected intrafamilial conflict, she diagnosed the problem as improper circulation of vāyu. She therefore almost seemed to confirm Obeyesekere's (1977, 159; 1982, 238) assessment of Ayurvedic treatment as somato-psychic, rather than psychosomatic, tracing mental illnesses to physical factors. In this as in other Ayurvedic narratives, however, the doṣa flow freely and indiscriminately between psyche and soma. Vāyu, after all, is typically associated with both nervous and digestive disorders.

In another therapy session on another day Dr. Nandi elaborated her own views on somatization. The one and only patient in that session was unusual in that he complained not only of his physical symptoms, tension and headache, but also of extreme depression. This patient had previously visited the psychiatry department. Dr. Nandi explained that people seldom visit the psychiatry department unless they are screaming or exhibiting other extreme symptoms. In India, she said to me, there is not much awareness about psychological problems. Usually people with psychological disorders come to the OPD complaining of physical ailments and are diagnosed with depression and/or anxiety. She said that many young people are concerned that their chest pain is a heart symptom when in fact it is a psychological symptom. There are so many family problems in this society, she added. In her psychotherapeutic discourse, then, there is a complex interplay of psyche, soma, and community that goes beyond the interpretation of illness as psychosomatic or somato-psychic. Somatic complaints are interpreted as mental concerns that are both traced to family and social difficulties and reinterpreted as doṣic disturbances.

To return to the psychotherapy session: Dr. Nandi uncovered the hidden emotion she was seeking when the first young man admitted that his dreams about religious themes were interspersed with dreams of taking exams. Yet her and her colleague's repetition of "anxiety, anxiety" seemed to rest in a satisfaction with naming the feeling. When the patient resisted her further inquiry about family conflict, the conversation veered into a long narrative of appropriate diet. The reference to anxiety therefore proved to be only a brief detour into interiority before a return to behavioral advice. Then the patient introduced yet another complaint: piles. Here the confessional structure of the session was broken by the participation of the office assistant, which seemed to mark the session as a semipublic conversation structured around a multidirectional flow of advice. Dr. Nandi again speculated on the source of the patient's worry. It was then finally that he told the story—a sexual scene no less—that would seem, in a standard psychotherapeutic narrative, to be a crucial clue to the origin of his psychological problem. Yet having identified his fear—without, however, inducing him to express it—what Dr. Nandi offered was diminution of the problem and calendula ointment. Here she practiced two of the nine techniques of sattvāvajaya, reassurance and replacement of emotions. A North American psychotherapist, on the other hand, would more commonly practice an elicitation of emotions. In the Ayurvedic psychotherapy, the consideration of interiority, like the consideration of emotions, ends in its naming.

In some ways, Dr. Nandi's psychotherapy sessions are not very different from everyday consultations in Ayurvedic clinics. One day a young man visited Dr. Pathi, complaining of mental strain. Dr. Pathi asked him to leave the room for a few minutes while he spoke with the young man's brother. The brother reported that the young man was suffering from sexual inadequacy, guilt, suicidal tendencies, and hallucinations. When the young man returned to the room, Dr. Pathi told him that hallucinations occur because of "impressions" made on the "subconscious mind." He said he must use two methods to train the mind: meditation and recitation of mantras. He added that certain medicines could also be used to strengthen the mind in relation to the subconscious mind. The young man said that if he was reading, he might perceive a word as "dead," even though it was a different word. Dr. Pathi told him he had not yet reached the stage of schizophrenia, but "your subconscious mind is dominating your mind." Describing some of his other hallucinations, the young man said, "It is like a set of voices; I can't describe it any other way." A little later he said that he "brooded" over small matters such as whether or not to have tea. Dr. Pathi advised the boy not to "brood" on his failures, saying that when one broods, the "subconscious mind starts giving you instructions how to behave." He told him, "Forgetting is very important. When you learn to forget, you will be able to live in present tense." He said that shock treatment was one way to break the dominance of the subconscious mind and that meditation was another. Medicine is like petrol, he said. "I will put petrol in the car, but you will have to drive it carefully." Electroshock, on the other hand, is the equivalent of having the car towed away by the police. "Don't go for shocks," he said. Instead, repeat the Gayatri mantra. Reciting the mantra a specific number of times would keep the patient's mind absorbed in numbers. After reciting the mantra for ten or fifteen minutes, he would forget about his problems. "Your duty is to meditate with the Gayatri mantra," he said. "That is the best mantra." Later he told me that the mantra was used to "divert attention." It might have some "power" also, he added, but that was a "different science." In this consultation Dr. Pathi demonstrates the use of yogic techniques to treat subconscious disturbances. Notice, however, that his aim is not to release the impressions in the subconscious mind but to prevent them from moving over into the conscious mind. He advocates the use of mantras and meditation to divert awareness away from the material that is surfacing from the subconscious. On other occasions Dr. Pathi advocated the use of mantras for older patients or students who were concerned about their memory.

According to Jacques Lacan (1977, 159), the meaning of the dream images of the unconscious mind lies less in the objects or concepts represented than in the positions of these images in relation to other images. In this respect the images tossed up by the unconscious are like linguistic signs: they do not refer to a preexistent terrain of meaning, but rather carve out a meaningful terrain through a process of differentiation. (Consider, for instance, the word "anxiety" used by Dr. Nandi. This word does not so much refer to a preexistent emotional state as it carves out an emotional state by means of a differentiation from other emotion words.) Therefore Lacan argues that the unconscious is "neither primordial nor instinctual" but a play of linguistic signs. The interior self is not authentic but rather rhetorical, "a thread woven with allusions, quotations, puns, and equivocations" (1977, 169–170). Lacan further argues that the linguistic structure of the unconscious is disguised in Freud's work by the "pseudo-biological glosses with which it is decked out for popular consumption" (1977, 167). Fooled by this pseudo-biology, professional psychoanalysis has failed to acknowledge the "self's radical ex-centricity to itself" (1977, 171). Professional psychotherapy is similarly oriented toward the search for a true self at the center of the personality structure. The unconscious is still taken to be not a play of signifiers but the repository of the signified, a web of instincts, feelings, and conflicts that have been repressed and call out to be expressed. In the Ayurvedic psychotherapy session, however, the unconscious appears not so much as the signified, a prior inner depth to be sounded, as a name, a mere sign, empty of any vaster terrain of reference than its commensurability with and difference from two other signs, the conscious mind and the mysterious "in between." Like the Lacanian unconscious, this interior self seems more rhetorical and "ex-centric" than authentic. It is not any complex syntax of unconscious images that suggests the rhetoric of the self in this case but, strikingly, the word "unconscious" itself. While Dr. Nandi invokes the unconscious as evidence for hidden anxiety, she does not look to it for either the source or the solution to this anxiety. She traces patients' fears ex-centrically to career pressures in their families.

In Dr. Pathi's informal psychotherapy, the subconscious is more extensively referenced as carrying impressions that give rise to hallucinations and guilt. Here also, however, he is concerned not so much to draw these impressions into consciousness as to draw consciousness away from them. The healing process is almost the reverse of what we might expect in North American psychotherapy, where subconscious material is defused by being dragged into consciousness. Even though Dr. Pathi compares meditation to careful driving and shock treatment to having the car towed, he also notes that meditation is similar to shock treatment in that it breaks the link between the subconscious and the conscious mind. While a North American psychotherapy might extensively interpret a patient's disturbed mentation, meditation, like shock treatment, simply interrupts it. In both these sessions, it is not so much the expressive talk of the patients, exteriorizing their fear or delusion, that facilitates the cure as it is the dietary, medicinal, and yogic advice and reassurance of doctors (and office assistant).

Selfhood Deferred

In yet another session a young man complained of gas, stomach pain, constant burping, lethargy, and sadness. After inquiring about his diet, Dr. Nandi asked about his economic situation and career plans. The patient revealed that he had twice failed to pass the exams for engineering school. The subject he found difficult was chemistry. Dr. Nandi suggested that he take time to notice the birds in the trees outside his window. She described this practice as a form of yoga. She predicted that if his chemistry score improved, his sadness would disappear. She told him to gaze at the birds and say to himself, "I have to pass the engineering exam." She said that this was a form of meditation or concentration (dhyān). They discussed the young man's diet in detail. At one point the office assistant listed the vegetables that were currently seasonal and would help his condition. Dr. Nandi suggested that the patient hire a tutor, study in the morning when he was fresh, and exercise by jogging on the roof of his apartment building. When the young man's father arrived, she told them both that the patient should not eat sweets. The young man asked if he could eat mangoes, and she said not during the monsoon. His father asked if his son could drink milk, and she said yes because he needed mental strength. Milk is considered a sattvic food that can therefore improve the mind. It also replenishes the tissues, especially semen, the *śukra* dhātu.

Again in this session Dr. Nandi was concerned to trace the patient's emotion to an external cause, his low chemistry score. The solution to the low score is to be found in mental discipline, tutoring, exercise, and milk. In addition to redirecting the patient's mind with reassurance and replacement of his emotion, she advised him to redirect his own mind with a form of meditation. While meditation techniques also invoke an interior self, it is a self that is not so much personal (as in the psychotherapeutic formulation) as depersonalized. In fact, it might be argued that the deeper one goes in meditation, the less one identifies with oneself as an individual and the more one identifies with something beyond one's individuality. Thus the meditation technique advocated by Dr. Nandi encouraged the patient to pursue a sense of oneness with other creatures as opposed to a sense of his own personal identity. Whereas in North American psychotherapy, the key to worldly success would be individuation, in this psychotherapeutic setting, the key to worldly success was deindividuation.

In yet another session, a return patient in her early twenties complained of pain in her lower back. Dr. Nandi inquired after her sister and explained to the other doctor that the sister had many mental problems. Dr. Nandi, the doctor, and the office assistant took several minutes to discuss anxiety and depression while the patient sat silently. Dr. Nandi spoke of the need for a counseling and guidance center for students. Then she examined the patient's case form and commented that she was extremely "sensitive," using the English word (*bahut zyāda sensitif*). The young woman reported that she was sleeping fitfully. Dr. Nandi recommended that she maintain a positive outlook and tell herself that everything will be okay. She reassured her that the physical pain she was experiencing would go away. They discussed the patient's career plans. She would like to get a job and live alone; then, she said, she would feel happy and peaceful. Dr. Nandi told her that remaining unmarried was out of the question for Indian women. Men will harass you, she said; you have to compromise. If you don't marry, who will you talk to? They discussed the placement of planets in the patient's birth chart. Mars was poorly positioned (*kharāb*). The conversation turned then to the young woman's stomach problems. Dr. Nandi and the office assistant launched into a long discussion of the patient's diet. They recommended pomegranate and milk with cardamom. The young woman talked to us of her fantasy of living in a village. Dr. Nandi told her she would never be able to adjust; villagers, she said, are very "orthodox," using the English word. They discussed further details of the young woman's diet. After she left, Dr. Nandi commented, "*Bahut* emotional *hai*"—i.e., she is very emotional. She diagnosed the young woman with "secondary depression" due to physical problems.

Another young woman complained of insomnia, nervousness, and chest pain. After some talk Dr. Nandi ascertained that she was a very successful student who would like to continue with school rather than marry. The young woman's symptoms first arose after a teacher was displeased with one of her papers. Worried that she would fail the class, she had developed a fever and chest pains. She was still concerned that she might have a heart ailment. Dr. Nandi told her, "You don't have any heart problem, understand?" She recommended to the young woman that she write down her daydreams and experiences in a diary. When the young woman's mother was shown in, Dr. Nandi reassured her that her daughter did not have a heart problem. She asked if the young woman had any friendship with a young man and the mother said no. The patient reiterated that she did not want to marry. She enjoyed peace and quiet. Dr. Nandi said that it was good to be alone, but she should socialize more. She did not have to excel all the time. Dr. Nandi referred to the *Bhagavad Gita,* saying that we should leave the fruits of our actions in

God's hands. She again recommended to the young woman that she write in a diary and then commented to the mother that the girl was very "emotional," again using the English word. She repeated that the young woman's problem was not heart disease but simply worry. Because of worry she could not sleep. She told the daughter to stop studying at night, and she told her mother to give her warm milk with cardamom. Milk was necessary for heavy mental work. Dr. Nandi and the mother agreed that the girl's worries were due to her schoolwork. Dr. Nandi reassured the girl that everything would be okay. When the conversation turned again to the topic of marriage, the daughter spoke passionately against the dowry system. Dr. Nandi responded that she must pay a dowry in order to be married. We humans, she said, must follow the example of Śiva and Parvati (Śiva's consort). If a daughter did not marry, the parents would worry. At the end of the session Dr. Nandi said to the mother, "Your daughter is fine. She is very 'emotional,' very 'sensitive.'" She turned to the daughter and reiterated, "You have to pay a dowry," then turned back to the mother and listed off the family problems that were affecting her daughter. The mother nodded in agreement. Dr. Nandi told the mother, "Inside she is suppressed" (Hindi verb *dabnā,* to be pressed down).

In these two narratives, as in the others, there is a vacillation between the triumphant naming of interior states (the young women are emotional, sensitive, or suppressed) and the offering of advice sprinkled with moral caution and spiritual inspiration. From the signs of the interior self, the worry or sensitivity, we are instantly deflected out again into home remedies, astrological forces, and social issues. Moreover, developing one's female identity is not here a matter of an inner struggle to define one's personal womanhood, but rather a practical recognition of what women must do in order to survive set against a political impulse to rebel. In a private conversation Dr. Nandi also said that the excess emotions that cause mental illness arise from overflowing triguṇa, the three qualities of sattva, rajas, and tamas that permeate not just mind, but also every other material substance. Thus the emotionality is both interior and exteriorized as a form of matter. This discovery of emotionality again seems to glide over the nominative surface. It seems less the recovery of a real self than the creative production of a psychological self, the kind of self expected from psychotherapy.

It is telling that the words on which interior selfhood is hinged—emotional, unconscious, sensitive, anxiety—are largely English, clearly imported from European psychological discourse. Their value derives primarily from their association with other signs charged with a potent modernity, such as "psychology" and "repression," rather than from their apprehension of a referent in the patient's experience. An interior self is also invoked in Dr. Nandi's advice to the patient to write in her diary. Again the English word (diary) carries modern European associations of individuality and the revelation of private lives. It is questionable, however, whether the diary Dr. Nandi recommended is any more pursuant of "authentic" interiority than the Indian diaries discussed by Chakrabarty. The point of identifying the patient's inner states seems to be not to seize the signified, to pursue a prior personality, but to savor the signs themselves, to proliferate character traits in the present. The construction of the interior self in the very instant of the awareness of its repression is not so much mystified, in this context, as relished.

I come to this insight, of course, through my own modern, North American disconcertion at the seemingly cavalier and unexplorative use of words such as anxiety, sensitivity, and unconscious. When I would expect the discussion to turn to analysis, it rests in characterization. Just as the colonial mimicry of European national institutions had the effect (for the colonist) of mocking "the monumentality of history," its "power to be a model" (Bhabha 1984, 128), so the mimesis of European psychotherapy has the effect, for the anthropologist, of mocking the monumentality of the interior self and *its* power to be a model. This self becomes, in these narratives, not an endpoint, a stable signified, but only another touchstone, another sign in a narrative of nervousness, strung together with stories about Śiva, vāyu, and the virtues of warm milk. The interior self is not privileged as authentic but passed over as one more rhetorical moment in a psychological discourse.

Two drawings from an Ayurvedic textbook sketch some of the ironies involved in the incorporation of modern concepts into Ayurvedic theories of the mind. In the first (figure 14), the mind is labeled as the "prime minister" and dressed in modern clothing. Like a master technician, he sits at a switchboard, adjusting the dials for buddhi, *medhā*, smṛti, and dhṛti, while meters register their activity overhead, emitting a continuous "beep, beep." From this control station he directs the five *karmendriya*, or

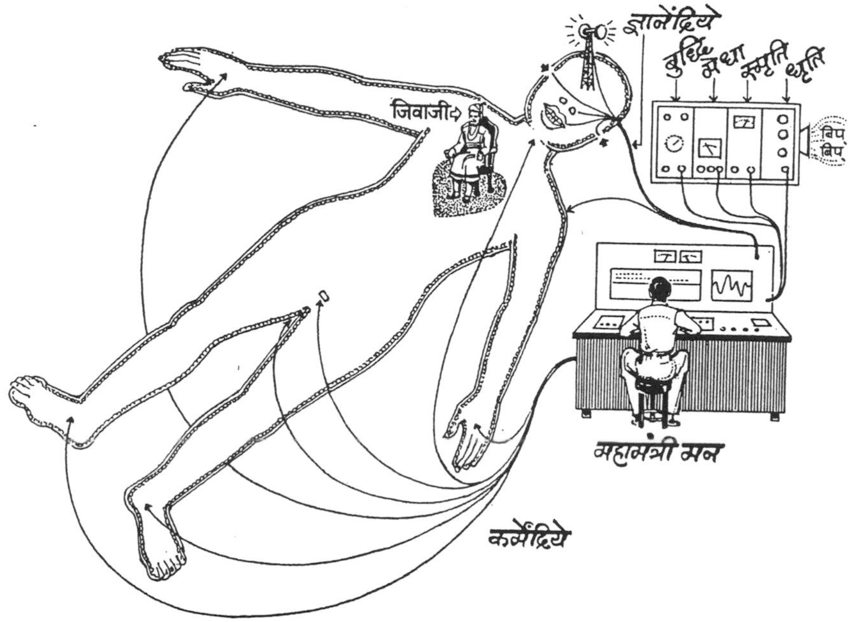

Figure 14. Master Technician. The "prime minister mind," dressed in modern clothing, sits at a switchboard controlling the mental functions and motor and sensory organs (Padyegurjar 1985, 28).

organs of action (hands, feet, larynx, reproductive organs, and organs of excretion) and the five sensory organs (hearing, sight, smell, taste, and touch), all of which are connected by wires to his switchboard. In this drawing, then, a classical Indian concept of mind is made analogous to the modern industrial nation-state: both are rational administrators. Meanwhile, the soul, dressed in the garments of an Indian prince or avatar, resides in the heart. Similarly, in the second drawing a person dressed for the twentieth century speaks over the phone lines to his *anta-rātma,* the inner self or soul residing in his heart, through the switchbox or transformer of his ego (figure 15). While his voice is transmitted through the telephone of his intellect, the voice of his inner self is transmitted through the telephone of the mind. Once again the soul is dressed in a royal costume reminiscent of representations of Kṛṣna or some other god. Beyond its immediate text of the relationships among aspects of the self, this drawing suggests yet other subtexts: a modern Ayurveda com-

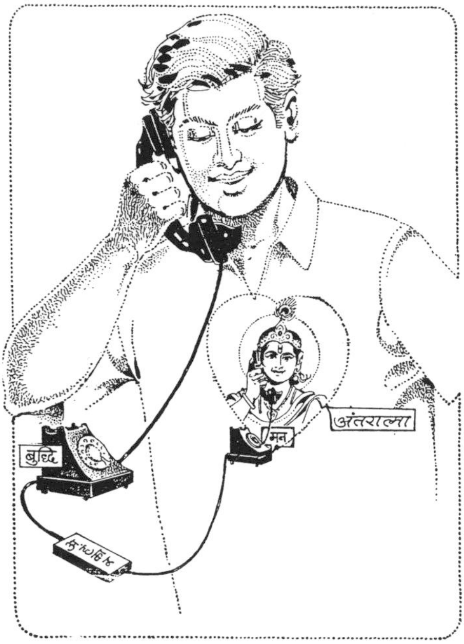

Figure 15. Telecommunicating Soul.
The generic subject speaks to his "inner self" over the telephone (Padyegurjar 1985, 108).

municating with an ancient Ayurveda, or science consulting (consorting) with the sacred. The telecommunication metaphor suggests a distance between the modern self and his Indian soul that is mediated by translations of indigenous concepts (such as *ahaṃkāra* as ego) and by the miracle of modern technologies. One of the most interesting puzzles of the drawing is the unlabeled larger body, which seems almost to offer a generic subject as a container to enframe "traditional" Indian facets of self. Yet for all their industrial metaphors and essentialist imagery of Indian culture, both these drawings ultimately work to displace modern psychology's hyperpersonal innermost self, scarred by its specific memories, with an image of a transpersonal, quasi-divine, and cosmic self, unmarked by colonial history.

Bharati has suggested that a Hindu vegetarian can eat meat or a Hindu Communist can be avowedly religious because there is no empirical ground of selfhood within which such identities would appear to contradict or cancel one another. The self that can be characterized is necessarily mutable and fluctuating in its identifications. The only "real" self, he argues, is the self that cannot be characterized, the ātmā: "The Self is the *sat,* the one and only existing being; it is the *paramartha,* the absolute; everything else about a person is *vyavahāra,* ephemeral, conventional, relative . . . superimposed upon the true self which is in no way touched by or susceptible to these modifications. Such is a pervasive Indian interpretation of persons, actions, and ideas, and it is so axiomatic that no one really talks about it unless pressed to do so" (1985, 198). We might read this argument as a phonocentrism wherein the statements of certain acquaintances are taken to transparently represent an essential Hindu self, an avatar seated in the heart. We might also read it, however, as a gesture toward the unrepresentable, the "not this, nor yet this" of the Upaniśads (Mascaro 1965, 12). Under this reading, the "self" of Ayurvedic psychology becomes, like Ayurveda itself, a signified forever deferred.

epilogue

I began this story with Dr. Vijayan's remark that he had learned the "true essence" of Ayurveda by treating foreign patients. Now that I have traced certain moments in the modernization of Ayurveda, this statement is perhaps no less ironic but more clearly linked to a particular political logic. Twentieth-century Ayurvedic practitioners redirected their practice to a nationalist task of healing particular wounds of colonialism and postcoloniality. In so doing, they sustained a tension between the modern modes of medical knowledge that are meaningful to a national modernity, and signs of "tradition" that are meaningful to a notion of Indian culture. Since the cannon blast that ideologically excluded Ayurveda from a universal medicine, practitioners have alternately used and "ab-used," resisted and renegotiated, embraced and wrestled with the construction of Ayurveda as culture. Upon considering a new job with an Ayurvedic pharmaceutical company, Dr. Upadhyay commented to me that the company executives had not yet realized the importance of Ayurveda as a "concept." By this he meant nothing less than the importance of Ayurveda, not just as effective medicine, but as cultural and philosophical difference.

At the time of Dr. Upadhyay's job interview, this pharmaceutical company was working to expand its markets in Europe and North America. Increasingly, it is as much the consumerist desires of late capitalism as the political desires of postcolonial nationality that encourage the development of Ayurveda as a cultural product. When I questioned students and practitioners about the future of Ayurveda, many of them replied that it depended on Ayurveda's acceptance by the "West." In closing, therefore, I return to my conversations with Dr. Vijayan, who offers Ayurveda as both healing and cultural commodity for new generations of foreigners engaged in medical tourism. For Dr. Vijayan's patients, the commodification of Ayurveda as both cure and culture occurs through a process of fetishization whereby Ayurveda has an enfolded value as both physical therapy and ethnospiritual capital. If understood as medicine, Dr. Vijayan's Ayurveda cures not only the illnesses, but also the cultural or spiritual emptiness of Europeans and North Americans. Conversely, if understood as cultural artifact, his Ayurveda lends an enlivening exoticism and antiquity to the medical treatments undergone by these foreigners. Dr. Vijayan's treatment of foreigners is a longer story, one that can only be prefigured here, but one that suggests possible futures for Ayurveda as a healing force, not only for postcolonial national culture, but also for neocolonial nostalgia. In the early twentieth century, as discussed in chapter 3, the first intimations of the idea of Ayurveda as culture were heard in an argument that Ayurveda was uniquely suited to Indian bodies. Now, in Dr. Vijayan's practice, the idea of Ayurveda as culture is developed through a claim of its specific curative value for Western bodies.

We were sitting again in my room at his family's hospital when Dr. Vijayan explained to me why Westerners have more psychological problems than Indians. Westerners, he said, feel less secure and loved as children. Indians, by contrast, are very secure and loved in early childhood. So when Indians have mental problems, they are more apt to be "real diseases," like schizophrenia. For foreigners, on the other hand, mental problems are simply endemic to their upbringing. He noticed that the facial expression of one German patient changed when he massaged her belly. When he asked what she was feeling, she said she was angry. She added that when her boyfriend touched her there, she felt like killing him. Dr. Vijayan wondered if perhaps her mother had had violent feelings when she was pregnant that were then passed to the daughter through the umbilicus. Eventually the patient told him that three days before she was born, her father had kicked her mother in the stomach. The next day when Dr. Vijayan massaged the patient's belly, he saw in her face that she was no longer angry. In classical Ayurvedic theory, he emphasized, this kind of occurrence is "totally omitted." Sometimes when Westerners tell him their painful memories, he feels very embarrassed. Sometimes the patients he treats in a nearby resort hotel cry loudly. He has to ask them to stop because they may disturb the other occupants of the hotel. Because of such experiences, Dr. Vijayan's treatment of Westerners has radically changed the way he thinks about Ayurveda. It has "altered my path," he said.

Colonial knowledge practices often obscured the way that identity—whether personal, cultural, or national—is constructed via difference (Mitchell 1988). The identities of the colonizers were understood to be self-consistent, self-present, integrated. Such undivided selves, however, could only be sustained by projection. Nandy (1983) and Taussig (1993), from very different theoretical orientations, have demonstrated how the parameters of European identity were defined through colonial projections of certain qualities onto the colonized. In the colonization of South America it was the qualities of barbarity and wanton violence that were projected onto colonial subjects, while in the colonization of India it was the qualities of passivity and effeminacy that were projected onto the colonized. Today these images are rerecruited by neocolonial knowers and consumers as techniques of healing. Thus North Americans seek out the wild savagery of a virtual South America via shamanism and the gentle introversion of a virtual India via yoga and Ayurveda. If such images of indigenous practices were recruited by colonialism to establish the orderliness of reason as against the disorderliness of superstition and recruited by the academy to establish the orderliness of healing as against the disorderliness of disease, they are now, through medical tourism, being recruited by European and North American popular culture to establish the orderliness of holism as against the disorderliness of systemic imbalance.

Zimmermann (1992) notes that the consumers of Ayurveda in Europe and North America associate it with the value of nonviolence (which is of course a favorite sign for India). Thus contemporary pancakarma, particularly in its "Westernized" versions, emphasizes nonviolent, "gentle" therapies, such as massage and bathing, over more violent, "evacuative" therapies, such as purgation, emetics, or bloodletting. Actually, even oil massage and sweat baths can be considered evacuative therapies in Ayurveda insofar as they draw the excess doṣa toward the digestive tract in preparation for its removal. Massage and sweat baths in contemporary Europe and North America are understood rather differently, however, as relaxation or revitalization therapies that reduce muscle tension and enhance circulation and elasticity. Zimmermann suggests that these latter images of massage and sweat baths have begun to influence Ayurvedic practice to such an extent that pancakarma treatment in certain parts of India and in Europe and North America has come to resemble the physical therapy of a health spa. My own observations in Ayurvedic hospitals indicate that practitioners have not completely embraced the health spa approach to pancakarma. In pancakarma departments, bloodletting with leeches is used to treat skin ailments, while oil massages and steam treatments are given as preparation for purgation or water-based vasti. One department had even organized a three-week camp in the city to demonstrate the value of vaman.

Dr. Vijayan, however, often begins his treatment of foreign patients with massage alone. Most of them first visit him in his office at the hotel of a nearby tourist resort. They are on vacation, seeking sunbathing and relaxation. The signs advertising Ayurveda that they have seen along the beach and the back roads promote Ayurvedic massage, suntan lotion, and hair oil (see figure 16). It is only when these patients come to trust Dr. Vijayan that he suggests some medicines to be taken internally. Though he eventually offers them both oil and watery vasti, he never uses emesis or bloodletting. He describes himself as "liberal" with his foreign patients. He uses different vasti medicines for foreigners than for Indians because he feels that the usual medicines would be "too spicy" for Westerners, inducing a more violent evacuation. Dr. Vijayan has also streamlined his pharmacopoeia for foreign consumption. He now uses only three formulae—one to calm each of the three doṣa—plus one additional formula without sugar for diabetics. These simplified formulae enable self-treatment. The medicines are now designed for a "self-help" Ayurveda, allowing his foreign patients to use his medicines with a minimum of Ayurvedic knowledge.

Dr. Vijayan told me he has learned to communicate with Westerners very well. Indeed, his ways of talking about illness uncannily resemble the psychological and energeticist language of new age therapies. He told me, for instance, that the practice of sirodhāra is a particularly "powerful psychotherapy." It is impossible, he said, to explain its effects. People go into meditation. Many remember past events that turn out to be important for future directions. Typically people lose track of time. As mentioned above, Dr. Vijayan feels that sirodhāra disengages the conscious mind, allowing the subconscious to surface. When the issues that are accessed in sirodhāra arise again in people's lives, they are no longer upset about them. He believes, moreover, that sirodhāra works by a vibration that affects the nerves. He developed this idea after hearing from one of

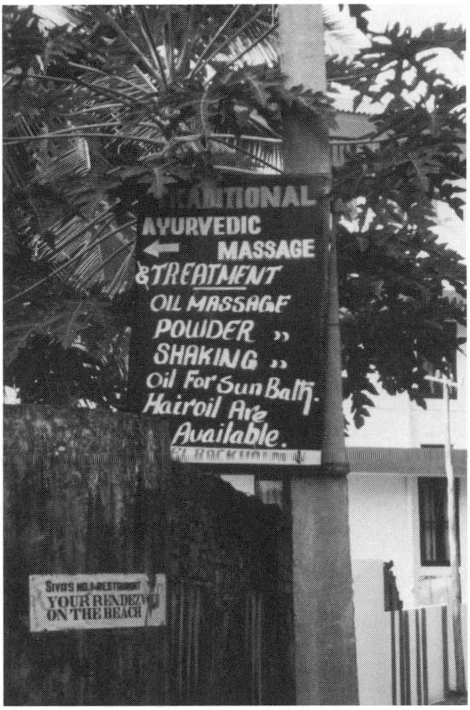

Figure 16. Global Marketing. A sign at a popular South Indian beach resort invites tourists to sample "traditional" Ayurvedic therapy as part of their vacation.

his European patients about a Swiss doctor who treats asthma by tapping a stick against a particular point of the nasal cavity. When the European said that the tapping must produce a resonance, it occurred to Dr. Vijayan that the rhythmic dripping of sirodhāra might also be producing a resonance. After experiencing this resonance of sirodhāra, moreover, people lose their materialist values. "Those patterns are totally out," he said.

When I asked Dr. Vijayan to explain my own health problems in doṣic terms, he told me that while I was basically pitta, there was a "kapha wall" in my system that prevented the natural movement between mental and physical levels. This wall, he said, prevents the emergence of pitta. The "kapha mask" is aloof. After treatment, he predicted, I would be more reactive. One woman with a kapha wall had a very puffy face. He told her to go to parties, wear red dresses, and mingle with pitta people. Not long after, she became involved with a man who rode a motorcycle. Soon the puffiness in her face disappeared. Dr. Vijayan said that people with kapha walls are sensitive but do not release their feelings as "natural pitta" people do. A kapha wall, he said, is something that has developed over many years. It is very difficult to explain in a rational way. A person with a kapha wall looks "inflated." In a sense the wall is simply water that is not able to disperse. The eyes of a kapha wall person are "sad and dull," while after treatment they become "lustrous and sharp." Kapha wall people are quiet, but it is not a "natural quietness." It is obvious that they are "holding a lot." "These people suffer silently," he said. During conversations they occasionally take a deep breath like a "heavy sigh." Because they cannot cry all the time, these people release their sadness in frequent laughter. Westerners' laughter, he said, often sounds like crying. When I asked him if he ever spoke to his Indian patients the way he spoke to me about my "kapha wall," he said no. "People don't understand," he said. Indian people "don't ask those kinds of questions." Whenever he uses such language with Indian patients, they look at him strangely or simply walk away. I, on the other hand, felt strangely exposed by his comments. I could not help but intuit that it was his astuteness as a healer of late-capitalist nostalgia that allowed him to place his hand on the precise feeling of cultural displacement that had flared up during fieldwork.

Slavoj Žižek observes that in late capitalism, the national community is "increasingly experienced as an external, purely formal frame . . . so that one is more and more looking for support in 'primordial,' usually smaller (ethnic, religious) forms of identification" (1997, 42). He notes that global capitalism makes every country a colony of multinational corporations: "In the long term, we shall all not only wear Banana Republic shirts but also live in banana republics." The quintessential ideology of this global capitalism, in his view, is multiculturalism, which " 'respects' the Other's identity, conceiving the Other as a self-enclosed 'authentic' community towards which he, the multiculturalist, maintains a distance rendered possible by his privileged universal position" (1997, 44). What Žižek does not emphasize here is that this peculiarly empty Eurocentrism is also infused with touristic desire. It is through catering to the intricacies of such desires that Dr. Vijayan has developed new variations of pancakarma that are particularly suited to Western bodies and new ways of communicating about illness that both resemble and deviate from the language of the late-capitalist "new age."

Even as he advocates a seemingly neo-orientalist construction of Ayurveda as spiritually enlivening, Dr. Vijayan also advances a construction of foreign bodies and subjectivities as fragile and uniquely damaged. For him, the bodies of Europeans and North Americans are overflowing with culturally aggravated doṣa. With his not-too-spicy pancakarma, he treats their late-capitalist illnesses of excess consumerism and troubled childhoods. His homemade powders and elixirs heal as much by their alterity as by their bitterness. As one of his Italian patients commented to me, "He has secrets." Ironically his cures for consumerism themselves satisfy a consumerist longing for ethnospiritual renewal. In Dr. Vijayan's practice the disciplinary signs forcibly inscribed on colonized bodies (Arnold 1993; Comaroff and Comaroff 1992) are answered by the doṣic signs benevolently inscribed on ex- and neocolonizers' bodies. Ayurveda, once offered as the cure for the cultural malaise of the colonized, is now offered as the cure for the cultural voids of ex-colonists.

interlocutors

Dr. Joshi: Practitioner in his forties who practices and teaches at a metropolitan hospital. Institutionally trained through M.D. Chapter 5.

Dr. Karnik: Private metropolitan practitioner in his sixties. Institutionally trained through M.D. Chapter 2 and cameos in chapter 5.

Kaviraj Kumar: Itinerant vaidya in his forties who diagnoses solely through pulse and guarantees a cure. Exact training uncertain. Chapter 6.

Dr. Lal: Private metropolitan practitioner in her thirties; partner to Dr. Mistry. Chapter 6.

Dr. Madhava: Private metropolitan practitioner in her forties. Institutionally trained through M.D. and through apprenticeship with her father. Chapter 5.

Dr. Mishra: Private practitioner in his forties who practices and teaches at a metropolitan hospital. Institutionally trained through M.D. Chapter 4.

Dr. Mistry: Private metropolitan practitioner in his forties who diagnoses solely through pulse, manufactures his own medicines, and is considered a quack by some of his colleagues. Exact training uncertain. Chapter 6.

Dr. Nandi: Ayurvedic psychotherapist in her thirties practicing at a metropolitan teaching hospital. Institutionally trained in both Ayurveda and psychology. Chapter 7.

Dr. Pathi: Private metropolitan practitioner in his sixties who acts as an examiner for Ayurvedic education. Trained in a gurukula-cum-college. Chapters 3, 4, and 7.

Vd. Rai: Practitioner in his thirties who practices out of a charitable dispensary in a Himalayan hill station. Trained by a correspondence course and a brief apprenticeship with another practitioner. Chapters 5 and 6.

Vd. Sharma: Private practitioner in his eighties working in a West Indian city. Trained in a gurukula through the All-India Ayurvedic Vidyapīṭh. Chapter 2.

Vd. Shastri: Private practitioner in his eighties practicing in a Himalayan hill station. Trained in a gurukula-cum-early-college and also by his father. Chapter 4.

Vd. Shukla: Retired urban practitioner in his eighties living in a West Indian city. Trained in a gurukula through the All-India Ayurvedic Vidyapīṭh. Chapters 1 and 4.

Dr. Singh: Practitioner in his fifties specializing in mental health who practices and teaches at a metropolitan hospital. Institutionally trained through M.D. Chapter 6.

Dr. Tiwari: Practitioner in his fifties who teaches at a metropolitan hospital. Institutionally trained through M.D. Chapter 5.

Dr. Trivedi: Private metropolitan practitioner in his sixties who diagnoses solely through pulse and manufactures his own medicines. Trained in both a gurukula and a college. Chapter 6.

Dr. Upadhyay: Private metropolitan practitioner in his forties. Institutionally trained through M.D. Chapters 2, 5, and 6, with cameos elsewhere.

Dr. Vijayan: Practitioner in his thirties working at a family-run clinic in South India with a large foreign clientele. Institutionally educated through B.A. Also trained by his father. Chapter 1, epilogue, and cameos elsewhere.

glossary

ācāryā: preceptor; teacher

adankal: marma points that can be stimulated to undo the negative effects of injury to other marma points

adharma: absence of dharma, unrighteousness

adhunik: modern

ādivāsī: indigenous, "tribal"

agadatantra: toxicology; one of the eight branches of Ayurveda

agni: fire; one of the five pancamahābhūta; also digestion; also an element in the body, of which there are thirteen types

ahaṃkāra: self-identification, ego

ākāsá: ether; one of the five pancamahābhūta

āma: undigested food residue that can contribute to illness

āmavāt: an illness similar to rheumatoid arthritis

amla: sour; one of the five flavors

amṛtasāgar: a book of medicinal formulae

anācār: improper conduct

anuloman: moving in the direction of the grain; in Ayurveda the proper downward direction of vāyu in the abdomen

anumān: inference; one of the means of knowledge within Ayurveda

anyadway: every other day, as in the fever that recurs every twenty-four hours

apāna: one of the five types of vāyu; it regulates downward motion in the abdomen

apasmāra: an illness similar to epilepsy

Arogyaśikśa: a turn-of-the-century Indian health manual

arth: entity, meaning, object of perception, wealth

āsana: posture, especially of hatha yoga

Aṣṭāṅga Saṃgraha: one of the three earliest Ayurvedic texts

asthi: bone; one of the seven dhātu

aśuddh: impure

aśvagandha: a well-known Ayurvedic herb used in the treatment of numerous ailments (*Withania somnifera*)

atīndriya: subtle, beyond the range of the senses
ātmā: self, soul
Āyurvedīy: Ayurvedic
Bhagavān: God
bhajan: devotional song
Bhārat: India
Bhāratakhaṇḍ: Indian land
bhasma: ash; a common form of certain Ayurvedic medicines
Bhāvaprakāś: a medieval Ayurvedic treatise
bhiṣak: physician, healing practitioner
bhūt: ghost; also element
bhūtavidya: knowledge of ghosts and spirits; one of the eight branches of Ayurveda
bīj: seed, embryo
bilwa: Ayurvedic medicinal herb (*Aegle marmelos*)
brahmācarya: sexual abstinence
brahmi: Ayurvedic herb used to treat mental dullness and other ailments (*Centella asiatica*)
buddhi: intellect
cakra: one of seven energy centers in the subtle body
Caraka Saṃhitā: one of the three earliest Ayurvedic texts
chadmacara: one who pretends to have expertise
cikitsā: therapy, treatment, medicine
cittaviṣāda: modern Sanskrit coinage used as a gloss for depressive illness
daivya: divine
dama: an illness similar to asthma
darśan: seeing, being in the presence of; also philosophy
davakhāna: dispensary
devī: goddess
dharma: righteousness, duty
dhātu: one or more of seven bodily "tissues" recognized by Ayurveda
dhī: intellect
dhṛti: mental fortitude, endurance
dhyān: meditation, concentration
divya: divine
divyadṛṣṭi: divine perception
doṣa: force in the body or mind responsible for illness; also trouble
dravyaguṇa: the properties of medicinal substances
dūṣti: disturbance, vitiation
dūṣya: disturbed dhātu

gandharva: celestial musician; one of several unseen entities by which a person may be possessed
gulma: tumor, nodule
guṇa: quality
gurukula: a center of learning consisting of a guru and his or her students
hakīm: practitioner of Unani medicine
hatha yoga: the aspect of yoga involving postures, breathing exercises, and so on
hetu: cause or origin of illness
hisāb: calculation, business account, price, transaction
indriya: organ, usually sensory organ
itihās: history
jaḍī-būṭī: medicinal flora, fauna, and minerals
jal: water; one of the five pancamahābhūta
jijñāsa: curiosity, inquiry
jñān: knowledge
jwar: fever
kal: time
kāliyug: the present age; the age of darkness and ignorance
kaniśṭha: junior, novice
kapha: one of the three bodily doṣa; associated with water/earth, phlegm, and mass or structure
kapikacchu: an Ayurvedic herb with multiple uses (*Mucuna pruriens*)
karma: action; also result of action
karmendriya: the five organs of action, which include hand, foot, larynx, genitalia, and excretory organs
kaṣāy: astringent; one of the six rasa
kastūrī: a medicine obtained from the navel of a deer
kaṭiśūl: lower back pain
kaṭu: pungent; one of the six rasa
kaumābhṛtya: pediatrics; one of the eight branches of Ayurveda
kāyacikitsā: one of the eight branches of Ayurveda; sometimes glossed as internal medicine
kriyākāla: stages of illness
kśay: wasting; sometimes used for tuberculosis
kuṭaj: Ayurvedic medicinal herb (*Holarrhena antidysenterica*)
laghu: the quality of lightness
lākh: one hundred thousand
lakṣaṇ: feature, characteristic, identifying sign or mark
lavaṇ: salty; one of the six rasa
liṅga/liṅgam: identifying sign, mark, or feature

lom: body hair
madhumeha: an illness similar to diabetes
madhur: sweet; one of the six rasa
mala: waste products of the body
mālā: circlet, such as a bracelet, necklace, or garland; often worn on the body
mala kriya: the eliminative processes of the body
mana/mānas: mind
manasik: mental; related to mānas
manodaihika/manośarīra: mental-bodily; usually glossed as psychosomatic
mans: muscle; one of the seven dhātu
marma: one of 107 or 108 specified vulnerable points on the body
medh: fat; one of the seven dhātu
medhā: intelligence
medhya: a medicine that strengthens the intelligence
miśra: mixed, integrated
mṛdaṅg: a two-headed drum
mūrti: image, especially of a god, goddess, or saint
nāḍī: pulse, vein, channel in the body
nāmamālā: garland of names, litany of names
nasya: nasal drops therapy; one of the five pancakarma
nidān: cause, etiology, diagnosis
nirām: without āma, the residue of undigested food
niṣiddh: forbidden
niyam: custom, routine, self-imposed restraint, moderation
oj/ojas: the most refined of the seven dhātu; associated with semen, strength, and overall health
padārth vijñān: knowledge of the meaning of words and objects; in Ayurveda, the subject that covers the basic principles and philosophical bases of Ayurveda; in secondary school, the subject of modern physics
pancakarma: five Ayurvedic purification treatments designed to remove disturbed doṣa from the body; they include nasal drops, emesis, purgation, oily enema, watery enema, and sometimes bloodletting
pancamahābhūta: the five great elements of which all creation is composed: air, water, earth, fire, ether
pandu: an illness similar to anemia
parampara: lineage, succession; usually translated as tradition
parikśan: examination
pāṭhaśāla: school, place of learning
pitta: one of the three bodily doṣa; associated with fire, bile, and metabolic processes

prabhav: effect, especially the specific effect of a medicinal substance on a particular physical part or function
prājñā: understanding, intelligence, wisdom
prājñaparādha: improper engagement with the objects of the senses; behavioral error that leads to illness
prakop: disturbance
prakriya: process
prakṛti: constitutional type, predominant doṣa of a person
prāṇa: breath, life breath
prāṇayāma: breathing exercises that are a part of hatha yoga
pratirūpaka: image, forgery, charlatan
pratyakṣa: direct observation; one of the means of knowledge recognized in Ayurveda
pravṛtti: application (of a practice), use
prayog: use, rational use
pṛthvī: earth; one of the five pancamahābhūta
pūjā: worship, prayer; also an altar where pūjā is performed
purūṣa: consciousness, soul; the twelfth tattva or level of phenomena in Saṃkhya; consciousness as distinct from "nature" or matter (prakṛti)
purvarūpa: early sign of not yet manifest illness
racana: formation, structure
rājā: king, prince
rajas: one of the three guṇa; related to desire, activity, initiative
rākṣasa: demon
raktmokśan: bloodletting
rasa: flavor; specifically one of six flavors according to which all ingested substances are classified
rasaśāstra: pharmacology; a subject in the contemporary Ayurvedic syllabus
rasāyan: rejuvenation or replenishment therapy; that which nourishes the dhātu
rog: disease, illness
ṛṣi: sage
rukśa: the quality of roughness, dryness
sabhā: association, organization
sadvṛtt: correct behavior
śālākya: one of the eight branches of Ayurveda; pertaining to illnesses located above the collarbone
sāma: with āma, undigested food residue
samādhi: deep state of meditation
Saṃkhya: a branch of Indian philosophy that arranges the phenomenological universe into thirty-six levels

saṃnyās: renunciation of worldly attachments
sampṛāpti: the course of illness organized into stages
samsāra: the cycle of worldly existence
saṃskāra: latent impressions left on the mind from the deeds and experiences of previous incarnations
samuccay: combination
sansthān: institution
sansthānik: institutional
śarīr: body
śarīr kriya: Sanskrit coinage for the subject of physiology
śarīr racana: Sanskrit coinage for the subject of anatomy
śarīrik: bodily, somatic
śāstra: scripture or scriptural knowledge
sattva: one of the three guṇa; associated with purity and virtue
sattvāvajaya: control over the mind, disciplining the mind; in contemporary Ayurveda, sometimes used to mean psychotherapy
satyayug: the age of truth, the golden age
siddhasādhita: those who have learned by experience rather than by study
siddhi: paranormal ability attained through yogic discipline
śilajīt: a medicinal mineral
sirodhāra: a process, considered to be part of pancakarma, in which a medicinal solution is dripped in a slow stream onto the forehead for up to an hour
śiṣya: student, disciple
ślok: verse
smṛti: memory
sneha: saturating the body with oil in preparation for pancakarma; also affection
snigdh: the quality of oiliness, unctuousness
śoth: swelling
śraddhā: faith, trust, confidence
śrota: channel within the body
sthūla: gross, dense
śuddh: pure
sūkśma: subtle, fine
Suśruta Samhita: one of the three earliest Ayurvedic texts
swanguli pramāṇ: a means of calculating the ideal proportions of the human body by calculating multiples of the measurement of a single finger; an aspect of Ayurvedic anatomy
śwās: an illness similar to asthma
swasthavṛtt: regimen for maintenance of one's health
tamas: one of three guṇa; associated with inertia, ignorance, and inhibition
tattva: element; level of the phenomenological universe

tikt: pungent; one of the six rasa
tol: a gathering of disciples and guru; a place of learning
tulsī: holy basil; a medicinal herb
unmād: insanity, especially psychosis
upacāra: remedy, treatment process
upaśāya: a means of Ayurvedic diagnosis that involves testing the patient's response to remedies
uṣṇa: "heat"; one of two types of effect produced by a food or medicine
vaidya: Ayurvedic practitioner
vaidyapavāda: one who is a vaidya in appearance only
vaidyaraṭna: healing manual composed primarily of formulae and recipes
vaijñānik: Sanskrit coinage for scientific
vājīkaraṇ: aphrodisiac or remedy to increase sexual power
vaman: emesis, therapeutic vomiting; one of the five pancakarma
vasti: one (or sometimes two) of the five pancakarma; similar to enema or douche; used to cleanse doṣa from the body with either an oil-based or water-based medicinal solution
vāta/vāyu: one of the three bodily doṣa; associated with air and movement
veda: knowledge
vidyapīth: center of scholarship
vijñān: specialized knowledge; usually translated as science
vikār: disturbance
vipāka: the rasa of a particular ingested substance after it has been metabolically transformed in the body
virecan: purgation; one of the five pancakarma
vīrya: the specific effect of a medicine, either "hot" or "cold"
viśarāda: an expert; one who is well-versed
yantra: a mystical diagram
yog: yoga, union, yoke, combination
yogakriya: use of medical compounds
yug: era, epoch
yukti: skill, technique, reasoning

notes

Chapter 1: (Re)inventing Ayurveda

1 The names of respondents in this work are pseudonyms. The descriptions of respondents who spoke with me about potentially sensitive subjects have also been fictionalized to some extent.

2 The five techniques of pancakarma, along with the various techniques, including massage, that are used to prepare a person for pancakarma, are discussed more fully in chapter 5.

3 I have parenthesized the "re" simply as a reminder that in redefining Ayurveda, practitioners and others simultaneously presume its prior existence, stabilizing an eclectic range of specific and local healing practices into a culturally bounded body of knowledge.

4 Jaggi (1981) estimates that the word Ayurveda was first coined between 800 and 600 B.C.

5 For a detailed account of this dual medical training and the biomedical training that succeeded it, see Jaggi (1996).

6 See Arnold (1993 and 1987) for a detailed account of the colonial disciplines imposed on Indian bodies, as well as for an account of resistance to these disciplines.

7 See Prakash (1992).

8 In his discussion of mimesis Taussig (1993) offers the valuable insight that such a sign draws not only essence but also power from the referent.

9 In Chatterjee's scheme, the nationalist forms compose the thematic, and the national content, the problematic. I am inspired here by his observation that the dynamic between the thematic and problematic can "produce at critical junctures a thoroughgoing critique of the thematic itself" (1986, 43).

10 The process is parallel to that documented by Cohn (1987b), who showed how the collection of cases in Indian juridical documents was reconceived by the colonialists as a civil code, rendering an assortment of situationally specific dispute practices as universalist statutes.

11 Each of these terms has particular political ramifications, particularly when used by practitioners or proponents of a certain type of medicine. "Modern"

or "cosmopolitan" medicine, used primarily by practitioners and allies of biomedicine or social researchers, implies that other types of medicine are either premodern or distinctly rural and locally specific. "Allopathy," used primarily by practitioners of Unani, Siddha, homeopathy, and Ayurveda, connotes a medicine that is more disease-oriented than health-oriented. "Biomedicine," used primarily by anthropologists, suggests a medicine that is based in biological science.

12 I am influenced here by David Scott's (1994) work, which suggests that we turn our attention from debunking particular social-scientific concepts to exploring how and why these concepts are generated and maintained.

13 It is worth noting that the very assumption of a fixed body of Ayurvedic knowledge that is changed by modernity overlooks previous historical work that traced the changes in the meaning of Ayurveda over the centuries. See, for instance, Zysk (1993).

14 Substitute terms for modernity such as the purely geographic "European" or the more specifically historical "post-Enlightenment" are no more politically neutral than "modern." It would conceivably be appropriate to use the phrase "colonial/neocolonial episteme" for a project of knowledge that has been at the same time a project of colonization and enclosure. Colonialism is not, however, unique to Europe, where the modern modes of knowledge analyzed by Foucault (1970, 1979), Fabian (1983), Mitchell (1988), and many others originated. I therefore continue to use the words "modern" and "modernity" under protest and under erasure.

15 Unani is the name given to healing practices of Islamic *hakīms* in South Asia, while Siddha is the name given to Tamil healing practices of South India and Sri Lanka.

16 Nostalgia, Stewart writes, is utterly dependent on the unsatisfied desire implicit in the discrepancy between "resemblance and identity," "the gap between sign and signified" (1993, 145). Put another way, nostalgia is dependent on the logic of the supplement (Derrida 1976).

17 The idea of enframing was developed in Mitchell (1988) and has been further elaborated ethnographically in Pemberton (1994).

18 While this irrelevance can sometimes be found in biomedical practices as well, I here explore the specificities of this irrelevance in Ayurvedic practice.

19 Taussig (1993) and Bhabha (1984) have each demonstrated that the mimicry of signs of European nationhood in colonies and postcolonies has a parodic effect.

20 Cohn (1985), Daniel (1984), and Ramanujan (1989) have each suggested that South Asian processes of signification themselves offer a challenge to the (European) cultural priorities of metaphoricity or arbitrariness. Inden (1990, 127), on the other hand, critiques the idea that icons are more crucial

to South Asian significations as a European attempt to access a lost and romanticized epistemology. Yet the compelling semiotics identified by Cohn, Daniel, and Ramanujan do not become products of European nostalgia simply because they are susceptible to being assimilated by it.

21 One caution about this danger appeared in a criticism of Mitchell by Coronil (1996). Mitchell (1988, 61) suggests that the distinctions between copy and original are meaningless in a precolonial Egyptian signification in which all phenomena both imitate and are imitated. Coronil argues that such an account reproduces the metaphysical binary of East and West. Similarly, Prakash (1990, 408) cautions against postorientalist histories that embed the study of Asia in a project of disturbing the European episteme. There is no easy resolution to this controversy. Mitchell (1990, 566) denies that he means to invoke an enchanted premodern world where words were not yet separate from objects. He clarifies that it is the very dualism of modern European thought that allows the imagination of an antecedent nondualism.

22 I take inspiration here from Pemberton's (1994) efforts to defer the enframing of Java.

Chapter 2: Ayurvedic Interiors

1 See Cohen (1999) for a brief but insightful discussion of the voyeurism involved in foreign accounts of labyrinthine Indian cities.

2 See chapter 5 for a more detailed discussion of how the effects of Ayurvedic medicines are understood.

3 In one study of the concept of person in India, Carter (1982) suggests that vyakti is a term used for a person with a definable social status. His consultants might comment, for instance, that a deceased infant was not yet a vyakti. Yet a deceased infant clearly could have been a "person" from the standpoint of social science.

4 Inden writes that "the representational theory of knowledge [claims that] taxonomic or typological knowledge . . . simply mirrors what exists out there." In contrast, Inden insists "that the knowledge of the knower is not a disinterested mental representation of an external, natural reality. It is a construct that is always situated in a world apprehended through specific knowledges and motivated by practices in it" (1990, 33). See Fabian (1983), Haraway (1991), and Mitchell (1988) for similar critiques of positivism.

5 Sattva is associated with qualities of calm, purity, and righteousness; rajas with energetic activity; and tamas with inertia.

6 See Pigg (1996) for a similar discussion of the way that Nepali villagers considered her a representative of modernity.

7 Even those doctors interviewed who were far more critical of biomedicine than Dr. Karnik considered their hospital experience an asset.

8 Although Vd. Sharma also correlates āmavāt and rheumatoid arthritis, he is, in general, less likely to make use of such correlations than Dr. Upadhyay.

9 See Zimmermann (1992) for an interesting discussion of some of the effects of the holistic movement on contemporary Ayurveda.

10 Similarly Baudrillard (1988, 13) has suggested that contemporary consumerism itself fosters the notion of being true to oneself.

11 See Wolffers (1989) for a related discussion of the range of Ayurvedic responses to competition from biomedicine.

Chapter 3: Healing National Culture

1 All translations of Hindi texts, lectures, and conversations are mine unless otherwise noted.

2 For a detailed consideration of images of aging in India, see Lawrence Cohen's excellent study (1998).

3 See Raju (1997) for a related discussion of temporality in medieval India.

4 D. P. Chattopadyaya (1996) has discussed the moral content of ancient Ayurvedic texts.

5 In this passage I have modified Sharma's translation in certain choices of word and phrase.

6 The difference in concern represents in part the different subject matters of the two books. The first book outlines rules for a healthy life; the second book is a vernacular edition of an important, and at that time somewhat neglected, medieval Ayurvedic text.

7 The word I have translated here as treatment is *yogakriya,* which connotes the use of medicinal compounds.

8 What Chatterjee wrote of Mrityunjay's Puranic history could also be said of these Ayurvedic texts: "Myth, history, and the contemporary—all become part of the same chronological sequence; one is not distinguished from another; the passage from one to another, consequently, is entirely unproblematical" (1993, 80).

9 This valorization, not unique to medicine, arose in the indigenous historiography of the late nineteenth century as a way to imagine the Indian nation (Chatterjee 1993; Prakash 1999).

10 Leslie (1976a) has referred to the "logic of a revivalist ideology," according to which Ayurvedic scholars perceive the medieval period as one of textual decline rather than practical innovation.

11 This trend sustains a privileging of text over practice that was notable in both British and Brahminical interpretations of Hinduism (see Mani 1989; Cohn 1985).

12 See Prakash (1999) for extensive discussion of Indian engagements with science during the late colonial and postcolonial eras.

13 In a related argument that does not, however, have recourse to a narrative of decline, Chattopadhyaya (1997) contends that the "sundry superstitions" mixed into *Caraka Saṃhitā* and other ancient texts were unwilling concessions to powerful spiritual authorities who still endanger scientific rationality in modern India.

14 See Chatterjee's (1993) by now familiar argument that Indian nationalists carved out a distinctive culture by separating society into "the material" and "the spiritual." Also related is Bhabha's (1990) argument that the nation operates like a Derridean supplement as both "presence and proxy," simultaneously embodying the presence of a prior community and substituting for a community that seems to be missing.

15 As Chakrabarty has written, "The practices that we [Indians] gather under the name 'religion' do not repeat the history of that European category of thought. I accept that in today's world such translations are unavoidable and often needed. But we need to recognize them for what they are: they are mistranslations" (1995, 755).

16 This is in contrast to most modern Indian historiography, which Chakrabarty (1995, 754) notes is characterized by a "hyperrationalism" that finds science and religion to be irrevocably opposed.

17 See Prakash (1999) for more extensive discussion of the ways that Indian science was cast in a Hindu idiom.

Chapter 4: The Effect of Externality

1 See chapter 2 for a discussion of enframing.

2 See Scheper-Hughes and Lock (1987) for a useful discussion of the relationships among three bodies: the physical body, the social body, and the body politic.

3 I have avoided the usual translation of parampara as tradition because of the loaded sense of that word in contemporary understandings of culture and modernity. The word "lineage" retains the sense of sequence and continuance held by the Sanskrit/Hindi word but without the sense of opposition to modernity.

4 When it appears in medical texts, the word lakṣaṇ is almost always translated as symptom or sign. See chapter 5 for a discussion of why this translation is problematic.

5 In that sense early Ayurvedic accounts of health and illness resembled medieval European natural history. See Foucault (1973, 39–40).

6 How far such a logo-cosmology may enter the modern Ayurvedic syllabus is considered in chapter 5.

7 Foucault (1979, 148) notes that in the eighteenth century "tables" were developed as a versatile tool of power/knowledge usable in operations rang-

ing from the classification of living creatures or diseases to the spatial arrangement of persons in a hospital or prison.

8 For more on the asceticism of ancient Ayurvedic practitioners, see Zysk (1991).

Chapter 5: Clinical Gazes

1 Modern medicine's reliance on an anatomical body has begun to be qualified by new somatic imageries, as instantiated in Martin's (1994) ethnography of the immune system. Nonetheless, as Farquhar observes, "We have a commonsense or 'textbook' knowledge of medicine in Europe and North America, in which we cling to the discreteness, mechanism, and anatomical architecture of the body" (1994, 79). I suggest that this body of gross anatomy continues to have an influence behind the "deconstructed" body of "cells and signal systems" (Farquhar 1994, 80), even as heavy industry continues to have an influence behind hi-tech manufacture.

2 Thongchai (1994) has coined the term "geo-body" to describe the way that the space of a modern nation is conceived.

3 In addition to the two mentioned here, the six rasa include *madhur* (sweet), *lavaṇ* (salty), *tikt* (bitter), and *kaṣāy* (astringent).

4 The six qualities pertaining to substances include, in addition to the four already mentioned, *śīt* (cool) and *guru* (heavy).

5 See Alter (1999) for a persuasive argument that Ayurveda is more focused on radical self-improvement than on the preservation of a norm.

6 A South Indian classification recognizes 108 marmas.

7 The projection is reminiscent of the later Spanish colonial projection, deftly traced by Taussig (1987), of the savage and bloody underside of civilizational grandeur onto a South American landscape.

8 In this work I am more concerned with how the concept of science is appropriated and retooled by Ayurvedic practitioners than with whether Ayurveda qualifies as science in the modern European sense of the word. For anthropological discussions of the latter issue, see Leslie (1976a), Obeyesekere (1992, 1982), Zimmermann (1987), and Trawick (1981).

9 See, for example, Stahl (1995) on the number of magical metaphors in articles about computers.

10 Taussig (1993, 22) refers us here to Marx's analogy between vision and commodification, in which the visual object seems to be "its own self-suspended self out there" and not the collision of light waves with the retina, just as the commodity seems to be an independent entity and not a thing shaped by labor. Thus the sensuosity of use value is swallowed up in and obscured by the arbitrariness of exchange value. It is arguable, however, that use value, which constantly shifts across a variety of uses, is no more

grounded in materiality than exchange value (see Keenan 1997). In Taussig's argument also, the distinction between exchange value and use value ultimately melts away. If use value, for Keenan, is only deceptively material, then exchange value, for Taussig, is only deceptively nonsensuous.

11 Auscultation, pulse taking, endoscopy, urine test results, and so on would all be considered indexical in Peircian terms because of their contiguity with their objects. On the other hand, sonograms and X rays would presumably, like photographs, be considered both indexical and iconic since their signifying value rests in both contiguity and resemblance. See Silverman (1983) for a clear discussion of Peirce's triadic typology of symbol, icon, and index.

12 As Barthes writes, "The mechanical guarantees objectivity" (1977, 44).

13 See Romanyshyn (1989) for a provocative discussion of this shift in artistic vision.

14 See the vast literature on laboratory knowledge practice and scientific image making—e.g., Amann and Knorr-Cetina (1988); Woolgar (1988); Lynch (1988); Latour and Woolgar (1979); Lynch and Woolgar, eds. (1988); Lynch and Woolgar (1990).

15 This same conflict between laboratory reports and clinical observations can and does arise in biomedicine. See, for example, Hahn's (1982) ethnography of a North American internist. In biomedicine, however, the laboratory technician and the physician work with closely aligned, if not identical, visions of the body.

16 In North America, by contrast, such research exercises are unquestionably directions in clinical practice. See Armstrong (1983) for a salient discussion of social surveillance in twentieth-century medicine.

17 Gordon's argument here is closely related to Bourdieu's (1977) argument that anthropological accounts of culture, devised to compensate for the anthropologist's lack of expertise, fail to grasp the complex maneuvers of actual cultural practice.

18 Thirteen types of agni are identified in classical Ayurveda. Six of these are related to digestion per se, and the other seven are related to the seven dhātu. See K. R. S. Murthy (1987) for a clear discussion.

19 Vaman and virecan are two of the five pancakarma. The others are usually counted as raktmokśan (bloodletting), vasti (a medicinal wash of the rectum and lower colon), and *nasya,* the administration of medicinal nose drops. Sometimes raktmokśan is excluded and two kinds of vasti (oily and watery) are counted instead.

20 Disturbed doṣa can be either *sāma* or *nirām*—that is, mixed with āma or not. For a detailed account of the role of āma in the conceptualization and treatment of disease at a modern institution in Gujarat, see Tabor (1981).

21 In a related argument Zimmermann (1995) notes that the importance of

language and rhetoric in Ayurveda is part of what differentiates it from medical science.

22 For a relatively clear explanation in English of numerous concepts involved in Ayurvedic conceptualizations of disease, see K. R. S. Murthy (1987).

23 In other contexts liṅga can refer to the distinguishing marks of gender.

24 I have modified Sharma's translation somewhat.

25 See, for example, the testimony in Government of Madras (1923, part 2:268).

26 This passage appears in "Nidānasthānam," chapter 4, verse 4.

27 See Young (1993 and 1995) for a detailed account of the construction of PTSD.

Chapter 6: Medical Simulations

1 While in this chapter I take a semiotic approach to quackery in order to interrogate the notion of authenticity, I do not mean to trivialize the problems of either medical malpractice (whether through ignorance, deceit, or error) or medical capitalism.

2 Ivy (1995, 21) has clarified that to insist that tradition is "invented" is to simultaneously imagine that it might have been "authentic." My practical no less than my theoretical reasons for distrust of "tradition" are traceable to the realization that disciplinary history itself as we know it is the reverberating play of a tradition-modernity binary.

3 P. V. Sharma (1997) argues that our current version of *Caraka Saṃhitā* has three layers of authorship, dating from periods ranging from 1000 B.C. to 500 A.D.

4 While this practitioner billed himself as Ayurvedic, his knowledge of tridoṣa was sketchy compared to that of Vd. Rai or Vd. Shastri.

5 A siddhi is a paranormal ability that appears to defy rational explanation.

6 See Kuriyama (1999) for an insightful discussion of the relationship between ancient Chinese pulse diagnosis and a language practice in which words signify not so much fixed referents as the motives and feelings of the speaker.

7 See the discussion of the Vidyapīth exam in chapter 4.

8 Scholarly literature is replete with documentation of the rituals, aesthetics, and historical contingencies that shape medical scientific "truth." For just a few examples see Young (1980), Hahn (1982), Arney and Bergen (1984), Haraway (1991), Rhodes (1990), and Martin (1994).

9 See Adams (1996) for a related discussion of encounters between transnational discourses of authenticity and local social practice.

10 Again, see Adams (1996) for an ethnography of the mimetic call and response between Tibetan sherpas and Western consumers of sherpa culture.

11 See chapter 4 for a list of the eight parts of Ayurveda.

12 In the United States such sales promotions take place when patients are absent. In Ayurvedic hospitals, however, they take place in crowded OPDs. The sliding of medical sign into advertising icon seems to lose some of its scandalous edge in Ayurvedic settings.

13 This is true for both allopaths and Ayurvedic doctors in urban India. It is less true in rural areas, where a more brazen performativity is sometimes an expected part of healing practice.

14 I have taken the liberty of associating magic with siddhis despite the connotative differences between the two words. While Dr. Mistry utters the English word "magic" in ironic and delighted tones, reflecting his awareness of the dismissive or performance registers in which the word would ordinarily be used, he utters the Hindi/Sanskrit word "siddhi," on the other hand, with great seriousness, reflecting his awareness of the philosophical and spiritual registers in which the word would be used.

15 There are interesting similarities between the touches of magic in Dr. Mistry's practice and those in certain post-Mao practices in China as discussed by Farquhar (1996). Both play on the unscientific longings of patients, but Mistry's use of "magic" is ambivalent, while that of the Chinese doctors is defiant of the exaggerated secularism of state socialism.

16 We learned in chapter 2 that Dr. Upadhyay was also concerned to induce faith in his patients—not, however, a faith in their own cure, but rather a faith in the general effectiveness of Ayurveda.

17 This is an example commonly given in Ayurvedic textbooks for the means of knowledge known as anumān (e.g., Tripāthi 1994, 158–159).

Chapter 7: Parodies of Selfhood

1 Sāṃkhya is extremely elaborate. Here I touch only on select aspects relevant to this discussion.

2 Some of the correlations made between psychiatric diagnoses and Ayurvedic illness categories in this institution are smoothly made, while others are awkward and contested. Psychosis is considered equivalent to the Ayurvedic illness *unmād,* but particular kinds of psychoses are not necessarily correlated with particular kinds of unmād. *Cittaviṣāda,* on the other hand, is simply a modern Sanskrit coinage for depression, formed from the words *citta,* meaning mind or soul, and *viṣāda,* meaning lassitude and despondence. When I asked a graduating M.D. student there if he felt that the Sanskrit term added anything to the modern concept, he said no, it had been invented only "to give it a name." One could say, however, that the coinage supplements the concept of depression by making it a decisively Ayurvedic illness treatable with Ayurvedic therapies.

3 Modern Ayurvedic scholars have struggled with the definition of hṛday. Some scholars argue that hṛday must be understood as the brain (Shukla 1992, 9; Agrawal 1980, 71); others simply note that there is controversy over the locus of the mind in Ayurveda (S. S. Mishra 1980, 37–38; Malviya 1976, 8).

4 These passages are found in chapter 9, verses 12 and 14, of "Cikitsāsthānam."

5 This passage is found in verse 54 of chapter 11 of the "Sūtrasthānam."

6 Kāyacikitsā is often translated as internal medicine or simply medicine. See chapter 4 for discussion of the eight branches of Ayurveda.

7 This list of methods for mental restraint may well be taken from chapter 10, verse 63, of the "Cikitsāsthānam" on the treatment of apasmāra (considered by contemporary practitioners to be the same as epilepsy); it states that close friends should turn the epileptic toward knowledge, fortitude, memory, and concentration (P. V. Sharma 1981, 2:177). Caraka wrote that the therapeutic measures for epilepsy should also be adopted for unmād (P. V. Sharma 1981, 2:171).

8 According to most Ayurvedic doctors and texts, prājñāparādha, which is also described as improper use of the senses, is a major etiological factor in physical illness as well.

9 These methods are discussed in verses 85–86 of chapter 9 of the "Cikitsasthānam" (P. V. Sharma 1981, 2:169–170).

10 Shocking the patient is discussed in verses 82–84 of chapter 9 of the "Cikitsasthānam" (P. V. Sharma 1981, 2:169–170).

11 Most of what was referred to as "group" psychotherapy at this hospital in 1995 involved no more than one or two patients at a time, always of the same gender.

12 In South Asia the last two complaints are frequently associated with one another since it is widely thought that loss of semen leads to loss of strength.

bibliography

Adams, Vincanne. 1996. *Tigers of the Snow and Other Virtual Sherpas: An Ethnography of Himalayan Encounters.* Princeton, N.J.: Princeton University Press.

Agrawal, V. V. 1980. "Neurohumoral Assessment of the Concept of Kriya-Kala with Special Reference to Some Psycho-Somatic Diseases." M.D. thesis, Department of Kayachikitsa, Institute of Medical Sciences, Benares Hindu University, Varanasi, India.

Ajaya, Swami. 1983. *Psychotherapy East and West: A Unifying Paradigm.* Honesdale, Pa.: Himalayan Institute.

Alter, Joseph S. 1999. "Heaps of Health, Metaphysical Fitness: Ayurveda and the Ontology of Good Health in Medical Anthropology." *Current Anthropology* 40:S43–S66.

Amann, K., and K. Knorr-Cetina. 1988. "The Fixation of Visual Evidence." *Human Studies* 11:133–169.

American Psychiatric Association. 1987. *Diagnostic and Statistical Manual of Mental Disorders: DSM-III-R.* Washington, D.C.: American Psychiatric Association.

Amṛtasāgar. 1899. Lucknow, India: Munśi Navalkiśar.

Anderson, Benedict. 1991. *Imagined Communities: Reflections on the Origin and Spread of Nationalism.* London: Verso.

Armstrong, David. 1983. *The Political Anatomy of the Body: Medical Knowledge in Britain in the Twentieth Century.* Cambridge: Cambridge University Press.

———. 1987. Bodies of Knowledge: "Foucault and the Problem of Human Anatomy." In *Sociological Theory and Medical Sociology,* ed. Graham Scambler, 59–76. New York: Tavistock.

Arney, William Ray, and Bernard J. Bergen. 1984. *Medicine and the Management of Living: Taming the Last Great Beast.* Chicago: University of Chicago Press.

Arnold, David. 1987. "Touching the Body: Perspectives on the Indian Plague, 1896–1900." In *Subaltern Studies V: Writings on South Asian History and Society.* Ranajit Guha, ed., Oxford University. 55–90.

———. 1993. *Colonizing the Body: State Medicine and Epidemic Disease in Nineteenth Century India.* Oxford: Oxford University Press.

Athavale, V. B. 1977. *Bala-Veda: Pediatrics and Ayurveda.* Bombay: Municipal Medical College.

Āyurveda Mahāsammelan. 1950. "Āyurveda kā Bhaviśya." *Āyurved Mahāsammelan Patrika* 36(10): 532–534.

Bakhtin, Mikhail. 1968. "The Grotesque Image of the Body." In *Rabelais and His World.* Trans. Helene Iswolsky, 303–367. Cambridge, Mass.: MIT Press.

Banerji, D. 1981. "The Place of Indigenous and Western Systems of Medicine in the Health Services of India." *Social Science and Medicine* 15A:109–114.

Barker, Francis. 1995. *The Tremulous Private Body: Essays on Subjection.* Ann Arbor: University of Michigan Press.

Barthes, Roland. 1977. *Image, Music, Text.* Trans. Stephen Heath. New York: Hill and Wang.

——. 1988. "Semiology and Medicine." In *The Semiotic Challenge.* Trans. Richard Howard, 202–213. Berkeley: University of California Press.

Bates, Don, ed. 1995. *Knowledge and the Scholarly Medical Traditions.* Cambridge: Cambridge University Press.

Baudrillard, Jean. 1981. *For a Critique of the Political Economy of the Sign.* Trans. Charles Levin. St. Louis, Mo.: Telos.

——. 1988. *Selected Writings.* Ed. Mark Poster. Stanford: Stanford University Press.

Benjamin, Walter. 1968. *Illuminations.* Trans. Harry Zohn. New York: Schocken Books.

Bhabha, Homi. 1984. "Of Mimicry and Man: The Ambivalence of Colonial Discourse." *October* 28:125–133.

——. 1990. "DissemiNation: Time, Narrative, and the Margins of the Modern Nation." In *Nation and Narration,* 291–322. New York: Routledge.

Bharati, Agehananda. 1985. "The Self in Hindu Thought and Action." In *Culture and Self: Asian and Western Perspectives,* ed. Anthony Marsella, George DeVos, and Francis Hsu, 185–226. New York: Tavistock.

Bourdieu, Pierre. 1977. *Outline of a Theory of Practice.* Trans. Richard Nice. Cambridge: Cambridge University Press.

Brass, Paul. 1972. "The Politics of Ayurvedic Education: A Case Study of Revivalism and Modernization in India." In *Education and Politics in India: Studies in Organization, Society and Policy,* ed. Susanne Hoeber Rudolph and Lloyd I. Rudolph, 342–371. Cambridge, Mass.: Harvard University Press.

Carrithers, Michael, Steven Collins, and Steven Lukes, eds. 1985. *The Category of the Person: Anthropology, Philosophy, History.* New York: Cambridge University Press.

Carter, Anthony T. 1982. "Hierarchy and the Concept of the Person in Western India." In *Concepts of Person: Kinship, Caste and Marriage in India.* Akos Ostor,

Lina Fruzzetti, and Steven A. Barnett, eds., 118–142. Cambridge, Mass.: Harvard University Press.

Central Council for Research in Ayurveda and Siddha. 1987a. *Aetiopathogenesis and Treatment of Timira (Errors of Refraction) with Saptamrita Lauha and Mahatriphala Ghrita.* New Delhi: Ministry of Health, Government of India.

———. 1987b. *Study of Health Statistics under Mobile Clinical Research Programme* (Ayurveda). New Delhi: Government of India.

———. 1988. *Clinical Studies on Kamala (Jaundice) and Yakrt Rogas (Liver Disorders) with Ayurvedic Drugs.* New Delhi: Ministry of Health, Government of India.

Chakrabarty, Dipesh. 1992a. "The Death of History? Historical Consciousness and the Culture of Late Capitalism." *Public Culture* 4(2):47–65.

———. 1992b. "Postcoloniality and the Artifice of History: Who Speaks for 'Indian' Pasts?" *Representations* 37:1–26.

———. 1992c. "Provincializing Europe: Postcoloniality and the Critique of History." *Cultural Studies* 6(3):337–357.

———. 1995. "Radical Histories and Question of Enlightenment Rationalism: Some Recent Critiques of *Subaltern Studies.*" *Economic and Political Weekly* 30 (14): 751–759.

———. 2000. *Provincializing Europe: Postcolonial Thought and Historical Difference.* Princeton, N.J.: Princeton University Press.

Chatterjee, Partha. 1986. *Nationalist Thought and the Colonial World: A Derivative Discourse?* London: Zed Books.

———. 1993. *The Nation and Its Fragments: Colonial and Postcolonial Histories.* Princeton, N.J.: Princeton University Press.

Chattopadhyaya, D. P. 1996. "On the Nature of Interconnection between Science, Technology, Philosophy and Culture." In Chattopadhyaya and Kumar, eds., part 1, 35–57.

———. 1997. "Science Menaced." In Chattopadhyaya and Kumar, eds., part 2, 1–26.

Chattopadhyaya, D. P., and Ravinder Kumar, eds. 1996 and 1997. *Science, Philosophy and Culture: Multidisciplinary Explorations,* parts 1 and 2. Delhi: Project of History of Indian Science, Philosophy and Culture.

Cohen, Lawrence. 1995. "The Epistemological Carnival: Meditations on Disciplinary Intentionality and Āyurveda." In Bates, ed. 320–343.

———. 1998. *No Aging in India: Alzheimer's, the Bad Family, and Other Modern Things.* Berkeley: University of California Press.

———. 1999. "The History of Semen: Notes on a Culture-Bound Syndrome." In *Medicine and the History of the Body,* 113–138. Tokyo: Ishiyaku EuroAmerica.

Cohn, Bernard. 1985. "The Command of Language and the Language of Command." In *Subaltern Studies IV: Writings on South Asian History and Society,* Guha, ed., 4:276–329.

———. 1987a. "The Census, Social Structure and Objectification in South Asia." In *An Anthropologist among the Historians and Other Essays,* 224–254. New Delhi: Oxford University Press.

———. 1987b. "Some Notes on Law and Change in North India." In *An Anthropologist among the Historians and Other Essays,* 554–574. New Delhi: Oxford University Press.

Comaroff, Jean. 1983. "The Defectiveness of Symbols or the Symbols of Defectiveness? On the Cultural Analysis of Medical Systems." *Culture, Medicine and Psychiatry* 7:3–20.

Comaroff, Jean, and John Comaroff. 1992. *Ethnography and the Historical Imagination.* Boulder, Colo.: Westview.

Coronil, Fernando. 1996. "Beyond Occidentalism: Toward Nonimperial Geohistorical Categories." *Cultural Anthropology* 11(1):51–87.

Dahiya, Jaiprakash. 1983. *Studies on Switra and Its Ayurvedic Management.* Jamnagar, India: Gujarat Ayurvedic University.

Daniel, E. Valentine. 1983. "The Pulse as an Icon in Indian Systems of Medicine." In *South Asian Systems of Healing,* ed. E. Valentine Daniel and Judy F. Pugh. *Contribution to Asian Studies* 18:207–214.

———. 1984. *Fluid Signs: Being a Person the Tamil Way.* Berkeley: University of California Press.

Derrida, Jacques. 1976. *Of Grammatology.* Trans. Gayatri Chakravorty Spivak. Baltimore, Md.: Johns Hopkins University Press.

Devalla, Ramesh Babu. 1989. "A Clinical Study of Ama and Its Possible Biological Correlates with Reference to the Effect of Pancakola Kasaya in the Management." M.D. thesis, Department of Kayachikitsa, Institute of Medical Sciences, Benares Hindu University, Varanasi, India.

Dhyani, Sivacarana. 1987. *Salient Features of Ayurveda.* Varanasi, India: Chaukhambha Orientalia.

Dreyfus, Hubert J., and Paul Rabinow, eds. 1982. *Michel Foucault: Beyond Structuralism and Hermeneutics.* Chicago: University of Chicago Press.

Dubey, G. P., and R. H. Singh. 1970. "Human Constitution in Clinical Medicine." In Udupa, Chaturvedi, and Tripathi, eds., 305–356.

Fabian, Johannes. 1983. *Time and the Other: How Anthropology Makes Its Object.* New York: Columbia University Press.

Farquhar, Judith. 1994. "Multiplicity, Point of View, and Responsibility in Traditional Chinese Healing." In *Body, Subject and Power in China,* ed. Angela Zito and Tani E. Barlow, 78–99. Chicago: University of Chicago Press.

———. 1996. "Market Magic: Getting Rich and Getting Personal in Medicine after Mao." *American Ethnologist* 23(2):239–257.

Felman, Shoshana. 1983. *The Literary Speech Act: Don Juan with J. L. Austin, or Seduction in Two Languages*. Trans. Catherine Porter. Ithaca, N.Y.: Cornell University Press.

Foucault, Michel. 1970. *The Order of Things: An Archaeology of the Human Sciences*. New York: Vintage.

——. 1973. *The Birth of the Clinic: An Archaeology of Medical Perception*. Trans. A. M. Sheridan. New York: Vintage.

——. 1979. *Discipline and Punish: The Birth of the Prison*. Trans. Alan Sheridan. New York: Vintage.

——. 1982. "The Subject and Power." In Dreyfus and Rabinow, eds., 208–226.

Frawley, David. 1989. *Ayurvedic Healing: a Comprehensive Guide*. Salt Lake City, Utah: Passage.

Gair, D. S., and L. P. Gupta. 1970. "A Study on Drug Evaluation in Ancient India." In Udupa, Chaturvedi, and Tripathi, eds. 357–385.

Geertz, Clifford. 1973. *The Interpretation of Cultures*. New York: Basic Books.

Ghanekar, Bhaskar Govinda. 1962. *Aupasargika Roga (Infectious Diseases)*. Varanasi, India: Caukhamba Vidyabhavana.

Gordon, Deborah R. 1988. "Clinical Science and Clinical Expertise: Changing Boundaries between Art and Science in Medicine." In Lock and Gordon, eds., 257–295.

Government of India (Ministry of Health). 1948. *Report of the Committee on Indigenous Systems of Medicine* [Chopra Report]. New Delhi: Government of India.

——. 1959. *Report of the Committee to Assess and Evaluate the Present Status of Ayurvedic System of Medicine* [Udupa Report]. New Delhi: Government of India.

Government of Madras. 1923. *The Report of the Committee on the Indigenous Systems of Medicine*. Madras: Government Printing.

Guha, Ranajit, ed. 1985, 1987. *Subaltern Studies IV, V: Writings on South Asian History and Society*. Oxford: Oxford University Press.

Gupta, Akhil. 1995. "Blurred Boundaries: The Discourse of Corruption, the Culture of Politics and the Imagined State." *American Ethnologist* 22(2):375–402.

Gupta, Brahmananda. 1976. "Indian Medicine in Nineteenth and Twentieth Century Bengal." In Leslie, ed., 368–378.

Gupta, Giri Raj, ed. 1981. *The Social and Cultural Context of Medicine in India*. New Delhi: Vikas.

Gupta, Nagendra Nath Sen. 1919. *The Ayurvedic System of Medicine,* vol. 1. New Delhi: Logos Press.

Hahn, Robert A. 1982. "'Treat the Patient, Not the Lab': Internal Medicine and the Concept of Person." *Culture, Medicine and Psychiatry* 6:219–236.

Haraway, Donna. 1991. *Simians, Cyborgs, and Women: The Reinvention of Nature*. New York: Routledge.

Hegel, G. W. F. 1902. *Lectures on the Philosophy of History*. Trans. J. Sibree. London: George Bell.

Hoad, T. F. 1986. *The Concise Oxford Dictionary of English Etymology*. New York: Oxford University Press.

Inden, Ronald. 1990. *Imagining India*. Cambridge, Mass.: Blackwell.

Ivy, Marilyn. 1995. *Discourses of the Vanishing: Modernity, Phantasm, Japan*. Chicago: University of Chicago Press.

Jaggi, O. P. 1981. *Ayurveda: Indian System of Medicine*. Vol. 4 of *History of Science, Technology and Medicine in India*. New Delhi: Atma Ram and Sons.

——. 1996. "Advent of Western Medical Education in India." In Chattopadhyaya and Kumar, eds., part 1, 427–464.

Johnson, Thomas M., and Carolyn F. Sargent, eds. 1990. *Medical Anthropology: Contemporary Theory and Method*. New York: Praeger.

Kakar, Sudhir. 1982. *Shamans, Mystics and Doctors: A Psychological Inquiry into India and Its Healing Traditions*. New York: Alfred A. Knopf.

Keenan, Thomas. 1997. "The Point Is to (Ex)Change It: Reading 'Capital,' Rhetorically." In *Fables of Responsibility: Aberrations and Predicaments in Ethics and Politics*. Stanford, Calif.: Stanford University Press.

Kenghe, C. T. 1976. *Yoga as Depth-Psychology and Para-Psychology*. Varanasi, India: Bharata Manisha.

Kirmayer, Laurence J. 1988. "Mind and Body as Metaphors: Hidden Values in Biomedicine." In Lock and Gordon, eds., 57–93.

Knorr-Cetina, Karin, and Klaus Amann. 1990. "Image Dissection in Natural Scientific Inquiry." *Science, Technology and Human Values* 15(3):259–283.

Kumar, Pal. 1966. *Yoga and Psychoanalysis: A Comparative Study of Indian Systems of Yoga and Western Schools of Psychotherapy*. Delhi: Bhagavan Das.

Kumar, Rajiv. 1994. "Development of an Ayurvedic Therapeutic Regimen for the Management of Depressive Illness." M.D. thesis, Department of Kayachikitsa, Institute of Medical Sciences, Benares Hindu University, Varanasi, India.

Kumar, Suresh, Sriram, Sharma, and Rananath Dwivedi. 1985. "Advances in Research and Education in Ayurveda." *Journal of Research and Education in Indian Medicine*. Varanasi, India: Benares Hindu University.

Kuriyama, Shigehisa. 1992. "Between Mind and Eye: Japanese Anatomy in the Eighteenth Century." In Leslie and Young, eds., 21–40.

——. 1999. *The Expressiveness of the Body and the Divergence of Greek and Chinese Medicine*. New York: Zone Books.

Kutty, Ramkumar. 1994. "Knowledge, Attitudes and Practice vis-à-vis Indigenous Systems of Medicine." Paper presented at conference on Priorities in the Studies of Indian Medicine and Relevant Research Methods. Pune, India, May 1994.

Lacan, Jacques. 1977. "The Agency of the Letter in the Unconscious or Reason since Freud." In *Ecrits: A Selection*. Trans. Alan Sheridan, 146–178. London: Tavistock.

Langford, Jean M. 1995. "Ayurvedic Interiors: Person, Space and Episteme in Three Medical Practices." *Cultural Anthropology* 10(3):330–366.

——. 1998. "Ayurvedic Psychotherapy: Transposed Signs, Parodied Selves." *Political and Legal Anthropology Review* 21(1):84–98.

——. 1999. "Medical Mimesis: Healing Signs of a Cosmopolitan Quack." *American Ethnologist* 26(1):24–46.

Latour, Bruno, and Steve Woolgar. 1979. *Laboratory Life: The Construction of Scientific Facts*. Princeton, N.J.: Princeton University Press.

Lele, R. D. 1986. *Ayurveda and Modern Medicine*. Bombay: Bharatiya Vidya Bhavan.

Leslie, Charles. 1973. "The Professionalizing Ideology of Medical Revivalism." In *Entrepreneurship and Modernization of Occupational Cultures in South Asia*, ed. Milton Singer, 216–242. Durham, N.C.: Duke University Press.

——. 1974. "The Modernization of Asian Medical Systems." In *Rethinking Modernization: Anthropological Perspectives*, ed. John J. Poggie Jr. and Robert N. Lynch. Westport, Conn.: Greenwood.

——. 1976a. "The Ambiguities of Medical Revivalism in Modern India." In Leslie, ed., 356–367.

——. 1976b. "Pluralism and Integration in the Indian and Chinese Medical Systems." In *Medicine in Chinese Cultures*, ed. Arthur Kleinman et al., 401–417. Washington, D.C.: Government Printing Office. National Institute of Health DHEW pub. no. (NIH) 75–653.

——. 1992. "Interpretations of Illness: Syncretism in Modern Ayurveda." In Leslie and Young, eds., 177–208.

——. 1994. "The Blind Anthropologist and the Elephant of Traditional Asian Medicine (or The Aesthetics of Humoral Practice)." Presentation at the International Congress of Traditional Asian Medicine 4. Tokyo, August 1994.

——, ed. 1976. *Asian Medical Systems: A Comparative Study*. Berkeley: University of California Press.

Leslie, Charles, and Allan Young, eds. 1992. *Paths to Asian Medical Knowledge*. Berkeley: University of California Press.

Lévi-Strauss, Claude. 1961. *Tristes tropiques*. Trans. John Russell. New York: Criterion Books.

——. 1963a. "The Effectiveness of Symbols." In *Structural Anthropology*, 186–205. New York: Basic Books.

——. 1963b. "The Sorcerer and His Magic." In *Structural Anthropology*, 167–185. New York: Basic Books.

Lindenbaum, Shirley, and Margaret Lock, eds. 1993. *Knowledge, Power and Prac-*

tice: The Anthropology of Medicine and Everyday Life. Berkeley: University of California Press.

Lock, Margaret, and Gordon, Deborah R., eds. 1988. *Biomedicine Examined.* Boston: Kluwer Academic Publishers.

Lutz, Catherine A. 1988. *Unnatural Emotions: Everyday Sentiments on a Micronesian Atoll and Their Challenge to Western Theory.* Chicago: University of Chicago Press.

Lynch, Michael. 1988. "The Externalized Retina: Selection and Mathematization in the Visual Documentation of Objects in the Life Sciences." *Human Studies* 11:201–234.

Lynch, Michael, and Steve Woolgar. 1988. "Introduction: Sociological Orientations to Representation Practice in Science." *Human Studies* 11:99–116.

——, eds. 1990. *Representation in Scientific Practice.* Cambridge, Mass.: MIT Press.

Malviya, P. C. 1976. "Clinical Studies on Cittadvega vis-à-vis Anxiety Neurosis and Its Treatment with the Rasayana Drug, Asvagandha." M.D. thesis. Varanasi: Department of Kayachikitsa, Institute of Medical Sciences, Benares Hindu University.

Mani, Lata. 1989 [1987]. "Contentious Traditions: The Debate on Sati in Colonial India." In *Recasting Women: Essays in Indian Colonial History,* ed. Kumkum Sangari and Sudesh Vaid, 88–126. New Brunswick, N.J.: Rutgers University Press.

Marriot, McKim. 1976. "Hindu Transactions: Diversity without Dualism." In *Transaction and Meaning: Directions in the Anthropology of Exchange and Symbolic Behaviour,* ed. Bruce Kapferer, 109–142. Philadelphia, Pa.: Institute for the Study of Human Issues.

Marriott, McKim, and Ronald Inden. 1973. "Toward an Ethnosociology of South Asian Caste Systems." In *The New Wind: Changing Identities in South Asia,* ed. Kenneth A. David, 227–238. The Hague: Mouton.

Martin, Emily. 1990. "Toward an Anthropology of Immunology: The Body as Nation State." *Medical Anthropology Quarterly* (n.s.) 4:410–426.

——. 1994. *Flexible Bodies: Tracking Immunity in American Culture: From the Days of Polio to the Age of AIDS.* Boston, Mass.: Beacon.

Mascaro, Juan. 1965. "Introduction." In *The Upanishads.* Trans. Juan Mascaro, 7–44. New York: Penguin Books.

McGregor, R. S. 1995. *The Oxford Hindi–English Dictionary.* Delhi: Oxford University Press.

Mehta, A. K. 1976. "Studies on the Psychotropic Effect of the Medhya Rasayana Drug, Sankhapuspi (Convolvulus Pluricaulis Chois)." M.D. thesis, Department of Kayachikitsa, Institute of Medical Sciences, Benares Hindu University, Varanasi, India.

Mehta, Shantilal J. 1986. Foreword to *Ayurveda and Modern Medicine,* by R. D. Lele, vii–ix. Bombay: Bharatiya Vidya Bhavan.

Mehta, V. R. 1989. "Teaching Methods in Ayurvedic Education." *Sachitra Ayurved* 41(9):479–483.

Meulenbeld, G. Jan, and Dominik Wujastyk, eds. 1987. *Studies on Indian Medical History.* Groningen, Netherlands: Forsten.

Mishra, S. S. 1980. "An Operational Study on the Status of Mental Health of a Rural Population near B.H.U. Campus and a Longitudinal Followup Study of the Role of Traditional Mental Health Promoting Practices." M.D. thesis, Department of Kayachikitsa, Institute of Medical Sciences, Benares Hindu University, Varanasi, India.

Mishra, Satyendra Prasad. 1986. *Yoga and Ayurveda: Their Alliedness and Scope as Positive Health Sciences.* Varanasi, India: Chaukhambha Sanskrit Sansthan.

Mitchell, Timothy. 1988. *Colonizing Egypt.* Berkeley: University of California Press.

——. 1990. "Everyday Metaphors of Power." *Theory and Society* 19:545–577.

Monier-Williams, Monier. 1993 [1899]. *A Sanskrit–English Dictionary.* New Delhi: Motilal Banarsidass.

Mukharjee M. K., and D. Narayanorow. 1954. "History of Ayurveda." In Pathi, ed., vol. 1, 257–360.

Mukhopadhyaya, Girindranath. 1994 [1922–1929]. *History of Indian Medicine: Containing Notices, Biographical and Bibliographical, of the Ayurvedic Physicians and Their Works on Medicine from the Earliest Ages to the Present Time.* 3 vols. Calcutta: Munshiram Manoharlal Publishers.

Mumbai Vaidya Sabhā. 1990. *Mumbai Vaidya Sabhā Shatābdi Smaranika (1890–1990)* [Bombay Vaidya Society centennial commemoration 1890–1990]. Bombay: Mumbai Vaidya Sabhā.

Murthy, A. R. V. 1986. "Non-Pharmacological Approach to the Management of Irritable Bowel Syndrome with Special Reference to Group Sattvavajaya." M.D. thesis, Department of Kayachikitsa, Institute of Medical Sciences, Benares Hindu University, Varanasi, India.

Murthy, K. R. Srikantha. 1987. *Doctrines of Pathology in Āyurveda.* Varanasi, India: Chaukhambha Orientalia.

Murthy, P. Himasagara Chandra. 1990. Curriculum Development and Methods of Teaching in Ayurved with Special Reference to Rasa Shastra. *Sachitra Ayurved* 43(1):45–48.

Nandy, Ashis. 1983. *The Intimate Enemy: Loss and Recovery of Self under Colonialism.* London: Oxford University Press.

Nespor, Karel, and R. H. Singh. 1986. Experiences with Ayurvedic Psychotherapy. *International Journal of Psychosomatics* 33(3):29–30.

Nichter, Mark. 1978. "Patterns of Resort in the Use of Therapy Systems and

Their Significance for Health Planning in South Asia." *Medical Anthropology Quarterly* 2(2):29–58.
———. 1980. "The Layperson's Perception of Medicine as Perspective into the Utilization of Multiple Therapy Systems in the Indian Context." *Social Science and Medicine* 14B(4):225–233.
———. 1981a. "Idioms of Distress: Alternatives in the Expression of Psychosocial Distress: A Case Study from South India." *Culture, Medicine and Psychiatry* 5:379–408.
———. 1981b. "Negotiation of the Illness Experience: Ayurvedic Therapy and the Psychosocial Dimension of Illness." *Culture, Medicine and Psychiatry* 5:5–24.
———. 1992a. "Kyasanur Forest Disease: An Ethnography of a Disease of Development." *Medical Anthropological Quarterly* (n.s.) 1:406–423.
———. 1992b. "Of Ticks, Kings, Spirits and the Promise of Vaccines." In Leslie and Young, eds., 224–253.
Nichter, Mark, and Carolyn R. Nordstrom. 1989. "A Question of Medicine Answering: Health Commodification and the Social Relations of Healing in Sri Lanka." *Culture, Medicine and Psychiatry* 13:367–390.
Nordstrom, Carolyn R. 1988. "Exploring Pluralism: The Many Faces of Ayurveda." *Social Science and Medicine* 27(5):479–489.
———. 1989. "Ayurveda: A Multilectic Interpretation." *Social Science and Medicine* 28(9):963–970.
Obeyesekere, Gananath. 1976. "The Impact of Ayurvedic Ideas on the Culture and the Individual in Sri Lanka." In Leslie, ed., 201–226.
———. 1977. "The Theory and Practice of Psychological Medicine in the Ayurvedic Tradition." *Culture, Medicine and Psychiatry* 1(2):155–181.
———. 1982. "Science and Psychological Medicine in the Ayurvedic Tradition." In White and Marsella, eds., 235–248.
———. 1992. "Science, Experimentation and Clinical Practice in Ayurveda." In Leslie and Young, eds., 160–176.
Olok, S. K. 1987. Preface to *Aetiopathogenesis and Treatment of Timira (Errors of Refraction),* with Saptamrita Lauha and Mahatriphala Ghrita. New Delhi: Ministry of Health, Central Council for Research in Ayurveda and Siddha, Government of India.
Padyegurjar, B. K. 1985. *Dehi Ārogya Nāndate.* Mumbai, India: Samant.
Palkhivala, Nani A. 1994. "People Not Basically Corrupt but Corrupted: The Phenomenon of Khairnar." *Indian Express* (Bombay), July 3, 1994.
Pathi, A. Lakshmi, ed. 1954. *A Textbook of Ayurveda* Ayurveda shiksha, vol. 1. Jamnagar, India: Jain Bhaskarodaya.
Patterson, T. J. S. 1987. "The Relationship of Indian and European Practitioners of Medicine from the Sixteenth Century." In Meulenbeld and Wujastyk, eds., 119–129.

Pemberton, John. 1994. *On the Subject of "Java."* Ithaca, N.Y.: Cornell University Press.

Pigg, Stacy Leigh. 1996. "The Credible and the Credulous: The Question of 'Villagers' Beliefs' in Nepal." *Cultural Anthropology* 11(2):160–201.

Prakash, Gyan. 1990. "Writing Post-Orientalism Histories of the Third World: Perspectives from Indian Historiography." *Comparative Studies in Society and History* 32(2):383–408.

——. 1992. "Science 'Gone Native' in Colonial India." *Representations* 40:153–178.

——. 1999. *Another Reason: Science and the Imagination of Modern India.* Princeton, N.J.: Princeton University Press.

Rahman, M. 1994. "Khairnar's Crusade: Striking a Chord." *India Today,* July 31, 1994: 26–32.

Rai, N. P., S. K. Tiwari, and S. D. Upadhya. 1981. "The Origin and Development of Pulse Examination in Medieval India." *Indian Journal of History of Science* 16(1):77–88.

Raju, C. K. 1997. "Time in Medieval India." In Chattopadhyaya and Kumar, eds., Part 2, 253–278.

Ramanujan, A. K. 1989. "Is There an Indian Way of Thinking? An Informal Essay." *Contributions to Indian Sociology* (n.s.) 23(1):41–58.

Rhodes, Lorna A. 1990. "Studying Biomedicine as a Cultural System." In Johnson and Sargent, eds., 159–173.

——. 1993. "The Shape of Action: Practice in Public Psychiatry." In Lindenbaum and Lock, eds., 129–144.

Roland, Alan. 1988. *In Search of Self in India and Japan.* Princeton, N.J.: Princeton University Press.

Romanyshyn, Robert D. 1989. *Technology as Symptom and Dream.* New York: Routledge.

Said, Edward. 1978. *Orientalism.* New York: Vintage.

Śarma, Maheśamanda. 1910. Introduction to *Vṛndavaidyak,* by Siropanibhut Vrnda. Bombay: Khemrāj Śṛīkṛṣnadas.

Śarma, Muralidhar. 1908. Arogyaśikśa [Health Education]. Bombay: Khemrāj Śṛīkṛṣnadas.

Sastri, M. Mahadeva. 1989. "Nadee Pareeksha or Examination of Pulse." *Sachitra Ayurved* 41(12):673–676.

Savnur, H. V. 1984 [1950]. *Ayurveda Materia Medica with Principles of Pharmacology and Therapeutics.* Delhi: Sri Satguru.

Scheper-Hughes, Nancy. 1992. *Death without Weeping: The Violence of Everyday Life in Brazil.* Berkeley: University of California Press.

Scheper-Hughes, Nancy, and Margaret Lock. 1987. "The Mindful Body: A Prolegomenon to Future Work in Medical Anthropology." *Medical Anthropology Quarterly* (n.s.) 1(1):6–41.

Scott, David. 1994. *Formations of Ritual: Colonial and Anthropological Discourses on the Sinhala Yaktovil.* Minneapolis: University of Minnesota Press.

Sen, M. M. Gananath. 1916. *Hindu Medicine.* Address delivered at ceremony for foundation of Benares Hindu University. Calcutta: Sushil Kumar Sen.

Seshu, Geeta. 1994. "Striking Back at the Empire." *Indian Express* (Bombay), July 10, 1994.

Sharma, H. L. 1979. *Yoga Technique of Psychotherapy.* New Delhi: GDK Publications.

Sharma, Priya Vrat. 1972. *Indian Medicine in the Classical Age.* Varanasi, India: Chowkhamba Sanskrit Series.

———. 1997. "Development of Āyurveda from Antiquity to A.D. 300." In Chattopadhyaya and Kumar, eds., part 2, 127–163.

———, ed. and trans. 1981. *Caraka Saṃhitā.* 2 vols. Varanasi, India: Chaukhambha Orientalia.

Sharma, Shiv. 1929. *The System of Ayurveda.* Bombay: Khemraj Shrikrishnadas.

Shetty, Ashwini. 1991. "Effect of Medhya Rasayana Drug in Psychomotor Epilepsy vis-à-vis Apasmara and Its E.E.G. Correlates." M.D. thesis, Department of Kayachikitsa, Institute of Medical Sciences, Benares Hindu University, Varanasi, India.

Shukla, K. P. 1992. *An Introduction to Indian Psychiatry.* Varanasi, India: Prateek.

Shweder, Richard, and Edmund Bourne. 1982. "Does the Concept of a Person Vary Cross-Culturally?" In White and Marsella, eds., 97–137.

Silverman, Kaja. 1983. *The Subject of Semiotics.* Oxford: Oxford University Press.

Singh, Ramaharś. 1986. *Āyurvediy Manas Vijñān.* Varanasi, India: Caukhamba Amarabharati Prakasan.

Singh, S. P. c. 1900. *Nutanamṛt Sāgar.* Bombay: Khemrāj Śṛīkṛṣnadas.

Singh, Śivanāth. 1912. *Śivanātha Sāgar.* Bombay: Brijawalabha Hariprasād.

Singh, Tavleen. 1994. "The Myth of the One-Man Demolition Squad." *Indian Express* (Bombay), July 10, 1994.

Spivak, Gayatri Chakravorty. 1992. *Thinking Academic Freedom in Gendered Post-Coloniality.* Capetown, South Africa: University of Capetown Press.

Stahl, William A. 1995. "Venerating the Black Box: Magic in Media Discourse on Technology." *Science, Technology and Human Values* 20(2):234–258.

Stewart, Susan. 1993. *On Longing.* Durham, N.C.: Duke University Press.

Śukla, Vidyadhar, and Ravidatt Tripāthī. 1993. *Āyurveda ka Itihās: Evam Paricay* [History of Ayurveda: Part one]. Delhi: Chaukhamba Sanskrit Pratishthan.

Śuklan, Amol Candra. 1990. *Adhunik Āyurved Gayd* [Modern Ayurvedic guide]. New Delhi: Hindi Pustak Bhandar.

Sullivan, Mark. 1986. "In What Sense Is Contemporary Medicine Dualistic?" *Culture, Medicine and Psychiatry* 10:331–350.

Tabor, Daniel C. 1981. "Ripe and Unripe: Concepts of Health and Sickness in Ayurvedic Medicine." *Social Science and Medicine* 15B:439–455.

Taussig, Michael. 1980. "Reification and the Consciousness of the Patient." *Social Science and Medicine* 14B:3–13.

———. 1987. *Shamanism, Colonialism and the Wild Man: A Study in Terror and Healing.* Chicago: University of Chicago Press.

———. 1992. "Homesickness and Dada." In *The Nervous System,* 149–182. New York: Routledge.

———. 1993. *Mimesis and Alterity: A Particular History of the Senses.* New York: Routledge.

Taylor, Charles. 1985. "The Person." In Carrithers, Collins, and Lukes, eds., 257–281.

———. 1989. *Sources of the Self: The Making of the Modern Identity.* Cambridge, Mass.: Harvard University Press.

Thakkur, Chandrashekhar G. 1965. "Introduction." In *Ayurveda (Basic Indian Medicine).* Bombay: *Times of India* Press.

Thatte, D. G. 1988. *Acupuncture, Marma and Other Asian Therapeutic Techniques.* Varanasi, India: Chaukhambha Orientalia.

Thongchai, Winichakul. 1994. *Siam Mapped: A History of the Geo-Body of a Nation.* Honolulu, Hawaiʻi: University of Hawaiʻi Press.

Trawick, Margaret. 1981. "The Ayurvedic Physician as Scientist." *Social Science and Medicine* 24(12):1031–1050.

———. 1991. "An Ayurvedic Theory of Cancer." *Medical Anthropology* 13:121–136.

———. 1992. *Notes on Love in a Tamil Family.* Berkeley: University of California Press.

Tripāthī, Ravidatt. 1994. *Padārth Vijñān.* Varanasi, India: Caukhamba Sanskṛt Pratiṣṭhan.

Tripathy, Rajkishore. 1981. "A Study of the Scope of Rasayana-Vajikarana Therapy in Manas Roga with Special Reference to Anxiety and Depression." M.D. thesis, Department of Kayachikitsa, Institute of Medical Sciences, Benares Hindu University, Varanasi, India.

Turner, Victor. 1967. *The Forest of Symbols: Aspects of Ndembu Ritual.* Ithaca, N.Y.: Cornell University Press.

Udupa, K. N., G. N. Chaturvedi, and S. N. Tripathi, eds. 1970. *Advances in Research in Indian Medicine.* Varanasi, India: Benares Hindu University.

Upadhyaya, Sarva Dev. 1986. *Nāḍī Vijñāna Ancient Pulse Science.* Delhi: Chaukhambha Sanskrit Pratishthan.

Vaiśya, Śaligrama. 1919. Introduction to *Bhāvaprakāś,* by Miśra Bhav. Bombay: Khemrāj Śrīkṛṣnadas.

von Schmadel, D., and B. Hochkirchen. 1987. "The Results of an Analysis Based on a Video of Consultations in Five Ayurvedic Medical Practices." In Meulenbeld and Wujastyk, eds., 225–232.

Waxler, Nancy E. 1984. "Behavioral Convergence and Institutional Separation: An Analysis of Plural Medicine in Sri Lanka." *Culture, Medicine and Psychiatry* 8:187–205.

Weiss, Mitchell, Amit Desai, Sushrut Jadhav, Lalit Gupta, S. M. Channabasavanna, D. R. Doongaji, and Prakash B. Behere. 1988. Humoral Concepts of Mental Illness in India. *Social Science and Medicine* 27(5):471–477.

White, Geoffrey, and Anthony Marsella, eds. 1982. *Cultural Conceptions of Mental Health and Therapy*. Boston: D. Riedel.

White, Hayden V. 1990 [1987]. *The Content of the Form: Narrative Discourse and Historical Representation*. Baltimore, Md.: Johns Hopkins University Press.

Wise, Thomas. 1986 [1845]. *The Hindu System of Medicine*. Delhi: Mittal Publications.

Wolffers, Ivan. 1989. "Traditional Practitioners' Behavioural Adaptations to Changing Patients' Demands in Sri Lanka." *Social Science and Medicine* 29(9):1111–1119.

Woolgar, Steve. 1988. "Time and Documents in Researcher Interaction: Some Ways of Making Out What Is Happening in Experimental Science." *Human Studies* 11:171–200.

Young, Allan. 1980. "The Discourse on Stress and the Reproduction of Conventional Knowledge." *Social Science and Medicine* 14B:133–146.

———. 1993. "A Description of How Ideology Shapes Knowledge of a Mental Disorder (Post-Traumatic Stress Disorder)." In Lindenbaum and Lock, eds., 108–128.

———. 1995. *The Harmony of Illusions: Inventing Post-Traumatic Stress Disorder.* Princeton, N.J.: Princeton University Press.

Zimmermann, Francis. 1978. "From Classic Texts to Learned Practice: Methodological Remarks on the Study of Indian Medicine." *Social Science and Medicine* 12:97–103.

———. 1987. *The Jungle and the Aroma of Meats: An Ecological Theme in Hindu Medicine*. Berkeley: University of California Press.

———. 1992. "Gentle Purge: The Flower Power of Ayurveda." In Leslie and Young, eds., 209–223.

———. 1995. "The Scholar, the Wise Man, and Universals: Three Aspects of Āyurvedic Medicine." In Bates, ed., 297–319.

Žižek, Slavoj. 1997. "Multiculturalism, or, the Cultural Logic of Multinational Capitalism." *New Left Review* 225:28–51.

Zysk, Kenneth G. 1991. *Asceticism and Healing in Ancient India: Medicine in the Buddhist Monastery*. New York: Oxford University Press.

———. 1993. "The Science of Respiration and the Doctrine of Bodily Winds in Ancient India." *Journal of the American Oriental Society* 113(2):198–224.

index

Bhagavad Gita, 51, 256
Bharati, Agehananda, 233, 260–261
Bhāvaprakāś, 81, 84, 106
Bhūtavidya (knowledge of ghosts): conceptions of, 85, 87; conceptions of bhūt, 85, 95
Biomedicine: and the body, 98, 145; clinical methods of, 13, 168, 184; conceptions of, 2, 11, 281 n.11; and disease nomenclature, 186; and mental illness, 237, 245, 252; militarism of, 140–141; and model of disease, 12–13; 34; in relation to Ayurveda, 167. *See also* Allopathy
Bodies: and conceptions of mind-body split, 234–235; as disciplined, 98, 123–124 (*see also* Personhood); dosic v. docile, 141–147; fluent, 22, 141; grotesque, 146–147; national, 20, 140; as sites of disease, 12–13
Borges, Jorge Luis, 117, 118
Bourdieu, Pierre, 287 n.17
Buddhi, 233

Cancer, 185
Caraka Saṃhitā, 4; aim of medical treatment in, 41; conceptions of disease in, 181, 183–184; and discourse of revival, 85–89; 91–92; discussion of medical incompetence in, 73–77, 83; emphasis on doṣa in, 172, 174; poetic language in, 44, 117, 120–123; psychological treatment in, 217, 236, 240, 242–244
Caraka. See *Caraka Saṃhitā*
Carter, Anthony T., 283 n.3
Central Council for Indian Medicine. (CCIM), 115, 122–123
Central Council for Research in Ayurveda and Siddha, 163–167
Chakrabarty, Dipesh, 64, 249, 258, 285 nn.15–16
Chatterjee, Partha, 281 n.9, 284 nn.8–9, 285 n.14
Chattopadhyaya, D. P., 284 n.4, 285 n.13
Chopra Report, 112, 114, 116
Cikitsā (treatment), 16, 105; anuloman, 160; marma, 212–217; śuddh Ayurvedīy, 81
Cohen, Lawrence, 283 n.1, 284 n.2
Cohn, Bernard, 136, 281 n.10, 282 n.20
Colonialism: Ayurveda as remedy for, 63–64, 263–264, 269 (*see also* Ayurveda: and postcoloniality); and knowledge practices, 265 (*see also* Orientalism); and mimicry of colonial power, 6–10, 22–23, 63, 88 (*see also* Mimesis); and policy on Indian medical education, 5–6, 45, 102–103
Coronil, Fernando, 283 n.21
Culture. *See* Nationalism: and national-cultural identity

Daniel, E. Valentine, 35, 157, 282 n.20
Darśan (seeing), 29–30, 40, 48
Derrida, Jacques, 10, 127, 180, 186, 282 n.16
Deshmukh, M. G., 151
Dharma, 34, 78–79, 84, 141
Dhātu: conceptions of, 22, 28, 33–34, 69, 170; hypothetical diagram of, 35; in medical treatment, 169–170; standardization of, 126–127
Discipline, 97–98; medical records as, 36, 48–49; temporal, 123. *See also* Foucault, Michel
Doṣa: biomedicalization of, 150–152, 154–155; conceptions of, 4, 28–29, 33–34, 37–39; creative ambiguity of, 172–177; dosic body, 141–147; hy-

pothetical diagram of, 35; as identity, 57–59; in medical treatment, 170–172. *See also* Vata/vāyu, pitta, kapha
Drugs: allopathic vs. Ayurvedic, 52–53, 56; in clinical research, 43–44, 164–166; medhya rasāyan (for mental problems), 239–240; standardization vs. non-standardization of, 31–32

Education, Ayurvedic: corruption in, 98–99, 132–139; institutionalization of, 7, 20, 108–116; modern curriculum, 122–126; śuddh-miśra controversy, 112 (*see also* Miśra Ayurveda; Śuddh Ayurveda); textbooks, 116–122
Enframing: of Ayurveda, 43, 45, 61–62, 138; of bodily phenomena, 37–38, 124; as modern knowledge practice, 25–26, 97–98
Ethnographic representation: issues of, 19–20, 24–25, 27–28, 37, 61, 69, 100–101
Ethnomedicine. *See* Anthropology: of "ethnomedicine"
Expressivism, 58, 246–247

Fabian, Johannes, 282 n.14, 283 n.4
Farquhar, Judith, 286 n.1, 289 n.15
Felman, Shoshana, 228–229
Fetishism: commodity, 208–209
Foucault, Michel: on concepts of disease, 158, 180, 285 n.5; on disciplinary power, 20–22, 97–98, 124–125, 282 n.14, 285 n.7; on interiority, 246; on the medical gaze, 30
Freud, Sigmund, 231, 253

Geertz, Clifford, 100
Gordon, Deborah, 168, 287 n.17
Guṇa (quality), 31, 35, 119, 166
Gupta, Akhil, 133
Gupta, Nagendra Nath Sen, 116, 117, 121, 155–156
Gurukula (learning centers), 101, 104–108, 116, 123, 134–136, 138–139. *See also* Education, Ayurvedic
Guruparampara. *See* Guru-śiṣya parampara
Guru-śiṣya parampara (teacher-student lineage), 76, 97, 101, 104–107, 109, 115, 117, 134–135, 139, 285 n.3

Hahn, Robert, 287 n.15, 288 n.8
Hakīms (Unani practioners), 79, 94
Haraway, Donna, 283 n.4, 288 n.8
Himasagara Chandra Murthy, P., 130
History: historicism, 64–65; homogenous empty time, 64, 67, 71, 90; mythic, 89–90
Holistic medicine: Ayurveda as, 43–44, 53; European and North American interest in, 56–60, 62, 219, 248

Inden, Ronald, 283 n.4
India National Congress, 7, 108–109
Ivy, Marilyn, 288 n.2

Jaḍī-būṭī, 104–105, 206, 210
Jaggi, O. P., 281 nn.4–5
Joshi, Dr., 152–153, 159–162, 167–176, 183–185, 192–193, 237, 244, 248

Kakar, Sudhir, 153
Kāliyug (era of darkness), 16, 89
Karmendriya, 258–259
Karnik, Dr., 25–26, 38–45, 47–48, 53, 55, 60–63, 135, 185
Keenan, Thomas, 286 n.10
Kenghe, C. T., 231–232
Kirmayer, Laurence, 234–235

Śāstri, Mahadeva, 197
Sattva, rajas, tamas: conceptions of, 35; in relation to mental illness, 170–172, 233, 236–237, 257
Sattvāvajaya (psychotherapy), 240–246, 252. *See also* Psychotherapy: Ayurvedic conceptions of
Satyayug (era of truth), 16, 89
Savnur, H. V., 149, 152
Scheper-Hughes, Nancy, 235, 285 n.2
Science: in Ayurvedic discourse, 4, 6, 86–87, 93, 147–150, 152–153
Scott, David, 282, n.12
Semiotics: dangers of contrasting European and South Asian, 24, 282 n.20; of diagnosis, 21, 40, 179–180, 182; of exchange value, 202; of pulse reading, 198; of sonographic technology, 157
Sen, Gananath, 85–87, 149, 151–152, 167–168
Sharma, Vd., 25–38, 40–43, 47–49, 52, 60–63
Sharma, Shiv, 93–94, 111–112, 115, 150, 153–154
Shastri, Vd., 104–107, 191
Shetty, Ashwini, 239
Shukla, Vd., 7–8, 104, 106, 109–110
Siddhi (paranormal power), 74, 223, 289 n.14
Śilajīt (medicinal mineral), 207–210
Silverman, Kaja, 287 n.11
Singh, Dr., 239–246
Singh, Śivanāth. See *Sivantha Sagar*
Śivanātha Sāgar : the body in, 143; discussion of the loss of vaidyak knowledge in, 65–67, 72–73, 76–77, 80, 83; poetics of, 67–71, 87–88, 120
Sphygmograph, 162–163
Spivak, Gayatri Chakravorty, 101
Stahl, William A., 286 n.9
Stewart, Susan, 18, 282 n.16
Śuddh Ayurveda, 109–112, 114. *See also* Sharma, Shiv
Śuddh-miśra controversy, 109–116
Supplementarity: of Ayurveda, 10; of disease nomenclature, 186; of modern body, 157
Surgery, 41–42
Suśruta Saṃhitā, 4, 89, 105, 123; as anticipating modern science, 6, 152, 172; discussion of marmas in, 145; and discourse of revival, 86; and idea of divine vision, 91–92
Suśruta. See *Suśruta Saṃhitā*
Swanguli pramān (self-finger measurement), 144–145, 147

Tabor, Daniel C., 287 n.20
Taussig, Michael, 14, 155–157, 189, 208–209, 216, 220, 230, 265, 281 n.8, 282 n.19, 286 nn.7–10
Taylor, Charles, 247
Technology, modern: diagnostic, 29–30, 40, 155–161; dosa-oriented, 162–163; as magical, 155–157, 159; statistical methods as, 167
Thongchai, Winichakul, 286 n.2
Tiwari, Dr., 173
Tourism. *See* Ayurveda; and medical tourism
Tradition, 188, 190–191; nostalgia for, 18–19 (*see also* Modernity)
Trawick, Margaret, 100, 286 n.8
Triguṇa. *See* sattva, rajas, tamas
Trivedi, Dr., 192–231
Turner, Victor, 14

Udupa Report, 87, 102, 104, 114, 116, 127, 221
Unani (healing practice), 18, 86, 94, 108, 282 n.15

Jean M. Langford is Assistant Professor of Anthropology at the University of Minnesota.

Library of Congress Cataloging-in-Publication Data
Langford, Jean.
Fluent bodies : Ayurvedic remedies for postcolonial imbalance / by Jean M. Langford.
p. cm. — (Body, commodity, text)
Includes bibliographical references and index.
ISBN 0-8223-2931-X (cloth : alk. paper)
ISBN 0-8223-2948-4 (pbk. : alk. paper)
1. Medicine, Ayurvedic — Social aspects.
2. Traditional medicine — India. I. Title. II. Series.
R605 .L36 2002 615.5′3 — dc21 2002004597